Encyclopedia of
Public Health

Editorial Board

Encyclopedia of Public Health

Edited by Lester Breslow

Volume 4
S-Z
Appendix
Index

MACMILLAN REFERENCE USA

GALE GROUP

THOMSON LEARNING

New York • Detroit • San Diego • San Francisco
Boston • New Haven, Conn. • Waterville, Maine
London • Munich

Macmillan Reference USA
1633 Broadway
New York, NY 10019

Macmillan Reference USA
Gale Group
27500 Drake Road
Farmington Hills, MI 48331-3535

Gale Group and Design is a trademark used herein under license.

Library of Congress Catalog in Publication Data
Encyclopedia of public health / edited by Lester Breslow.
     p. cm.
     Includes bibliographical references and index.
     ISBN 0-02-865354-8 (set : hardcover : alk. paper) — ISBN 0-02-865350-5 (v. 1 : alk. paper) — ISBN 0-02-865351-3 (v. 2 : alk. paper) — ISBN 0-02-865352-1 (v. 3 : alk. paper) — ISBN 0-02-865353-X (v. 4 : alk. paper)
     1. Public health—Encyclopedias.   I. Breslow, Lester.

RA423 .E53 2001
362.1'03—dc21   2002031501

Printed in the United States of America

10 9 8 7 6 5 4 3 2 1

S

SAFETY

Safety consists of "attempts to minimize the risk of injury, illness, or property damage from the hazards to which one may be exposed" (Edlin et al. 1999, p. 522). Safety for one's home, one's community, and oneself is best achieved through a joint effort involving individuals, schools, law enforcement, and other private and public agencies.

Home safety can be improved by exterior lighting around doors and windows, secure locks that are consistently used, block watch programs, and informing neighbors of unusual individuals or events. Internal home safety is optimized by lighting on stairways, lack of clutter, and consistent maintenance of home and contents.

The National Crime Prevention Council has identified several strategies to improve community safety. Community mobilization is the process of bringing individuals together so that they can jointly guard property, report suspicious behavior to the police, combat criminality, and form a spirit of community. Examples of community-mobilization efforts include neighborhood watch groups, mobilizing senior citizens as volunteers, business watch groups, and early warning arson prevention. These efforts are a cost-effective way to combat crime and reduce fear.

Violence prevention at the local level recognizes the need to punish violent offenders, support victims, and teach nonviolence. Strategies can include teaching conflict management, public dialogue, and dispute resolution; combating teen dating violence; court-based programs for victims of domestic violence; mentoring; and parent education.

Communities should also make efforts to assure safe public places. Thriving communities need parks, downtown shopping areas, business districts, schools, and public-housing communities where residents can feel protected from the threat of crime and violence. There are several ways to create such places through joint efforts with government agencies, businesses, law enforcement, and citizens' groups. Poverty, discrimination, lack of education, and lack of employment opportunities are important risk factors for violence and must be addressed as part of any comprehensive solution to the epidemic of violence in urban communities. Strategies for reducing violence should reach children early in life, before violent beliefs and behavioral patterns can be adopted.

A new concern for parents and teachers is the concept of cybersafety. The Internet has many sites devoted to pornography, hate literature and excessive violence, and parents and teachers need to monitor the web sites that children visit. The best defense for children is for adults to educate them about issues that can cause them harm. Parents and teachers should carefully select an online service that offers control features to block out different types of sites, and children should be taught to not give out personal information, to never agree to meet anyone without their parent's consent, and to never send a photo of themselves over the Internet to someone they do not know.

The reduction of intentional (deliberate) and nonintentional (accidental) injuries is the concern of both individuals and communities. Such injuries include nonfatal head injuries, nonfatal spinal cord injuries, firearm-related injuries and deaths, motor vehicle-related injuries, poisonings, and deaths from suffocation. Prevention strategies for unintentional injuries include the use of safety belts, child restraints, motorcycle and bicycle helmets, graduated driver licensing, and functioning smoke alarms in residences.

Understanding the factors that cause injuries allows for development and implementation of effective prevention interventions to improve safety. Some interventions can reduce injuries from both unintentional and violence-related causes. For instance, efforts to promote proper storage of firearms in homes can help reduce the risk of unintentional shootings in the home. Higher taxes on alcoholic beverages are associated with lower death rates from motor vehicle crashes and lower rates for some categories of violent crime, including rape.

Women face special threats to their safety. Date rape (acquaintance rape) occurs when a date, boyfriend, or someone that a woman knows forces sexual relations. Women can help protect their safety while dating by openly discussing sexual expectations. Women also need to be very careful not to become intoxicated or be under the influence of any substance that will lessen their ability to make rational decisions while on a date.

Although recent tragedies and mass murders at schools have led to the conclusion that schools are becoming less safe, it is important to remember that 90 percent of the schools in the United States are free of violent crimes and serious safety issues (U.S. Department of Education and the U.S. Department of Justice, 1998). In recent years there has been a decrease in criminality and the number of children carrying weapons to school. Some of the reasons for this change are due in part to increases in school security measures, zero-tolerance policies, and the implementation of school violence prevention programs (U.S. Department of Education and the U.S. Department of Justice, 1998). Children are more likely to be the victim of a crime or seriously harmed in their own home or in the community than at school. Despite these facts, children are more fearful of school today than what has historically been reported.

To continue the decrease in school criminality and hopefully lessen the incidents of school shootings/mass murders, the U.S. Department of Education and the U.S. Department of Justice (1998) recommend the following for schools to do the following:

1. Provide strong administrative support for assessing and enhancing school safety.

2. Redesign the school facility to eliminate dark, secluded, and unsupervised spaces.

3. Devise a system for reporting and analyzing violent and noncriminal incidents.

4. Design an effective discipline policy.

5. Build a partnership with local law enforcement.

6. Enlist school security professionals in designing and maintaining the school security system.

7. Train school staff in all aspects of violence prevention.

8. Provide all students access to school psychologists or counselors.

9. Provide crisis response services.

10. Implement school-wide education and training on avoiding and preventing violence.

11. Use alternative school settings for educating violent and weapon-carrying students.

12. Create a climate of tolerance (address racism and discrimination).

13. Provide appropriate education services to all students.

14. Reach out to communities and businesses to improve the safety of students.

15. Actively involve students in making decisions about school policies and programs.

16. Prepare an annual report on school crime and safety.

Some specific measures that a school can initiate quickly are the following: "hiring security personnel, installing security devices, conducting random inspections, and providing students/staff with identification cards" (U.S. Department of Education and the U.S. Department of Justice 1998, p.

25). With these continued efforts, schools can continue to be a safe place for America's youth.

KATHY AKPOM
TAMMY A. KING

(SEE ALSO: *Behavioral Change; Community Organization; Crime; Domestic Violence; Family Health; Legislation and Regulation; Occupational Safety and Health; Street Violence; United States Consumer Product Safety Commission; Violence*)

BIBLIOGRAPHY

Eldin, G.; Golanty, E.; and Brown, K. M. (1999). *Health and Wellness,* 6th edition. Sudbury, MA: Jones and Bartlett.

National Crime Prevention Council (2000). *Cybersafety for Kids Online: A Parent's Guide.* Washington, DC: Bureau of Justice Assistance, Office of Justice Programs, U.S. Department of Justice. NCPC information is available at http://www.ncpc.org.

—— (2000). *Date Rape Is a Power Trip.* Washington, DC: Bureau of Justice Assistance, Office of Justice Programs, U.S. Department of Justice.

—— (2000). *Invest in Home Security.* Washington, DC: Bureau of Justice Assistance, Office of Justice Programs, U.S. Department of Justice.

U.S. Department of Education and the U.S. Department of Justice (1998). *Annual Report on School Safety.* (Pamphlet released by Richard W. Riley, Secretary of Education and Janet Reno, Attorney General.)

U.S. Department of Health and Human Services (2000). *Health People 2010.* Available at http://web.health.gov/healthypeople/.

SAFETY ASSESSMENT

Safety assessment is the process that results in an "acceptable daily intake" (ADI) of specific chemicals. Safety assessment has been carried out in the United States and much of the Western world since the late nineteenth century. Since the 1950s it has become much more formalized in its use by regulatory agencies to incorporate animal toxicology studies and potential exposures. Safety assessment starts with the underlying premise that exposure to a chemical, be it a drug, food additive, cosmetics ingredients, or consumer product, will occur. It also relies on animal toxicology studies. The assumption made is that humans are more sensitive to these chemicals than the most sensitive animal species tested.

Acute toxicity studies are used to determine the potential for poisoning, as well as possible antidotes. The acute LD50 (that dose that is lethal to 50% of the animals tested) is seldom directly extrapolated from animals to man, but many occupational exposure standards and categorizations of household chemicals are based on the LD50. Safety assessment for direct food additives, such as colorants or flavors, is based on the no observable effect level (NOEL) in laboratory animals, or on an approximation of that level. The ADI is determined from the NOEL (with appropriate safety factors) and is based on the percentage of any dietary component that contains the chemical, so that if a person consumes a kilogram of food per day and the compound of interest is only found in 10 percent of the food products generally consumed, that 10 percent becomes the exposure maximum that is used in the calculations.

Safety assessment for therapeutic agents is also based on animal toxicity, but it is also a function of the doses to be used, the diseases to be treated, and the conditions of the treated populations. As an example, the safety assessment of an over-the-counter (OTC) drug is more stringent than for a drug to be used for the treatment of a life-threatening situation. A therapeutic index (TI) is developed for almost all drugs and is based on the ratio of the toxic dose to the efficacious dose: The greater the ratio, the greater the margin of safety in use of the drug. A drug being used for cancer chemotherapy can have a greater toxicity and a much smaller TI than a drug for the common cold. A cancer patient may be in a life-threatening situation, but a doctor or nurse is monitoring his or her signs and symptoms of toxicity. In contrast, an individual may be taking uncontrolled amounts of a cold preparation and is probably not being monitored by a health professional. The other issue in this example is that there is a much larger consumer population for OTC products than for chemotherapeutic products, and the risks of OTC drugs may not be as well appreciated. Hence, the "involuntary" risk taker must be more protected.

Consumer products present a different challenge for safety assessment. The assumption here is that the consumer of a household product will ingest or touch the product, or inhale vapors from the product. The product is manufactured for something other than consumption, and the packaging has to be part of the safety assessment. For example, a household cleanser may be caustic and highly oxidizing. This product will cause extreme damage to tissues, and the risk is known from animal studies or by analogy to other chemicals of the same class. The only way to assure less risk to the user is through strong, vivid, unequivocal labeling, and childproof packaging.

Pesticides present a special case in safety assessment. First, most pesticides are designed to control and/or kill pests. By definition, pesticides, especially insecticides, are moderately or highly toxic when compared to most other consumer products. The safety assessment and toxicology package for a pesticide depends on whether it is going to be registered as a crop chemical, a chemical for ornamental flowers, a home-use pesticide, or some other use. The crop chemicals, be they insecticides, herbicides, fungicides, or growth regulators, complete a battery of tests from in vitro through carcinogenicity. The logic being that consumers could be exposed to minute amounts of residues from application to the crops, and there must be a large margin of safety between potential exposure and toxicity. Again, an ADI is established based on the toxicity of the chemical, the NOEL, the shape of the dose-response curve, the amount of a particular crop in a food product, how much may be eaten or drunk, and the body weight or surface area of the consumer (children are special cases). This information allows the regulators to establish an ADI expressed in milligrams (or micrograms) of a chemical that can be consumed safely in a day. ADIs are also set for different durations of exposure, but usually for a greater part of the lifetime.

Safety assessment differs from cancer risk assessment in several ways. Safety assessments are for multiple endpoints, not just cancer, and can be for multiple time points. Threshold limit values (TLVs) are examples of safety assessments that can be set for acute toxicity, eye irritation, or systemic toxicity. Safety assessments arrive at an exposure or dose limit and are not expressed as a probability, which cancer risk assessments are. Safety assessments are similar throughout the world.

MICHAEL GALLO

(SEE ALSO: *In Vivo and In Vitro Testing; Risk Assessment, Risk Management; Safety Factors; Toxicology*)

SAFETY FACTORS

Safety factors have been used to protect the public health since the advent of modern safety assessment. Originally based on very little experimental data, the concept of safety factors was based on the premise that humans are more sensitive to chemicals and environmental agents than the most sensitive laboratory animal. By the time of World War I, experimental evidence with laboratory animals was being directly compared with findings in humans. It was evident that the original premise had little basis in fact, but was still a prudent approach for public health. As novel organic molecules were being developed as drugs and insecticides in the 1930s and 1940s, the concept of safety factors gave scientists and regulators some comfort that the public was being protected. Actual data on safety factors is still incomplete.

For many highly toxic compounds, humans are almost identical to laboratory animals in sensitivity. However, there are startling examples, such as thalidomide and some retinoic acid analogs, where humans are much more sensitive than laboratory animals. Several attempts have been made to quantify the physiological and toxicological differences across species. For the basic physiological systems that are essential for all mammalian species, the responses to many classes of chemicals, drugs, and physical agents are similar.

The basic assumptions underlying the use of safety factors is that by using these factors the public health is protected and special populations are also protected. Further assumptions hold that humans are somewhere between 10 and 1,000 times more sensitive to some toxic agents than are animals, adults are less sensitive than children, and the aged are more sensitive than younger individuals. Hence, a safety assessment can be conducted using the proper toxicological evaluation with multiple species of animals to establish the NOEL (no observable effect level) or its equivalent. The assessor can then use safety factors for species to species extrapolation (usually a factor of ten or more), which involves multiplying the NOEL by a tenfold factor for age differences, and perhaps a tenfold factor for special populations. Hypothetically if a NOEL established for Chemical A at 1,000 milligrams per kilogram body weight of the laboratory rat per day, the assessor could compute the safety factors and conclude that a safe dose would be 1 milligram per kilogram per day.

This is a simple case, and many other variables can be added. For an occupational exposure one might add a factor for hours worked compared to hours used in the tests. For an immunotoxic agent there might be a greater safety factor used for species or age comparison, particularly if children or the aged are exposed. The uncertainties surrounding testing for adverse birth outcomes usually result in the use of greater safety factors.

The rationale for additional safety factors for children has evolved over several years. Originally, children were looked on as small adults and their physiological differences, especially the rapid development and remarkable tissue and organ systems changes of children, were not given as much as attention as necessary. Recently, the emphasis has been on understanding how seemingly modest or small changes in a developing system can permanently alter that system when it matures. Greater care is now going into using safety factors for children. More basic research is still necessary to protect children, and until that work is completed the prudent approach has been to increase the safety factors for children.

Safety factors are widely used by regulators throughout the world. Some countries use safety factors for assessing the exposures to some carcinogens. The United States generally uses a quantitative risk assessment (QRA) approach to carcinogens, but uses a modification of the original safety factor approach for most other toxic endpoints. Safety factors were used exclusively until the late 1960s and early 1970s when the QRA methodologies were developed. The U.S. National Academy of Sciences/National Research Council has, through its many studies on drinking water,

food additives, and others types of chemicals, published a rich history of the rationale and use of safety factors.

MICHAEL GALLO

(SEE ALSO: *Environmental Determinants of Health; Risk Assessment, Risk Management; Safety Assessment; Toxicology*)

SAFETY STANDARDS

During the twentieth century many countries began to develop requirements for manufacturers and service industries to reduce high rates of injury, illness, and fatality in both the working environment and in consumer products. Led by professional organizations and by the United Nations, safety standards set criteria for the construction of machinery to prevent injury to operators of the machines, and for the production of consumer products to avoid injury to purchasers. Through such standards, dramatic improvements have occurred throughout the world in industrial health and accident prevention. Not all countries have well-developed or enforced standards, however, and standards continue to be refined and developed.

BARBARA TOEPPEN-SPRIGG

(SEE ALSO: *Occupational Safety and Health; Prevention; Primary Prevention*)

SALMONELLOSIS

Salmonellosis is a common enteric disease caused by rod-shaped, gram-negative bacteria. The name is derived from the American veterinary surgeon, Daniel A. Salmon, who described *Salmonella choleraesuis* as the cause of hog cholera in 1885. Since then over 2,200 *Salmonella* serotypes have been described; each is distinguished by its unique combination of cell wall, flagella, and capsular antigens. Many serotypes are further subdivided, usually for epidemiological studies, by their sensitivity to standard sets of bacteriophages (phage typing), and DNA fingerprinting methods. *Salmonella* are found in the intestinal tract of animals and birds, including domestic species (e.g., cattle, poultry), wild animals, and pets. Most human infections are caused by a few serotypes, commonly *S. typhimurium* and *S. enteritidis*. In most countries that keep national statistics, the majority of human cases are due to only five to ten common serotypes.

Salmonellosis is characterized by diarrhea, headache, abdominal pain, fever, and vomiting, beginning 6 to 72 hours (usually 6 to 36 hours) after infection. Healthy people normally recover within a week. Some individuals, however, are more susceptible to serious illness (see Table 1), and there is increasing evidence of longer-term sequelae occurring in a small proportion of cases.

Specific *Salmonella* serotypes are adapted to specific hosts, in which they usually cause septicaemia. For example, *Salmonella typhi*, is the cause of typhoid in man. Human infection is linked to a diverse variety of foods, possibly contaminated by animal or human feces during slaughter or during cultivation, harvesting, and preparation. Foods most commonly linked to illness include those of animal origin, such as meat products, unpasteurized milk, poultry, and eggs; foods contaminated during cultivation or preparation including vegetables, salads, fruit; and, less commonly, processed foods such as chocolate and snack products. Human infection has also been linked to exotic pets such as turtles, reptiles, and small mammals. People recovering from infection or with mild symptoms excrete salmonellae in their feces, and they may become a source of infection for others. Person-to-person spread is a particular risk where hygiene standards are difficult to maintain, as in institutions, day-care facilities, nursing homes, and households with ill individuals.

Most cases are apparently sporadic, though outbreaks occurring in the general population are not unusual and may be linked to a social event or institution such as a hospital or nursing home, or large-scale catering issues such as hotels, restaurants, and canteens. More rarely, large national and international outbreaks have been associated with manufactured or processed food products—in 1998 over 800 cases of *S. enteritidis* in Canada were associated with a pre-packed lunch product. Probably the largest recorded *Salmonella* outbreak affected an estimated 185,000 individuals who drank improperly pasteurized milk in the United States in 1985. It is recognized that even in countries which keep national statistics most cases are not reported. For example, only an estimated 1

Table 1

Individuals Susceptible to Severe Disease or Complications	
Susceptible Individuals	Possible Complication
Very young and elderly.	Rapid and severe dehydration.
Individuals with low stomach acid.	Increased susceptibility to infection.
Individuals with cancers and depressed immune systems, including HIV-infected persons.	Increased risk of *Salmonella* septicaemia.
Individuals with sickle-cell disease.	Risk of internal abscesses and bone-joint infections.

SOURCE: Courtesy of author.

percent of cases in the United States are reported, and the estimated morbidity and economic burden is high. Current public health concern centers around the emergence of multiple antibiotic resistant salmonellae, which make serious illness, such as blood infection, difficult to treat.

PAUL N. SOCKETT

(SEE ALSO: *Food-Borne Diseases*)

BIBLIOGRAPHY

Old, D. C. (1992) "Nomenclature of *Salmonella.*" *Journal of Medical Microbiology* 37:361–363.

Roberts, J. A., and Sockett, P. (1994) "The Socioeconomic Impact of Human *Salmonella Enteritidis* Infections." *International Journal of Food Microbiology* 21:117–129.

Rodrigue, D. C.; Tauxe, R. V.; and Rowe, B. (1990). "Increase in *Salmonella Enteritidis*: A New Pandemic?" *Epidemiology and Infection* 1:21–27.

Saeed, A. M.; Gast, R. K.; Potter, M. E.; and Wall, P. G., eds. (1999). *Salmonella enteritidis serovar enteritidis in Humans and Animals: Epidemiology, Pathogenesis, and Control.* Ames, IA: Iowa State University Press.

Sockett, P. N. (1991). "The Economic Implications of Human *Salmonella* Infection." *Journal of Applied Bacteriology* 71:289–295.

SAMPLING

In many disciplines, there is often a need to describe the characteristics of some large entity, such as the air quality in a region, the prevalence of smoking in the general population, or the output from a production line of a pharmaceutical company. Due to practical considerations, it is impossible to assay the entire atmosphere, interview every person in the nation, or test every pill. Sampling is the process whereby information is obtained from selected parts of an entity, with the aim of making general statements that apply to the entity as a whole, or an identifiable part of it. Opinion pollsters use sampling to gauge political allegiances or preferences for brands of commercial products, whereas water quality engineers employed by public health departments will take samples of water to make sure it is fit to drink. The process of drawing conclusions about the larger entity based on the information contained in a sample is known as statistical inference.

There are several advantages to using sampling rather than conducting measurements on an entire population. An important advantage is the considerable savings in time and money that can result from collecting information from a much smaller population. When sampling individuals, the reduced number of subjects that need to be contacted may allow more resources to be devoted to finding and persuading nonresponders to participate. The information collected using sampling is often more accurate, as greater effort can be expended on the training of interviewers, more sophisticated and expensive measurement devices can be used, repeated measurements can be taken, and more detailed questions can be posed.

DEFINITIONS

The term "target population" is commonly used to refer to the group of people or entities (the "universe") to which the findings of the sample are to be generalized. The "sampling unit" is the basic unit (e.g., person, household, pill) around which a sampling procedure is planned. For instance if one wanted to apply sampling methods to estimate the prevalence of diabetes in a population, the sampling unit would be persons, whereas households would be the sampling unit for a study to determine the number of households where one or more persons were smokers. The "sampling frame" is any list of all the sampling units in the target population. Although a complete list of all individuals in a population is rarely available, an alphabetic listing of residents in a community or of registered voters are examples of sampling frames.

SAMPLING METHODS

The general goal of all sampling methods is to obtain a sample that is representative of the target population. In other words, apart from random error, the information derived from the sample is expected to be the same had a complete census of the target population been carried out. The procedures used to select a sample require some prior knowledge of the target population, which allows a determination of the size of the sample needed to achieve a reasonable estimate (with accepted precision and accuracy) of the characteristics of the population. Most sampling methods attempt to select units such that each has a definable probability of being chosen. Methods that adopt this approach are called "probability sampling methods." Examples of such methods include simple random sampling, systematic sampling, stratified sampling, and cluster sampling.

A random sample is one where every person (or unit) in the population from which the sample is drawn has some chance of being included in it. Ideally, the selections that make up the sample are made independently; that is, the choice to select one unit will not affect the chance of another unit being selected. The simplest way of selecting sampling units where each unit has an equal probability of being chosen is referred to as a simple random sample.

Systematic random sampling involves deciding what fraction of the target population is to be sampled, and then compiling an ordered list of the target population. The ordering may be based on the date a patient entered a clinic, the last surname of patients, or other factors. Then, starting at the beginning of the list, the initial sample unit is randomly selected from within the first k units, and thereafter every kth individual is sampled. Typically, the integer k is estimated by dividing the size of the target population by the desired sample size. This method of sampling is easy to implement in practice, and the sampling frame can be compiled as the study progresses.

A stratified random sample divides the population into distinct nonoverlapping subgroups (strata) according to some important characteristics (e.g., age, income) and then a random sample is selected within each subgroup. The investigator can use this method to ensure that each subgroup of interest is represented in the sample. This method generally produces more precise estimates of the characteristics of the target population, unless very small numbers of units are selected within individual strata.

Cluster sampling may be used if the study units form natural groups or if an adequate list of the entire population is difficult to compile. In a national survey, for example, clusters may comprise individuals in a localized geographic area. The clusters or regions are selected, preferably at random, and the persons are enumerated in each selected region and random samples are drawn from these units of the population. Because sampling is performed at multiple levels, this method is sometimes referred to as multistage sampling.

With nonprobability sampling methods, the probability of being included in the sample is unknown. Examples of this sampling method include convenience samples and volunteers. These types of samples are prone to bias and cannot be assumed to be representative of the target population. For example, people who volunteer are frequently different in many respects from those who do not. Tests of hypothesis and statistical inference concerning the sampled units and the target population can only be applied with probability sampling methods. That is, there is no way to assess the validity of the samples obtained using nonprobability sampling strategies.

VALIDITY AND SOURCES OF ERROR

The distribution of values in any sample, no matter how it is selected, will differ from the distribution in sample chosen by chance alone. The larger the sample, the more likely it is that the sample reflects the characteristic of interest in the target population. However, there are sources of error not related to sampling that may bias comparisons between the sampled units and the target population. First, coverage error (selection bias) may arise when the sampling frame does not fully cover the target population. Second, nonresponse bias may occur when sampled individuals cannot be reached or will not provide the information requested. Bias is present if respondents differ systematically from the individuals who do not respond. Finally, the measuring device may not be able to accurately determine the characteristics being measured.

PAUL J. VILLENEUVE

(SEE ALSO: *Statistics for Public Health; Stratification of Data; Survey Research Methods*)

BIBLIOGRAPHY

Kelsey, J. L.; Thompson, W. D.; and Evans, A. S. (1986). *Methods in Observational Epidemiology.* New York: Oxford University Press.

Pagano, M., and Gauvreau, K. (2000). *Principles of Biostatistics,* 2nd edition. Pacific Grove, CA: Duxbury.

SANGER, MARGARET

Born in Corning, New York, Margaret Sanger (1883–1966) became a public health nurse and a pioneer in the birth-control movement when contraception and any publications dealing with it were illegal. Her concern about prevention of repeated pregnancies and the heavy toll of sickness and premature deaths they caused among working-class women was aroused when she worked in the poorest neighborhoods of New York early in the twentieth century. She traveled to Europe and trained in aspects of human sexuality with Havelock Ellis. Upon returning to the United States, she embarked on a campaign to improve access to family-planning information for women in their childbearing years. In 1915 she was indicted for sending birth-control pamphlets through the U.S. mails, and in 1916 she was arrested for conducting a birth-control clinic in Brooklyn. She set out her manifesto on family planning in many books and pamphlets, including *What Every Girl Should Know* (1913). This contained chapters on girlhood; puberty; the sexual impulse; reproduction; some consequences of ignorance and silence (such as venereal diseases); and menopause. There were oblique but not direct references to ways that the risk of pregnancy could be reduced, but these and her frankness about taboo topics such as masturbation were enough to make her reviled among leaders of the medical and nursing professions of the day.

However, her enlightened attitudes ultimately prevailed. Her first family planning clinic opened in New York in 1923; she organized national (1921) and international (1925) conferences on family planning. She founded the National Committee on Federal Legislation for Birth Control and presided over this committee until it was disbanded after federal birth control legislation was enacted in 1937. She traveled widely, lecturing on birth control on many countries in Europe, Africa, and Asia and helping to establish family planning clinics in many of them. Her life's work immensely enhanced the lot of women everywhere.

JOHN M. LAST

(SEE ALSO: *Abortion; Condoms; Contraception; Family Planning Behavior*)

BIBLIOGRAPHY

Sanger, M. (1927). *What Every Boy and Girl Should Know.* New York: Bretano's.

—— (1938). *Margaret Sanger: An Autobiography.* New York: W. W. Norton and Company.

SANITARIAN

A sanitarian is a person who is trained in the sanitary sciences, biology, chemistry, geology, physics, and math, and who operates as an inspector or health official in the public sector or private industry, reviewing programs and enforcing local laws to protect the public's health. She or he is a public health professional whose responsibilities may include food sanitation and safety; air, water, and environmental protection; inspection of water-well and sewage-disposal systems; control of insect pests, and animals; disease control and epidemiology; housing, occupational, and institutional safety and sanitation; and nuisance control. Many states require sanitarians to be registered and to maintain registration and continuing education.

DONALD J. MANSON

(SEE ALSO: *Environmental Determinants of Health; Regulations Affecting Housing; Regulations Affecting Restaurants; Vector-Borne Diseases; Waterborne Diseases*)

SANITATION

Sanitation is a basic, as well as a long-standing, public health issue. When early peoples settled in communities and started to cultivate crops and raise animals, sanitation became a primary concern for society. The Book of Leviticus, in the Torah, includes specific guidelines regarding the disposal of wastes, the placement and disinfection of wells, and related issues. Today, as urban areas grow, more pressure has been put on local water supplies, for the quality of the water that is available to a community greatly impacts all aspects of health. Worldwide, 40 percent of the population does not have ready access to clean, safe drinking water, and approximately 60 percent does not have satisfactory facilities for the safe disposal of human waste. Infectious agents in drinking water and food cause the diarrheal deaths of several million children annually.

In the United States, every person uses almost 100 gallons of drinking water per day, though only a small portion of this amount is actually used for drinking. Other uses include toilet flushing, bathing, cooking, cleaning, and lawn watering.

SOURCES OF WATER

Water sources are manifold. Many communities get their water from reservoirs. In 500 B.C.E., the Greeks supplemented local city wells with water supplied from the mountains as far as ten miles away. In later times, the Romans built aqueducts that were many miles long—there are more than two hundred that are still standing in the year 2001. Cities and other communities often provide for their water supply by allocating an open area that is pristine and protected as a watershed. The water is usually of high quality and free from chemical and microbial contamination. These sources are referred to as surface water sources and include lakes, streams, and rivers. Some surface water requires extensive treatment before it can be distributed for human consumption.

In other parts of the country, water is supplied to communities from groundwater sources through deep wells, often many thousands of feet down. Water from these sources is also usually free of chemical and microbial contamination. Groundwater is the main source of drinking water for almost half of the population in the United States. While it is usually free of solids and bacteria, as well as other chemical pollutants, it has often become contaminated by disposal of liquid waste and agricultural runoff. Groundwater is relatively inexpensive, but it is limited in volume and irreplaceable if depleted. By providing protection to the source, either through buffers from the reservoirs or by protecting the well head for the deep wells, water is available without much treatment.

Because of the increasing population and the increased use of water by each individual in the United States, there are less uncontaminated water supplies available. Many sources of water must be treated prior to consumption. Disinfection is an important step in the water treatment process to destroy pathogenic bacteria and other harmful agents. Most water is treated with chlorine, as it is a very effective and economical method of treatment. An important advantage to using chlorine is that it has residual properties and continues to provide germ-killing potential as the water travels from the distribution point to the end users. There are concerns, however, about the formation of disinfection by-products from the reaction of the chlorine with humic substances in the water. These by-products are referred to as trihalomethanes, or THMs. The most common THM is chloroform, which is a carcinogen.

Sanitation includes the appropriate disposal of human and industrial wastes and the protection of the water sources. Waterborne agents are the cause of many diseases in the United States and elsewhere in the world. These diseases may be caused by bacteria, viruses, and protozoans. Bacterial diseases include typhoid, shigellosis, and cholera. Viral agents cause diseases such as include polio and hepatitis. Parasites include the protozoa *Entamoeba histolytica* and *Giardia lambdia*, which cause amebiasis and giardiasis, respectively. For the last decade the primary agents in waterborne disease outbreaks in the United States have been the protozoal parasite *Giardia*, and the bacteria *Shigella*. Another common agent is *Cryptosporidium*.

Another example of sanitation as it relates to waterborne diseases globally is schistosomiasis. Schistosomiasis is a chronic debilitating disease with significant morbidity and mortality that affects more than 200 million people worldwide. Sanitation and water supply are important issues in an integrated schistosomiasis control program.

SANITATION AND WATER POLLUTION

Sanitation is directly related to water quality and water pollution. Water quality usually describes the level of certain compounds that could present a health risk. The quality of water is usually defined by guideline values of what is suitable for human consumption and for all usual domestic purposes, including personal hygiene.

In relating sanitation to water pollution, one must examine both point and nonpoint source pollution, as these are the two routes of entry of the pollution into the water supply. Point-source pollutants enter the waterways at well-defined locations, such as a pipe or a sewer outflow. The discharges are usually even and continuous. Industrial factories, sewage treatment plants, and storm sewer outflows are common point sources of pollution. Nonpoint sources enter the water system from broad areas of land. It is estimated that 98 percent of the bacterial contamination and 73 percent of biological oxygen demand are due to nonpoint sources.

WASTEWATER

Water containing human waste is generally referred to as wastewater. In the United States, the disposal of human waste must be handled in a sanitary manner. Usually, this waste is disposed of via a sewer system that uses water as the vehicle for the disposal. Treatment of wastewater is required to prevent pollution of pristine surface waters and groundwater sources. Wastewater treatment consists of physical, chemical, and biological processes. In a typical suburban or urban setting, wastewater from the home enters a domestic or sanitary sewer system. The sanitary sewer is a system of pipes that collects the wastewater, and the waste is transported to a wastewater treatment plant. The water goes through a series of processes that removes the solids from the water. Solids are composted or removed and disposed of via landfill or land application as fertilizer. Sewage consists of more than 99.9 percent water by weight, and the average domestic sewage contains 600 ppm of total solids. The amount of solids present in water has been one of the major water pollution control criteria, due to the relationship of the solids to the oxygen demand.

Water reuse is an important concept that has only recently gained attention and interest in the United States. Water that is reused, commonly known as "gray water," cannot be used on food crops or in any type of domestic use. This water can be used to water landscape and turf. Water reuse will continue to expand as water resources become more and more limited.

Since approximately 1950, a common method of disposal of solids in the United States has been the use of a sanitary landfill. The landfill, which typically is located outside a populated area, is a place where wastes are dumped, compacted, and buried. Special care in siting the landfill must be taken to avoid runoff and leaching of the waste materials into surface water and groundwater. Landfills that are properly designed with the correct engineering and liners can provide adequate protection. In many locations in the United States, these landfills have been sited on marginal land that was unsuitable for industry or agriculture. Many of these sites are sensitive wetland areas that serve as habitat for plants and animal species.

The 1974 Safe Drinking Water Act established a set of primary standards to protect human health. These standards consist of maximum contaminant levels for specific inorganic contaminants, volatile organic chemicals, and radioactive materials, as well as limits for turbidity and coliform organisms. Secondary standards are set for temperature, color, taste, and odor. The Environmental Protection Agency has identified treatment via conventional coagulation, sedimentation, and filtration as effective processes in removing or reducing the levels of contaminants. Societal concerns for the quality of water resources continue as many streams and coastal waters do not meet water quality goals. States report that 40 percent of the waters surveyed are too contaminated for drinking, fishing, and swimming. Since the Clean Water Act was signed in 1972, it is estimated that more than $5 trillion has been spent on water pollution control in the United States.

MARK G. ROBSON

(SEE ALSO: *Ambient Water Quality; Biological Oxygen Demand; Chlorination; Clean Water Act; Disinfection By-Products in Drinking Water;* *Groundwater; Landfills, Sanitary; Municipal Solid Waste; Pollution; Wastewater Treatment; Water Quality; Water Reuse; Water Treatment; Waterborne Diseases*)

BIBLIOGRAPHY

McKenzie, J., and Pinger, R. (1997). *An Introduction to Community Health.* Sudbury, MA: Jones and Bartlett.

Merson, M.; Black, R.; and Mills, A., eds. (2001). *International Public Health: Diseases, Programs, Systems, and Policies.* Gaithersburg, MD: Aspen Publishers.

Morgan, M. T. (1997). *Environmental Health.* Madison, WI: Brown and Benchmark.

SANITATION IN DEVELOPING COUNTRIES

In 1999 the United Nations acknowledged that the development gap between rich and poor countries was widening: about three-fifths of the world's population lacked access to basic sanitation; and one-third did not have access to safe drinking water. Industrial development affects public health both favorably and unfavorably. Improved housing and social conditions and reductions in infectious diseases like gastroenteritis or pneumonia are often accompanied by increases in degenerative, noninfectious diseases like cancer and heart disease. In rapidly developing countries, such as Mexico, the People's Republic of China, and the Philippines, new public health problems often emerge before the old ones have been solved, and it is important to assess which problems pose the greatest risks to health, and which solutions are most cost-effective. Large funding organizations like the United Nations, the World Bank, and regional development banks now recognize that to solve priority health problems requires improvements in behaviors, attitudes, skills, services, products, and infrastructure that together yield lasting benefits long after external support is withdrawn.

In this global context, providing both safe drinking water and wastewater sanitation have long been recognized as priorities for the improvement of human health, especially in the prevention of infant and child mortality from diarrheas and dysenteries (e.g., *Amoebiasis*, caused by a protozoan; or *E. coli* diarrhea, caused by a bacterium). An estimated 4 billion cases of diarrheal disease occur worldwide every year, killing an estimated 3

Table 1

Major Water-Related Diseases and Sanitation Solutions

Disease	Infection route	Range	Cases[1]	Deaths per year	Problem → Sanitation Solution
Major Water-borne Diseases					
1. Amoebic dysentry	Protozoa (e.g. *Giardia* or *Cryptosporidium*) follow the fecal-oral route; i.e., feces contaminate water and/or food that is ingested.	Worldwide	500 million per year	included in 3. below	Unsanitary excreta disposal, poor personal and domestic hygiene, unsafe drinking water. → Low-cost sanitation such as latrines, pour-flush toilets, and septic tanks. Education to promote basic hygiene (e.g., washing food, handwashing before eating and preparing meals). Provide safe drinking water sources.
2. Bacillary dysentry	Bacteria by fecal-oral route	Worldwide	included in 3.	included in 3.	
3. Diarrheal disease (incl. Amoebic and Bacillary dysentry)	Various bacteria, viruses, and protozoa by fecal-oral route.	Worldwide	4 billion in 1998	3-4 million	
4. Cholera	Bacteria by fecal-oral route.	S. America, Africa, Asia	384,000 per year	20,000	
5. Hepatitis A	Virus by fecal-oral route.	Worldwide	600,000 to 3 million per year	2,400-12,000	
6. Paratyphoid & Typhoid	Bacteria by fecal-oral route.	Asia (80%), Africa, Latin America (20%)	16 million in 1996	600,000	
7. Polio	Virus by fecal-oral route.	India (66%), Near East, Asia, Africa (34%)	82,000 in 1996	9,000	
Major Water-based Diseases					
8. Ascariasis	Eggs in human feces – larvae develop in soil – soil on food – food eaten by humans and worm infects small intestine.	Africa, Asia, Latin America	250 million in 1996	60,000	Unsanitary excreta disposal, poor personal and domestic hygiene. → Low-cost sanitation. Education to promote basic hygiene, especially in children.
9. Clonorchiasis	Worms in snails – snails eaten by fish – raw/undercooked fish eaten by humans.	Southeast Asia	28 million in 1994	None reported	Unsanitary excreta disposal, poor personal and domestic hygiene → Low-cost sanitation. Education to promote basic hygiene.
10. Dracunculiasis (Guinea worm)	Human host has blister, immersion in water causes larvae to release, larvae eaten by crustacean, in turn eaten by humans.	Sudan (78%), sub-Saharan Africa	153,000 per year	None reported	Unsafe drinking water supply. → Provide safe drinking water supply.
11. Necatoriasis (Hookworm)	Eggs in feces hatch to larvae in soil and on grass, pass into humans through skin to infect small intestine.	Tropical and subtropical Africa and Asia	900 million in 1990	60,000 per year	Unsanitary excreta disposal, poor personal and domestic hygiene. → Low-cost sanitation such as latrines, pour-flush toilets, and septic tanks. Education to promote basic hygiene.
12. Paragonimiasis	Worms in human lungs lay eggs, coughed up and swallowed – eggs excreted in feces and break in freshwater. Larvae find snail host then move into crab or crayfish – humans eat raw seafood – worms move from stomach to lungs.	Far East, Latin America	5 million in 1994	None reported	
13. Schistosomiasis (Bilharzia)	Eggs passed out in feces to water, releasing parasites – pass into snail host to replicate – pass into water – pass through human skin and become worms.	Africa, Near East, Western Pacific, Southeast Asia	200 million in 1996	20,000	Unsanitary excreta disposal, unsafe bathing water. → Provide safe water. Low-cost sanitation such as latrines, pour-flush toilets, and septic tanks.

[CONTINUED]

Table 1 continued

Major Water-Related Diseases and Sanitation Solutions

Disease	Infection route	Range	Cases[1]	Deaths per year	Problem → Sanitation Solution
Major Water-related Vector Diseases					
14. Dengue	Virus passes to mosquito from infected person or animal – replicates and passes again into human by mosquito bite.	Tropical areas, Asia, Central and South America	50-100 million per year	24,000	Poor water management: poor operation of water sources, drainage and storage. Poor solid waste management.
15. Filariasis (includes Elephantiasis)	Worm larvae pass to mosquito and replicate – pass into humans by bite.	Africa, Eastern Mediterranean, Asia, South America	120 million in 1996	None reported	→ Combination of improved water management (drainage, preventing stagnant water bodies), physical barriers to hosts (bednets, screens at night), biological methods (introduce natural enemies of hosts), and chemical (pesticides). Best methods emphasize sanitation to reduce dependence on chemicals like DDT.
16. Malaria	Protozoa in mosquito gut pass to humans by bite.	Africa, Southeast Asia, India, South America	300-500 million per year (clinical)	2 million	
17. Onchocerciasis (river blindness)	Worm embryos eaten by black flies and become larvae – pass to humans by bite.	sub-Saharan Africa, Latin America	18 million in 1996	None reported but 270,000 cases of blindness per year	
18. Rift valley fever (RVF)	Virus passes to mosquito/other blood-sucking insects from infected person or animal – replicates and passes again into human by bite.	sub-Saharan Africa	No data	No data	
Water-washed Diseases					
19. Trachoma	Virus infects eye and infection is contagious.	Worldwide	150 million	None reported but 5.9 million cases of blindness or severe complications per year	Lack of face washing, bathing and safe water. → Provide safe water. Personal hygiene and education.
20. Flea, mite (e.g. Scabies), lice, and tick-borne diseases	Contagious skin infections caused by contact with fleas, mites, lice and ticks.	Worldwide	No data	No data	

[*] cases given as number per year (incidence) or as number of cases in existence at a given time/in a given year (prevalence)

SOURCES: Hinrichsen et al., 1998; World Health Organization at http://www.who.ch/

to 4 million people per year, most of them children (see Table 1). While it can be readily argued that a safe water supply plus wastewater sanitation is the most cost-effective public health goal for any given population, in practice, many social, cultural, technical, and economic factors govern whether the design and implementation of these systems will provide the long-term benefits sought.

To measure development and health progress, public health agencies use indicators such as access to water supply, access to sanitation, the under-five-year-old child mortality rate (U5MR), and per capita income. In 2000, the UN reported that the U5MR varied from 4 per 1,000 live births for developed countries like Sweden, Japan, and Norway, to 280,292, and 316 per 1,000 for Niger, Angola, and Sierra Leone, respectively. Figure 1 shows the relationship between the U5MR and access to safe water. Figure 2 shows the relationship between the U5MR and access to sanitation. These figures clearly show that improved water supply and/or sanitation can reduce child mortality (see Table 2).

WATER AND HEALTH

The uncontrolled pollution of water supplies by chemical and pathogens is one of the most serious threats to public health and the natural environment in developing countries. Standing water is a

Figure 1

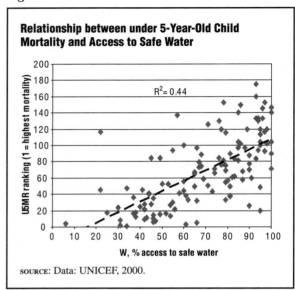

Relationship between under 5-Year-Old Child Mortality and Access to Safe Water

$R^2 = 0.44$

U5MR ranking (1 = highest mortality)

W, % access to safe water

SOURCE: Data: UNICEF, 2000.

medium for vector-borne diseases, and caused by poor water management, especially poor drainage. Table 1 shows the main water-related diseases from pathogens (viruses, bacteria, and protozoa), their relative geographical extent, numbers of cases, mortality rate, and sanitation solutions. Although the focus for remediation varies by disease and local conditions, all solutions include attention to four basic factors: 1) basic infrastructure (water supply and waste disposal); 2) personal and domestic hygiene; 3) better housing; and 4) primary health care and health promotion. Where basic infrastructure is lacking, pathogens are the priority contaminants, although the comparative risks posed by chemical pollutants should also be considered, especially in industrial areas and areas using pesticides. In dealing with pathogens in these areas, it is important to consider the life cycle of pathogens, pathogen infection routes, and pathogen susceptibility to treatment.

Chemical pollution of water from agricultural and/or industrial practices may include organic substances such as polychlorinated biphenyls (PCBs), chlorinated pesticides and herbicides, polyaromatic hydrocarbons (PAHs), solvents and disinfection by-products (DBPs), as well as inorganic substances like metals and nitrates. The risks posed by such chemicals to human health depend on three parameters: their concentrations in the

water; their specific toxicity for both cancer effects and noncancer effects (e.g., birth defects, reproductive effects, neurotoxicity); and dose rate (the amount of substance entering the body over time). Pollutants in water can enter the body by ingestion of the water in drinks and food, by bathing and skin contact with the water, and by inhalation of the water vapor while showering.

Sanitation solutions for chemical agents combine prevention and cure tactics. Prevention includes minimizing the sources of pollution by substituting nontoxic substances and using cleaner, more efficient technologies. Cure consists of treating water to appropriate quality standards according to use (domestic, industrial, or agricultural). Water supply and wastewater treatment systems in developing countries must be affordable, cost-effective, and able to be maintained by local people.

The monitoring and enforcement of appropriate water quality standards is a vital part of sanitation. Diverse chemical and microbial standards seek to regulate important known risk agents, and acceptable levels must be monitored. In the United States, the Primary ("legally enforceable") Drinking Water Standards cover 60 organic chemicals, 20 inorganics, and 8 microbes/indicator organisms. The World Health Organization's *Guidelines for Drinking-Water Quality* includes over 60 organic chemicals (31 of them pesticides), 19 inorganics, 17 disinfectants and their by-products, and pathogens. However, although water quality laws exist in many developing countries, their enforcement is either weak or nonexistent, most often due to a lack of resources and political will.

The 1980s were designated the International Drinking Water Supply and Sanitation Decade by the United Nations. Despite the efforts of this campaign, however, in many countries more than half the rural populations are without adequate water supply access and sanitation. Many of the failures can be explained by weaknesses in the design and implementation of projects, as evidenced by many abandoned water and wastewater treatment plants. Such weaknesses often stem from a lack of maintenance caused by failures in equipment or training. A widespread lack of community participation in projects also helps explain failures. In most developing countries, the public sector provides facilities to central urban areas but

Table 2

World Sanitation Status

Country	W(%)	S(%)	U5MR	P	Country	W(%)	S(%)	U5MR	P	Country	W(%)	S(%)	U5MR	P
Afghanistan	6	10	4	257	Ghana	65	32	49	105	Nigeria	49	41	15	187
Algeria	90	91	88	40	Guatemala	68	87	74	52	Oman	85	78	140	18
Angola	31	40	2	292	Guinea	46	31	14	197	Pakistan	79	56	33	136
Argentina	71	68	126	22	Guinea-Bissau	43	46	11	205	Palau	88	98	97	34
Bahamas	94	82	130	21	Guyana	91	88	60	79	Panama	93	83	133	20
Bahrain	94	97	133	20	Haiti	37	25	36	130	Papua New Guinea	41	83	45	112
Bangladesh	95	43	48	106	Honduras	78	74	81	44	Paraguay	60	41	100	33
Barbados	100	100	146	15	India	81	29	49	105	Peru	67	72	73	54
Belize	83	57	83	43	Indonesia	74	53	71	56	Philippines	85	87	81	44
Benin	56	27	22	165	Iran	95	64	100	33	Qatar	100	97	140	18
Bhutan	58	70	41	116	Iraq	81	75	37	125	St. Kitts and Nevis	100	100	90	37
Bolivia	80	65	57	85	Jamaica	86	89	149	11	St. Vincent/Grenadines	89	98	120	23
Botswana	90	55	77	48	Jordan	97	99	93	36	Sao Tome and Principe	82	35	61	77
Brazil	76	70	85	42	Kazakhstan	93	99	83	43	Saudi Arabia	95	86	113	26
Burkina Faso	42	37	22	165	Kenya	44	85	40	117	Senegal	81	65	38	121
Burundi	52	51	17	176	Korea, Dem. People's Rep.	100	99	104	30	Sierra Leone	34	11	1	316
Cambodia	30	19	24	163	Korea, Rep. of	93	100	175	5	Somalia	31	43	8	211
Cameroon	54	89	27	153	Kyrgyzstan	79	100	69	66	South Africa	87	87	58	83
Cape Verde	65	27	65	73	Lao People's Dem. Rep.	44	18	41	116	Sri Lanka	57	63	137	19
Central African Rep.	38	27	18	173	Lebanon	94	63	94	35	Sudan	73	51	43	115
Chad	54	27	13	198	Lesotho	62	38	33	136	Swaziland	50	59	53	90
China	67	24	79	47	Liberia	46	30	6	235	Syria	86	67	102	32
Colombia	85	85	104	30	Libya	97	98	117	24	Tanzania	66	86	32	142
Comoros	53	23	53	90	Madagascar	40	40	25	157	Thailand	81	96	90	37
Congo	34	69	47	108	Malawi	47	3	7	213	Togo	55	37	30	144
Congo, Dem. Rep.	42	18	9	207	Malaysia	78	94	153	10	Tonga	95	95	120	23
Cook Islands	95	95	104	30	Maldives	60	44	56	87	Tunisia	98	80	102	32
Costa Rica	96	84	145	16	Mali	66	6	5	237	Turkey	49	80	85	42
Côte d'Ivoire	42	39	28	150	Mauritania	37	57	16	183	Turkmenistan	74	91	66	72
Cuba	93	66	160	8	Mauritius	98	100	120	23	Tuvalu	100	78	71	56
Djibouti	90	55	26	156	Mexico	85	72	97	34	Uganda	46	57	35	134
Dominica	96	80	133	20	Micronesia	22	39	117	24	United Arab Emirates	97	92	153	10
Dominican Rep.	79	85	75	51	Rep. of Moldova	55	50	94	35	United States	100	100	160	8
Ecuador	68	76	89	39	Mongolia	45	87	28	150	Uzbekistan	90	100	70	58
Egypt	87	88	68	69	Morocco	65	58	67	70	Vanuatu	77	28	76	49
El Salvador	66	90	97	34	Mozambique	46	34	10	206	Venezuela	79	59	115	25
Equatorial Guinea	95	54	20	171	Myanmar	60	43	44	113	Viet Nam	45	29	85	42
Eritrea	22	13	45	112	Namibia	83	62	62	74	Yemen	61	66	38	121
Ethiopia	25	19	18	173	Nepal	71	16	51	100	Yugoslavia	76	69	130	21
Fiji	77	92	120	23	Nicaragua	78	85	77	48	Zambia	38	71	12	202
Gambia	69	37	59	82	Niger	61	19	3	280	Zimbabwe	79	52	55	89

W   percentage of population with access to safe drinking water 1990-98
S   percentage of population with access to adequate sanitation 1990-98
U5MR   world ranking of under-five-year-old mortality (1998 data)
P   1998 under-five-year-old mortality: probability of dying between birth and 5 years old expressed per 1,000 live births

SOURCE: UNICEF 2000, multiple data compilation

leaves rural and marginal urban areas underserved. A 1990 evaluation of water-decade achievements in rural Bangladesh revealed that even when safe water supply and sanitary latrines were provided, people did not always use them, while only a third of the household water supplies had adequate usage. This demonstrates the need for joint improvements in education and economic conditions to accompany investments in infrastructure.

A useful reference for the visualization of health-risk sources, diseases, and solutions is the water-wastewater cycle (see Figure 3). The cycle ideally consists of water supply parts and sanitation counterparts, with each stage (or lack of it) affecting others. It should be remembered that this engineered cycle operates within the natural constraints of a dynamic hydrological cycle that supplies water to plants and animals as well as

Figure 2

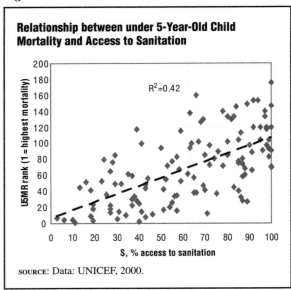

Relationship between under 5-Year-Old Child Mortality and Access to Sanitation

$R^2 = 0.42$

U5MR rank (1 = highest mortality)

S, % access to sanitation

SOURCE: Data: UNICEF, 2000.

people. Human beings have coevolved with other species in these ecosystems, while at the same time becoming super-modifiers of them. Logically, the health of people is influenced by the condition of these ecosystems.

ENVIRONMENTAL SANITATION

Holistic environmental sanitation has four main water-related aspects: water supply, rainwater drainage, solid waste disposal, and excreta disposal.

Water Supply. The major problem for poor people in most countries is access to safe water in adequate quantity, with reasonable convenience, and at an affordable cost. Solutions include local grants to install household gutters and rainwater capture tanks; local wells designed to resist pollution; and small networks of water points served by a local well, borehole, or spring. The supply problems of major cities require integrated approaches that combine demand management, leak repair, backflow prevention, wastewater reuse, and the efficient, sustainable exploitation of sources.

Rainwater Drainage. Without adequate control of rainwater to mitigate floods and soil erosion, other sanitation measures can be nullified. People safe from floods and mudslides are more willing to invest in sanitation for their homes; and

those in poor tropical urban areas attach a high priority to rainwater drainage. While local communities can build local drainage, downstream obstructions can cause the backing-up of channels and rivers, requiring a watershed-wide strategy.

Solid Waste Disposal. The interdependence of sanitation aspects is illustrated by the need for adequate solid waste removal to prevent the blockage of rainwater drains. Collection of refuse in hot climates must be frequent since piles attract flies and rats, and it should rely more on local labor-intensive methods rather than on expensive trucks. For the operation to be successful requires close cooperation between the users and providers of the service, and financing must come either from municipal recurrent funds and/or user fees.

Excreta Disposal. Large sewerage infrastructure projects tend to be too expensive for the vast majority of urban and rural people in developing countries, and it may be impossible to build a sewage network infrastructure in congested, narrow streets. On-site options include latrines, pour-flush toilets, and septic tanks. There should be evaluated at each location according to needs and priorities. As water use grows in villages and towns, wastewater from washing and bathing (sullage) can be cost-effectively handled by a separate drainage system coupled to on-site excreta disposal.

TOWARD LASTING SANITATION

Sanitation, including water supply, is a major part of the United Nation's 1992 Agenda 21, a "Blueprint for Sustainable Development." The paradigm of sustainable development focuses on how to satisfy the basic needs of the present human population, and also secure resources to satisfy the needs of future generations. Growing population pressure, persistent poverty, and ecological degradation call for new integrated solutions to sanitation problems that strengthen both socio-economic and technical elements, including the following:

1. Financial, political, and societal will to invest in public health and the environment.

2. Human resources and public awareness through education and training.

Figure 3

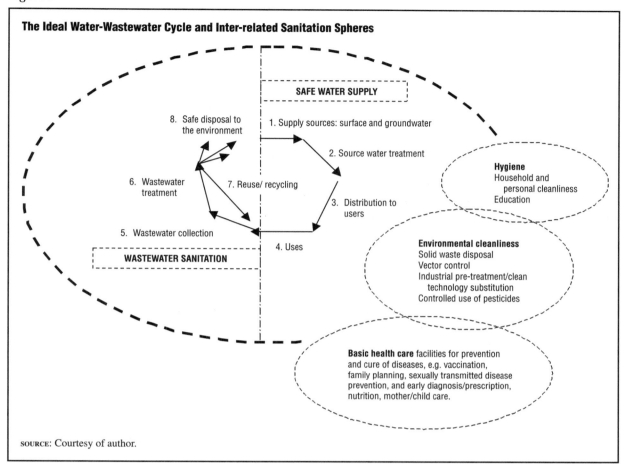

The Ideal Water-Wastewater Cycle and Inter-related Sanitation Spheres

SAFE WATER SUPPLY

8. Safe disposal to the environment

1. Supply sources: surface and groundwater

2. Source water treatment

6. Wastewater treatment

7. Reuse/ recycling

3. Distribution to users

5. Wastewater collection

4. Uses

WASTEWATER SANITATION

Hygiene
Household and personal cleanliness
Education

Environmental cleanliness
Solid waste disposal
Vector control
Industrial pre-treatment/clean technology substitution
Controlled use of pesticides

Basic health care facilities for prevention and cure of diseases, e.g. vaccination, family planning, sexually transmitted disease prevention, and early diagnosis/prescription, nutrition, mother/child care.

SOURCE: Courtesy of author.

3. Information resources—on health, water cycle, and ecological monitoring—for informed planning and actions.

4. Regulatory frameworks, enforcement, and compliance.

5. Basic sanitation infrastructure suited to local priorities and conditions.

6. A market for public health and environmental support goods and services that provide economically viable, effective, and lasting sanitation strategies.

These elements are interdependent. For example, adequate training improves monitoring and the operation and maintenance of infrastructure; and effective, enforced regulations stimulate a market and long-term investment. In India, state water boards were established to prevent pollution under the 1974 Water Act, closely modeled on

systems in Great Britain. However, despite good scientists and engineers on staff, the chronic shortage of funds means controls have a limited effect on sanitation.

Above all, the support and involvement of the local community are essential if sanitation is to work. Ideally, many social sectors should be involved, to varying degrees, in community-driven ("bottom-up") sanitation projects. Sanitation users, water and public health regulators and administrators, health professionals, sanitation engineers, ecologists, researchers and scientists, financing agencies and donors, nongovernmental organizations, and suppliers of health and sanitation products and services can all contribute to a successful project. These new approaches reflect the trend away from professionally centered, curative methods and towards multi-stakeholder preventive strategies. To face these challenges, public health professionals and institutions need to play an expanding role as facilitators and promoters of this trend, building new partnerships in developing and developed countries. Protecting public health and ecological integrity are ethical and practical imperatives to be viewed as opportunities for people from diverse cultures, social groups, and disciplines to work more closely together.

TIMOTHY J. DOWNS
I. H. SUFFET

(SEE ALSO: *Chlorination; Drinking Water; E. Coli; International Development of Public Health; Rural Public Health, Sanitation; Sewage System; Wastewater Treatment; Waterborne Diseases; Water Quality; Water Treatment*)

BIBLIOGRAPHY

Bell, M.; Franceys, R.; and Liao, M. (1995). "The International Water Decade and Beyond: New Public Health Interventions." In *Health Interventions in Less Developed Nations*, ed. S. J. Ulijaszek. Oxford: Oxford University Press.

Carter, R. C.; Tyrrel, S. F.; and Howsam, P. (1999). "The Impact and Sustainability of Community Water Supply and Sanitation Programmes in Developing Countries." *Journal of the Chartered Institution of Water and Environmental Management* 13(4):292–296.

Downs, T. J. (2000). "Changing the Culture of Underdevelopment and Unsustainability." *Journal of Environmental Planning and Management* 43(5): 601–621.

Downs, T. J.; Mazari-Hiriart, M.; Dominguez-Mora, R.; and Suffet, I. H. (2000). "Sustainability of Least Cost Policies for Meeting Mexico City's Future Water Demand." *Water Resources Research* 36(8):2321–2339.

Feachem, R. G.; McGarry, M.; and Mara, D., eds. (1977). *Water, Wastes, and Health in Hot Climates*. Chichester, Sussex: John Wiley.

Harpham, T.; Lusty, T.; and Vaughan, P., eds. (1988). *In the Shadow of the City: Community Health and the Urban Poor*. Oxford: Oxford University Press.

Hinrichsen, D.; Robey, B.; and Upadhyay, U. D. (1998). "Solutions for a Water-Short World." *Population Reports* Series M, No. 14.

Lewis, W. J.; Foster, S. S. D.; Read, G. H.; and Schertenleib, R. (1981). "The Need for an Integrated Approach to Water Supply and Sanitation in Developing Countries." *Science of the Total Environment* 21:53–59.

Listorti, J. A. (1993) *Environmental Health Components for Water Supply, Sanitation and Urban Projects* (World Bank Technical Paper 121). Washington, DC: The World Bank.

Muyibi, S. A. (1992). "Planning Water Supply and Sanitation Projects in Developing Countries." *Journal of Water Resources Planning and Management* 118(4): 351–355.

Phillips, D. R. (1990). *Health and Health Care in the Third World*. New York: John Wiley.

UNICEF. *The State of the World's Children 2000*. Available at http://www.unicef.org/sowc00.

World Health Organization. *Water-Related Diseases Bibliography*. Available at http://www.who.ch/.

Yusuf, M., and Hussain, A. M. Z. (1990). "Sanitation in Rural Communities in Bangladesh." *Bulletin of the World Health Organization* 68(5):619–624.

SCHISTOSOMIASIS

Schistosomiasis, also known as bliharzia or bilharziasis, is a parasitic infection caused by trematodes, also known as flatworms or flukes, of the genus *Schistosoma*. There are many species of animal schistosomes worldwide, with five responsible for the majority of human infections: *S. haematobium, S. mansoni, S. japonicum, S. intercalatum,* and *S. mekongi*. Schistosomiasis is the second most common human parasitic disease, malaria being the most common.

The World Health Organization estimates that 600 million people worldwide are at risk of infection, with 200 million already infected. Of these, over 120 million have a symptomatic infection. The disease is endemic in over seventy-five countries.

Schistosomes are blood flukes that have two distinct life-cycle stages: a sexual stage in mammals and an asexual stage in freshwater snails. Humans acquire infection when they come into contact with freshwater lakes and rivers containing infective schistosome larvae, called "cercariae." Cercariae penetrate the skin, migrate through the bloodstream and, in the case of *S .mansoni, S. japonicum, S. intercalatum,* and *S. mekongi*, come to rest in the mesenteric venous plexus. *S. haematobium* cercariae end up in venous plexus surrounding the urinary bladder. The male and female worms mature into adults and form a permanent mating pair that lives up to five years. Approximately six weeks after the initial infection, the females begin to produce between 200 and 3,000 eggs a day, depending on the species. Approximately half of the eggs are excreted in the urine or stool. If the excreted eggs reach freshwater, they hatch into free swimming miracidiae that will infect the appropriate snail species. Further development occurs within the snail and, after three to five weeks, a new generation of cercariae emerge from the snail ready to infect other mammalian hosts.

Most infections are asymptomatic. In a minority of cases, a transient illness may occur several weeks after the initial infection, known as Katayama fever, characterized by fever, cough, abdominal pain, and diarrhea.

Many eggs are not excreted and end up trapped in tissues. The host's granulomatous inflammatory response to these eggs is responsible for most of the damage associated with chronic schistosomiasis. S. haematobium eggs, which are mainly found around the bladder, can result in hematuria, ureteric obstruction, and bladder cancer. Eggs of the other species usually lodge in mesenteric vessels draining to the liver and cause periportal fibrosis, with the subsequent development of portal hypertension, splenomegaly, esophageal varices, and progressive liver dysfunction. Eggs in the bowel mucosa cause ulcerations and polyp formation leading to diarrhea and abdominal pain. When portal hypertension occurs, eggs are shunted to the lungs, where pulmonary hypertension may occur.

Diagnosis is made by finding the characteristic eggs in stool or urine. Because eggs may be excreted intermittently, several specimens should be examined. Occasionally, a rectal or bladder biopsy may be necessary. Serology is the most sensitive diagnostic tool and is particularly useful for detecting light infections. However, the antibody test does not distinguish between past and current infection, so it is not clinically useful in areas of high prevalence where individuals may have been successfully treated and then reinfected.

The drug of choice for treatment is praziquantel. Other options include oxamniquine for treatment of S. mansoni and metrifonate for S. haematobium. Treatment may reverse some of the long-term sequelae of infection, including fibrosis, especially in children.

Infection control is based on two strategies: reduction of transmission and reduction of morbidity. Reduction of transmission is accomplished by providing safe water supplies and proper sanitation facilities. Snail eradication is not an effective long-term strategy. Much of the focus of current schistosomiasis control strategies is to minimize the morbidity caused by the infection through mass treatment of at risk populations with praziquantel. This approach also leads to the reduction of egg output and transmission.

MARTHA FULFORD
JAY KEYSTONE

(SEE ALSO: *Communicable Disease Control; Tropical Infectious Diseases*)

BIBLIOGRAPHY

Ali El-Garem, A. (1998). "Schistosomiasis." *Digestion* 59:589–605.

Bica, I.; Hamer, D. H.; and Stadecker, M. J. (2000). "Hepatic Schistosomiasis." *Infectious Disease Clinics of North America* 14(3):583–604.

Dunne, D. W.; Hagan, P.; and Abath, F. G. C. (1995). "Prospects for Immunological Control of Schistosomiasis." *Lancet* 345:1488–1492.

Elliot, D. E. (1996). "Schistosomiasis, Pathophysiology, Diagnosis and Treatment." *Gastroenterology Clinics of North America* 25(3):599–625.

Lucey, D. R., and Maguire, J. H. (1993). "Schistosomiasis." *Infectious Disease Clinics of North America* 7(3):635–653.

Mostafa, M. H.; Sheweita, S. A.; and O'Connor, P. J. (1999). "Relationship between Shistosomiasis and Bladder Cancer." *Clinical Microbiology Reviews* 12(1): 97–111.

World Health Organization (1993). "The Control of Schistosomiasis: Second Report of the WHO Expert Committee." *WHO Technical Report Series* 803:1–86.

—— (1996). "Schistosomiasis." (Fact Sheet No. 115). Geneva: Author.

SCHIZOPHRENIA

Schizophrenia, often misunderstood as split personality, is a chronic mental illness characterized by psychosis, or loss of reality testing. It is a heterogeneous disease in its presentation, course, effect on functioning, response to treatment, and possibly even etiology. In 1990, the total cost of schizophrenia in the United States, including mental health and societal costs, was estimated at $32.5 billion. The risk of suicide in schizophrenia is at least 10 percent, which is twenty times the risk in the general population. Over 70 percent of persons with schizophrenia are unemployed. An estimated 30 to 50 percent of the homeless population has schizophrenia. As one of the most chronically disabling mental illnesses, it can be devastating for those afflicted and their families, and it has a significant impact on public mental health systems.

Schizophrenia presents as a syndrome. The symptoms are organized into three major categories: positive symptoms, negative symptoms, and cognitive impairment. Positive symptoms include hallucinations, delusions, thought disorders, and bizarre behaviors. Hallucinations are most commonly auditory, usually experienced as voices talking to or about the person. Delusions are false beliefs and tend to be paranoid, grandiose, or bizarre in nature. Disorganized speech is presumed to be a manifestation of an underlying thought disorder. The flow of ideas is illogical and may range from being mildly confusing to incomprehensible. Words may be strung together based on sound rather than meaning, or entirely new words may be created. Bizarre behavior may be observed as repetitive movements, unusual mannerisms, odd ways of dressing, and disregard for social norms.

Negative symptoms include flat affect (facial expression), avolition, and apathy. A flat affect is one revealing little emotion or expression. Generally, persons with schizophrenia seem emotionally disconnected and tend to be socially withdrawn. Avolition and apathy are characterized by a lack of motivation and poor grooming and hygiene. In addition to the positive and negative symptoms of schizophrenia, cognitive impairment with deficits in attention span, memory, and information processing is often present. Persons with schizophrenia experience varying constellations and severities of symptoms resulting in a range of impaired functioning.

The prevalence of schizophrenia is approximately 0.85 percent of the population worldwide and is fairly consistent across race and geographical regions. Men and women are equally affected. Average age of onset in men is 15 to 25 years of age, while in women it is 25 to 35 years of age. No clear risk factors for developing schizophrenia have been identified except a family history of the disease. The disease course is marked by relapses and remissions. Although some persons with schizophrenia regain their premorbid functioning, most experience chronic debilitating symptoms. Acute onset, female gender, being married, and good premorbid adjustment are factors associated with a better prognosis.

The etiology of schizophrenia is poorly understood. Prevailing theories propose a biological vulnerability to developing schizophrenia with both environmental and psychological factors contributing. The biological vulnerability is likely genetic and is suggested by twin studies, adoption studies, and an increased rate of schizophrenia in relatives of persons with the disorder. Immunological abnormalities, viral infections, and hypoxia have all been hypothesized as mechanisms of environmental assaults on the developing brain. Pathological theories focus on abnormalities in the neural circuitry and in neurotransmitters, particularly dopamine. The role of dopamine in schizophrenia is supported by studies showing that increased dopamine activity can induce psychotic symptoms, while blocking dopamine receptors can decrease psychosis.

Schizophrenia is a chronic illness that is managed, not cured. Treatment is most effective when elements of pharmacotherapy, supportive therapy, and psychosocial rehabilitation are integrated. Pharmacotherapy with antipsychotic medications, also called neuroleptics, is the mainstay of treatment and is crucial for diminishing the acute symptoms of schizophrenia as well as maintaining remission. The presumed mechanism of action of these medications is blockade of dopamine receptors in neural tissue. Due to the severity of symptoms and the functional impairments they produce, psychosocial supports and rehabilitation are important for individuals with schizophrenia and their families. Individual supportive therapy and group therapy can promote the development of strategies to manage psychotic symptoms and to manage stress, which can contribute to relapses. Rehabilitation targets the improvement of vocational and social skills. Case management facilitates access to social services, entitlements, housing, and medical care. Up to 25 percent of those with schizophrenia are too impaired to care for themselves in the community and require residential treatment programs or long-term hospitalization. Even when a person is able to live in the community, brief hospitalizations are often necessary to treat exacerbations of psychosis.

STUART J. EISENDRATH
KARA POWERS

(SEE ALSO: *Community Metal Health Centers*)

BIBLIOGRAPHY

Eisendrath, S. J., and Lichtmacher, J. E. (1999). "Psychiatric Disorders." In *Current Medical Diagnosis and Treatment 1999*, eds. L. M. Tierney, S. J. Mcphee, and M. A. Papadakis. Stamford, CT: Appleton and Lange.

Kaplan, H. I., and Sadock, B. J. (1998). *Kaplan and Sadock's Synopsis of Psychiatry: Behavioral Sciences/Clinical Psychiatry*, 6th edition. Baltimore, MD: Williams & Wilkins.

SCHOOL HEALTH

For more than 150 years, schools in the United States have addressed the health and safety needs of their students. Prior to the mid-1800s, public education was still in a formative state, and efforts to introduce health into the schools were isolated and sparse. In 1840, Rhode Island became the first state in the nation to require children to attend school, and other states adopted compulsory education soon afterwards. The foundation for school health programs is often credited to Lemuel Shattuck's report in 1850 for the Sanitary Commission of Massachusetts. Among other recommendations, the report described the value of using schools to control communicable diseases. Shattuck's report is applicable to current health problems, which often have their etiology in health risk behaviors established during childhood. According to the report: "Every child should be taught early in life, that, to preserve his own life and his own health and the lives and health of others, is one of the most important and constantly abiding duties." By the late 1860s, the New York City Board of Health had established sanitary inspections for communicable diseases in schools.

By the end of the nineteenth century, the era of medical inspection in schools became institutionalized, with school nurses gradually replacing medical inspectors.

In 1918, the Commission on the Reorganization of Secondary Education published a landmark report identifying the desired outcomes of education. Health was the first of seven cardinal outcome objectives, the other objectives were command of fundamental processes, worthy home membership, vocation, citizenship, use of leisure, and ethical character. As a result of the temperance movement of the late nineteenth and early twentieth centuries, schools incorporated lessons on the effects of alcohol, tobacco, and narcotics into the hygiene curricula. Physical education was also introduced into the school curricula during this time period.

Between 1918 and 1921, many U.S. states enacted laws requiring health education and physical education for school children. However, as a result of a report issued by the National Education Association and the American Medical Association, primary health care services were gradually replaced with preventive health care by school nurses. This report defined the role of schools in screening for health problems and referring students with problems to health professionals. By the 1970s, there was a reemergence of primary health care in schools, with the establishment of school-based clinics centered around the unique physical, emotional, and developmental needs of students. By 1999, there were over 1,100 school-based or school-linked health centers in forty-five states.

From the early 1900s through the 1980s, school health programs had three components: health education, health services, and a healthy school environment. In 1987, D. D. Allensworth and L. J. Kolbe proposed an eight-component model that included the original three components, but added physical education; nutrition and food services; counseling, psychological, and social services; health promotion for staff; and family and community involvement.

Health education consists of a planned, sequential, K-12 curriculum that addresses the physical, mental, emotional, and social dimensions of health. Health services are provided to students to appraise, protect, and promote health. These services include the provision of emergency and primary care, access and referral to community health services, and management of chronic health conditions. A healthy school environment attends to the physical and aesthetic surroundings, and to a psycho-social climate and culture that maximizes the health of students and staff. Physical education is a planned, sequential, K-12 curriculum that provides cognitive content and learning experiences from a variety of activities that students can enjoy all their lives, such as basic movement skills; physical fitness, rhythms and dance; games; and sports. School nutrition and food services promote the health and education of students through access to a variety of nutritious meals, an environment that promotes healthful food choices, and support for nutrition instruction in the classroom and cafeteria. Counseling, psychological, and social services provide broad-based individual and group assessments, interventions, and referrals that attend to the mental, emotional, and social health of students. Health promotion for staff provides health assessments, health education, and health-related fitness activities. These programs also encourage staff to become positive role models. Family and community involvement promotes an integrated school, parent, and community approach that establishes a dynamic partnership to enhance the health and well-being of students, with schools being encouraged to actively solicit parent involvement and engage community resources and services.

These eight components interact best when they focus on the behaviors that interfere with learning and long-term well-being; and when they foster support of family, friends, and community; use interdisciplinary and interagency teams to plan and coordinate the program; use multiple intervention strategies; promote student involvement; and provide staff development.

The eight-component model forms the basis of a coordinated school health program (CSHP), currently defined as "an integrated set of planned sequential, school-affiliated strategies, activities, and services designed to promote the optimal physical, emotional, social, and educational development of students. The program involves and is supportive of families and is determined by the local community based on community resources, standards and requirements. It is coordinated by a multidisciplinary team and accountable to the community for program quality and effectiveness" (Allensworth, 1997).

While no studies have evaluated the efficacy of the CSHP, there have been numerous studies that have evaluated the components individually and in combination with each other. These studies have shown that health education can improve the adoption of health-enhancing behaviors (Connell et al., 1985; Resnicow et al., 1991) and school achievement (Hawkins et al., 1999); and that nutrition services, and particularly school breakfast programs, have increased learning (Meyers et al., 1991; Powell et al., 1998). Health services have been associated with reduced absenteeism, academic achievement, and improved health status (U.S. General Accounting Office, 1983). Physical education has been shown to improve physical fitness, reduce stress, and enhanced student's self image (Dwyer, 1983; Pate et al., 1995). Involving family members and the community have been linked with improving health knowledge and behaviors (Pentz, 1997), and health promotion for faculty and staff have improved absenteeism rates for staff as well as improved their health status (Blair et al., 1984).

Public support is strong for health-related services and education in schools. According to a Gallup survey of U.S. adults in 1998, health ranked the highest of fifteen subject areas that were "definitely necessary" for schools to teach (Marzano et al., 1998). Business leaders are concerned about the "employability" of graduates and want schools to help provide a healthy, productive workforce. Voluntary health organizations and insurance companies support school health programs in order to prevent future chronic health conditions that lead to increased medical care costs.

During the 1990s in Europe, the concept of a health-promoting school has emerged, which incorporates policies, curriculum, psycho-social and physical environment, health services, and formal and informal partnerships between schools, parents, the health sector, and the local community to maximize successful outcomes in youth. With the support of the World Health Organizations, the European Network for Health Promoting Schools now has thirty-eight countries involved. WHO's Expert Committee on Comprehensive School

Health Education and Promotion has identified principles and priorities for actions to improve global school health, acknowledging that theories and frameworks for a coordinated and integrated approach to school health are relatively sophisticated, so application and adaptability to different nations and cultures may be far less developed. The WHO notes that school health policies, intersectoral collaboration, program implementations, financial support and administrative support could be enhanced in many countries.

Schools alone cannot be expected to solve the most serious health and social problems. However, schools can provide an ideal setting in which families, health professionals, and community agencies can work together to improve the well-being of young people.

DIANE D. ALLENSWORTH
LINDA S. CROSSETT

(SEE ALSO: *Child Care, Daycare; Child Health Services; Community Health; School Health Educational Media*)

BIBLIOGRAPHY

Allensworth, D. D., and Kolbe, L. J. (1987). "The Comprehensive School Health Program: Exploring an Expanded Concept." *Journal of School Health* 57(10): 408–41.

Allensworth, D.; Lawson, E.; and Nicholson, W. J., eds. (1997). *Schools and Health: Our Nation's Investment.* Washington, DC: Institute of Medicine.

Allensworth, D. (1998). "Improving the Health of Youth through a Coordinated School Health Programme." *Health Promotion and Education* 1.

Blair, S. N.; Collingwood, T. R.; Reynolds, T. C.; Smith, M.; Hagen, R. D.; and Sterling, C. L. (1984). "Health Promotion for Educators: Impact on Health Behaviors, Satisfaction, and General Well-Being." *American Journal of Public Health* 74:147–149.

Buddy, D., ed. (1999). *The Evidence of Health Promotion Effectiveness,* Brussels: European Commission and International Union for Health Promotion and Education.

Connell, D. P.; Turner, R. R.; and Mason, E. F. (1985). "Summary of Findings of the School Health Education Evaluation: Health Promotion Effectiveness, Implementation, and Costs." *Journal of School Health* 55(8):316–384.

Dwyer, T.; Coonan, W. E.; Leitch, D. R.; Hetzel, B. S.; and Baghurst, R. A. (1995). "An Investigation of the Effects of Daily Physical Activity on the Health of Primary School Students in South Australia." *International Journal of Epidemiology* 12:308–313.

Hawkins, J. D.; Catalano, R. F.; Kosterman, R.; Abbot, R.; and Hill, K. G. (1999). "Preventing Adolescent Health-Risk Behaviors by Strengthening Protection during Childhood." *Archives of Pediatric Adolescent Medicine* 153:226–233.

Marks, E.; Wooley, S. F.; and Northrop, D., eds. (1998). *Health Is Academic: A Guide to Coordinated School Health Programs.* New York: Teachers College Press.

Marzano, R.; Kendall, J.; and Cicchinelli, L. (1998.) *What Americans Believe Students Should Know: A Survey of U.S. Adults.* Aurora, CO: Gallup Survey for Mid-continent Research for Education and Learning.

Meyers, A.; Sampson, A.; and Weitzman, M. (1991). "Nutrition and Academic Performance in School Children." *Clinics in Applied Nutrition* 1:13–25.

Pate, R. R.; Pratt, M.; Blair, S. N.; Haskell, W. L.; Macera, C. A.; Bouchard, C. et al. (1995.) "Physical Activity and Public Health: A Recommendation from the Centers for Disease Control and Prevention and the American College of Sports Medicine." *Journal of American Medical Association* 273(5):402–407.

Pentz, M. A. (1997). "The School-Community Interface in Comprehensive School Health Education." In *Schools and Health: Our Nation's Investment,* eds. D. Allensworth, E. Lawson, and W. J. Nicholson. Washington, DC: Institute of Medicine.

Powell, C. A.; Walker, S. P.; Chang, S. M.; and Grantham-McGregor, S. M. (1998). "Nutrition and Education: A Randomized Trial of the Effects of Breakfast in Rural Primary School Children." *American Journal of Clinical Nutrition* 68(10):873–879.

Resnicow, K.; Ross, D.; and Wyner, E. L. (1991). "The Role of Comprehensive School-Based Interventions. The Results of Four 'Know Your Body' Studies." *Annals of the New York Academy of Sciences* (April 12):285–298.

U. S. General Accounting Office (1993). *School-Linked Human Services: A Comprehensive Strategy for Aiding Students at Risk for School Failure.* GAO/HRD-94-21. Washington, DC: Author.

WHO/UNFPA/UNICEF Study Group on Programming for Adolescent Health (1999). *Programming for Adolescent Health and Development.* Geneva: WHO.

SCHOOL HEALTH AND SAFETY

See School Health

SCHOOL HEALTH EDUCATIONAL MEDIA

Media in learning consists of environment educational formats and tools that appeal to the learner through the senses of sight, sound, touch, taste, and smell. Multiple media formats provide opportunities to enrich health topics in the classroom by providing more than one view of an issue, and by encouraging thinking. To be effective, such formats must be aligned with focused educational objectives. Health education is one important component of the comprehensive school health program that includes the development, delivery, and evaluation of a planned instructional program and related activities for students preschool through 12th grade. Both parents and school staff should have a role in such a program. Media formats contribute to the understanding and development of health knowledge, attitudes, and skills. Media aligned with school health education supports several dimensions of education, including curricula, school environment, health-related services, and community-based interactions.

School-based curricula are supported by a variety of media venues, including audio, visual, and electronic formats. They are selected based upon specific objectives relating to knowledge gain, attitude change, and behavior change. As an example, a video that depicts factual information about an infectious disease like chlamydia may work well if the objective is to impart knowledge. However, when the objective is to change attitudes, a medium may be selected which impacts on a person's perceived susceptibility to acquiring chlamydia (e.g., an audiotape or video which features interviews with infected peers).

In addition to addressing established objectives, media selections are also based upon audience age level, cultural sensitivity, accuracy of the information, duration of the media format, and cost. Personal computer (PC) technology is a medium that not only supports in-class activities, but can also assist in facilitating homework and project development. Some instructors use e-mail technology to interact with their students, possibly posing a hypothetical problem that needs resolution. Using this approach, a dialogue may be established between the instructor and the students while they are in a real world setting (e.g., home, community, school).

Media formats can also enhance healthful school environments and services. Developing an environment of support can be important in both the social and psychological dimensions, as well as in the physical school setting itself. Various colors, placement of artwork, pleasant sounds, and offering a safe environment for learning all can contribute to the development of a positive, supportive, and learning-conducive environment. Timely and well-placed print and electronic announcements regarding available health services provided by the school or outside agencies can generate a sense of caring. Such approaches also engender a sense that the school is a valued community resource.

Community-based interactions can be enhanced through a careful selection of media formats. A typical objective is to convey information to key community members (parents, agency representatives, government officials) about a major school-related issue. This may be achieved through printed reports that summarize and highlight school-based survey data, accomplishments in accordance with state, regional, or national standards, or other important information. Curricular revisions are often presented in printed and audiovisual formats. When requested revisions are presented in a clear and timely manner it can provide a sense of an orderly and consistent approach to change. It also enables community members to receive the information in advance of public hearings or discussions. Complementing the printed material, audiovisual formats can help clarify important health-related issues and trends in the school and community. Audiovisual formats can be enhanced using computer-based media, which can provide clear overviews and examples, incorporating static or movement-related visuals.

School health education plays a vital role, not just in education, but in improving public health throughout the community and the nation. Major negative issues such as violence, injury, and abuse;

as well as important positive aspects of both the school and community settings such as asset development, wellness enhancement, and achievement recognition, can be reviewed and addressed more completely and systematically through the selection of appropriate media formats.

GARY D. GILMORE

(SEE ALSO: *Communication for Health; Communication Theory; School Health*)

BIBLIOGRAPHY

Cortese, P., and Middleton, K. (1994). *The Comprehensive School Health Challenge.* Santa Cruz, CA: ETR Associates.

Gilbert, G., and Sawyer, R. (1995). *Health Education: Creating Strategies for School and Community Health.* Boston: Jones and Bartlett.

Joint Committee on Health Education Terminology (1990). "Report of the 1990 Joint Committee on Health Education Terminology." *Journal of Health Education* 22(2):97–108.

Meeks, L.; Heit, P; and Page, R. (1996). *Comprehensive School Health Education.* Blacklick, OH: Meeks Heit.

Read, D., and Greene, W. (1989). *Creative Teaching in Health.* Prospect Heights, IL: Waveland Press.

SCREENING

Screening is performed to identify the presence of a disease or a risk factor for a disease, typically among asymptomatic persons (those who do not already manifest symptoms of disease). In this way, a disease, or risk factors for a disease, can be detected early, allowing either early treatment or prevention, including preventing further spread of communicable or transmissible diseases. Screening tests are widely used by clinicians as part of the periodic health examination, as well as by public health officials. Examples of screening tests are as varied as blood tests to detect lead poisoning in young children, blood tests to detect the human immunodeficiency virus (HIV), measuring blood pressure to detect high blood pressure, mammography to detect breast cancer, sigmoidoscopy and colonoscopy to detect cancers of the rectum and colon, and questionnaires to identify persons with alcohol or other drug problems.

Table 1

Two-By-Two Table to Assess the Usefulness of a Screening Test			
	Disease	No Disease	
Positive Test	True Positive (TP)	False Positive (FP)	Total Positive
Negative Test	False Negative (FN)	True Negative (TN)	Total Negative
	Total with Disease	Total with No Disease	

SOURCE: Courtesy of author.

Several factors determine the usefulness of a screening test for use with any individual person. The first is the accuracy of the test itself, specifically its sensitivity and specificity. Sensitivity is the probability that a person with the disease or risk factor will test positive. Specificity is the probability that a person without the disease or risk factor will test negative. Sensitivity and specificity are illustrated in Table 1. The sensitivity of a screening test is determined by the number of true positives divided by the total number with disease (or TP/[TP+FN]). The specificity is the number of true negatives divided by the total number with no disease (or TN/[FP+TN]).

Because there is often some overlap in the distributions of test results among people with and without disease (i.e., some people without disease will have test results in the disease range, and some people with disease will have test results in the no disease range), a test's sensitivity and specificity usually trade-off against one another. As the sensitivity increases the specificity usually decreases, and vice versa. A screening test that identifies almost all people with a disease (high sensitivity) may also produce more false positives among those people without the disease who may have borderline results (results near the cut-off value defined for the test). Conversely, a screening test that correctly identifies almost all people without the disease (high specificity) usually misses more people who truly have the disease (false negatives). Tables 2 and 3 represent the characteristics of two hypothetical screening tests when applied to a sample of 100,000 people with a true prevalence of disease of 10 percent (e.g., a relatively common disease). Table 2 is for a test with a sensitivity of 95

Table 2

Screening Test with High Sensitivity (95%) and Moderate Specificity (65%) in a Sample with a 10% True Prevalence of Disease			
	Disease	No Disease	Total
Positive Test	9,500	31,500	41,000
Negative Test	500	58,500	59,000
Total	10,000	90,000	100,000

SOURCE: Courtesy of author.

Table 3

Screening Test with Moderate Sensitivity (65%) and High Specificity (95%) in a Sample with a 10% True Prevalence of Disease			
	Disease	No Disease	Total
Positive Test	6,500	4,500	11,000
Negative Test	3,500	85,500	89,000
Total	10,000	90,000	100,000

SOURCE: Courtesy of author.

percent and a specificity of 65 percent. Table 3 is for a test with 65 percent sensitivity and 95 percent specificity. The test with high sensitivity (Table 2) identifies more people who truly have the disease and misses fewer people who truly have the disease (false negatives). However, this test incorrectly classifies more than three people without the disease (false positives) for every one person it correctly identifies with the disease. In contrast, the test with high specificity (Table 3) incorrectly classifies many fewer nondiseased people as having the disease (false positives) but misses more truly diseased people (false negatives).

In addition to the accuracy of the test itself, another important factor is how well the test is implemented. Errors may be introduced that depend on who is performing the test or on variations in the way the test is performed. For example, not all radiologists are equally proficient at reading mammograms and not all laboratories will get the same result when measuring cholesterol levels from the same blood sample. Therefore, the test characteristics that are initially reported for a screening test often represent a best case scenario—the best that a test can be expected to perform. As a result, it is also important to evaluate test accuracy in the real world settings where the tests are being used.

The usefulness of a screening test also depends upon the probability that the individual being tested has the disease or risk factor of interest. This is termed the "prior probability" of disease. This issue is illustrated by comparing Table 2 and Table 4. Table 4 represents the same hypothetical test shown in Table 2, but applied to a

sample in which the true prevalence of disease is less common, only 1 percent instead of 10 percent. As shown, screening tests are more useful when they are used on people who are more likely to have the disease than people who are less likely to have the disease. When a screening test is used in a sample with a lower prior probability of disease, even more false positives are identified. In this example (Table 4), the test has incorrectly identified more than 36 people who do not really have the disease (false positives) for every one person correctly identified with the disease (true positives).

Prior probability is taken into account in calculating the predictive value of a test. The predictive value of a positive test is the probability that someone who tests positive truly has the disease. For the examples shown in Tables 2, 3, and 4, the predictive values of a positive test are 23 percent, 59 percent, and 3 percent, respectively. As can be seen, the predictive value of a positive test is increased when tests with higher specificity are used in samples of people with a higher prevalence of the disease.

Finally, the usefulness of a screening test depends on the existence of an effective and feasible treatment. This may include treatment for the disease or risk factor detected, and/or an intervention to prevent further spread of the problem to others, such as removing lead paint from homes or genetic counseling. If there are no feasible and effective responses to the results of a screening test (e.g., the result wouldn't change anything) then there is no reason to perform the test.

These issues are of particular concern for screening asymptomatic or healthy people. All

Table 4

Screening test with high sensitivity (95%) and moderate specificity (65%) in a sample with a 1% true prevalence of disease			
	Disease	No Disease	Total
Positive Test	950	34,650	35,600
Negative Test	50	64,350	64,400
Total	1,000	99,000	100,000

SOURCE: Courtesy of author.

testing involves risks. These risks might be acceptable to the small number of persons who turn out to have the disease. However, the risks of side-effects from the screening tests themselves, or from an incorrect or ambiguous diagnosis and the subsequent testing that an incorrect initial test result requires, may not be acceptable to the much larger number of people who do not have the disease or risk factor of interest. In addition, there are economic costs to screening large numbers of asymptomatic people to identify a small number of people with disease. Therefore, clinicians, patients, and public health professionals must weigh the risks and benefits when deciding to use a screening test for any individual or population.

THOMAS N. ROBINSON

(SEE ALSO: *Assessment of Health Status; Blood Lead; Blood Lipids; Breast Cancer; Cancer; Cholesterol Test; Colorectal Cancer; Diabetes; HIV/AIDS; Mammography; PAP Smear; Periodic Health Examination; Prevention; Preventive Medicine; Serological Markers; VDRL Test*)

BIBLIOGRAPHY

Kraemer, H. C. (1992). *Evaluating Medical Tests: Objective and Quantitative Guidelines.* Newbury Park, CA: Sage Publications.

U.S. Preventive Services Task Force (1996). *Guide to Clinical Preventive Services,* 2nd edition. Washington, DC: U.S. Department of Health and Human Services.

SECONDARY PREVENTION

Secondary prevention generally consists of the identification and interdiction of diseases that are present in the body, but that have not progressed to the point of causing signs, symptoms, and dysfunction. These preclinical conditions are most often detected by disease screening (and follow-up of the findings). Examples of screening procedures that lead to the prevention of disease emergence include the Pap smear for detecting early cervical cancer, routine mammography for early breast cancer, sigmoidoscopy for detecting colon cancer, periodic determination of blood pressure and blood cholesterol levels, and screening for high blood-lead levels in persons with high occupational or other environmental exposures.

ROBERT B. WALLACE

(SEE ALSO: *Prevention; Prevention Research; Primary Prevention; Screening; Tertiary Prevention*)

SEER PROGRAM

The Surveillance, Epidemiology, and End Results (SEER) Program of the National Cancer Institute is the most authoritative source of information on cancer incidence and survival in the United States. Established in 1973, SEER originally provided cancer incidence data for Connecticut, Iowa, New Mexico, Utah, and Hawaii, and for the metropolitan areas of Detroit and San Francisco-Oakland. Since then, a number of other areas have been added to the program, including the metropolitan areas of Atlanta, Seattle, and Los Angeles; counties in Georgia; Native-American populations in Arizona and Alaska; and the states of New Jersey, Louisiana, Kentucky, and California.

SEER registries routinely collect data on cancer patients, demographics, primary tumor site, morphology, stage at diagnosis, first course of treatment, and follow-up for vital status. SEER data, publications, and resources are available at http://www.seer.cancer.gov.

BRENDA K. EDWARDS

(SEE ALSO: *Cancer; Data Sources and Collection Methods; Demography; Epidemiology; National Institutes of Health; Vital Statistics*)

SEGREGATION

Segregation is the separation of people based on race, religion, ethnic group, sex, or social class. In the United States, racial segregation has been the most prevalent and visible form. After the abolition of slavery in 1865, laws, known as Jim Crow laws, were passed in most southern states. The term "Jim Crow" referred to an African-American character in a popular song composed in the 1830s, and these laws, already introduced after that time were designed to enforce racial separation. Segregation was not only enforced by law, but also by various forms of physical violence. African Americans were forced to sit only in the back of buses and trains, use "black only" water fountains, and enter through the back doors of hotels and restaurants—if allowed to enter at all. Laws forced blacks to live only in certain sections of a town or city, be educated in separate schools, and obtain health care in separate hospitals or wards. They were also excluded from some governmental jobs.

Segregation not only limited black people physically, but also economically and socially, by blocking access to schooling and jobs. It also served as a form of humiliation and degradation. The Supreme Court, however, upheld segregation laws as late as 1896, in *Plessy v. Ferguson*, ruling that "separate but equal" facilities were constitutional. This concept was argued against strongly by both African Americans and whites throughout the United States. Eventually, arguments by Thurgood Marshall before the Supreme Court in *Brown v. Board of Education of Topeka* in 1954 led the Court to declare school segregation unconstitutional. This started a series of legal battles, lobbying efforts, boycotts, and protests, which eventually brought an end to de jure, or legal, segregation and discrimination. Even so, de facto segregation, or segregation in fact, continues, and is evident in housing, education, and a number of other areas. Integration remains a continuous process in the United States.

The long-term impact of years of racial segregation persists even to this day. African Americans continue to live in the sections of cities and towns where they were initially forced to live, and they continue to suffer from a lack of economic and educational opportunities. The long and difficult experience of segregation has also resulted in deep mistrust of whites by African Americans. This has, at least in part, contributed to the noticeable disparities in health status and access to health services. In particular, African Americans appear to be more hesitant to seek medical attention. There are many potential reasons, such as previous bad experiences with white health care providers as well as the fact that they may not be as aware of their health problems as whites because of disparities in the provision of health education. Even after becoming aware of their need for services, however, African Americans may experience many barriers to accessing services (i.e., lack of insurance, transportation). They are also more likely to obtain inadequate care even after overcoming these barriers. These discrepancies are extensively documented in the health-services research literature.

RACHEL JEAN-BAPTISTE
DUNCAN NEUHAUSER

(SEE ALSO: *African Americans; Asian Americans; Cultural Appropriateness,; Cultural Identity; Ethnicity and Health; Ethnocentrism; Hispanic Cultures; Inequalities in Health; Prejudice; Race and Ethnicity*)

BIBLIOGRAPHY

Barnes, C. A. (1983). *Journey from Jim Crow: The Desegregation of Southern Transit*. New York: Columbia University Press.

Bhopal, R. (1998). "Spectre of Racism in Health and Health Care: Lessons from History and the United States." *British Medical Journal* 316(7149):1970–1973.

Feagin, J. R. "Segregation." *World Book Encyclopedia Millennium 2000*. Chicago: World Book.

Freeman, H. W.; Blendon, R. J.; Aiken, L. H.; Sudman, S.; Mullinix, C. F.; and Corey, C. R. (1987). "Americans Report on Their Access to Health Care." *Health Affairs* 6(1):6–8.

King, D. (1995). *Separate and Unequal: Black Americans and the U.S. Federal Government*. Oxford: Claredon Press.

Wasby, S. L.; D'Amato, A. A.; and Metrailer, R. (1977). *Desegregation from Brown to Alexander*. Carbondale: Southern Illinois University Press.

Wolf, J. H.; Breslau, N.; Ford, A. B.; Ziegler, H. D.; and Ward, A. (1983). "Access of the Black Urban Elderly to Medical Care." *Journal of National Medical Association* 75(1):41–46.

SELF-CARE BEHAVIOR

Self-care behavior, a key concept in health promotion, refers to decisions and actions that an individual can take to cope with a health problem or to improve his or her health. Examples of self-care behaviors include seeking information (e.g., reading books or pamphlets, searching the Internet, attending classes, joining a self-help group); exercising; seeing a doctor on a regular basis; getting more rest; lifestyle changes; following low fat diets; monitoring vital signs; and seeking advice through lay and alternative care networks, evaluating this information, and making decisions to act or even to do nothing. Self-care is generally viewed as a complement to professional health care for persons with chronic health conditions. Self-care behavior is, however, broader than just following a doctor's advice. It also encompasses an individual's learning from things that have worked in the past.

Presumed benefits of self-care include lower costs for the health care system; more effective working relationships between patients and physicians and other health care providers; increased patient satisfaction; and improved perceptions of one's health condition. Self-help behaviors have been shown to lessen pain and depression and to improve quality of life. However, a relationship between self-care behaviors and positive physiological outcomes has not been proven. Generally, health care practitioners encourage and support patients to practice self-care behaviors because patients then actively participate in their own care. However, many practitioners experience difficulty in offering advice on self-care behaviors because they are not aware of specific techniques, strategies, and supports that patients can use.

Within a health promotion context that views health as a resource for daily living, self-care is seen as empowering. Through acquisition of self-care skills, people are able to participate more actively in fostering their own health and in shaping conditions that influence their own health.

DEFINITIONS OF SELF-CARE

No single definition of self-care behavior has been broadly accepted. Definitions vary as to (1) who actually engages in self-care behavior (e.g., individual, family, community); (2) what prompts self-care behaviors (e.g., to practice health promotion, to prevent illness, to limit the impact of illness, to restore health); and (3) the extent to which health care professionals are involved.

The World Health Organization defines self-care as "activities individuals, families, and communities undertake with the intention of enhancing health, preventing disease, limiting illness, and restoring health. These activities are derived from knowledge and skills from the pool of both professional and lay experience. They are undertaken by lay people on their own behalf, either separately or in participative collaboration with professionals." Other experts define self-care in terms of individual behavior when a person functions on his or her own behalf in health promotion and prevention or in disease detection and treatment. In this definition, self-care behaviors occur without professional assistance, but individuals are informed by technical knowledge and skills derived from both professional and lay experience. Still others define self-care as involving activities to enhance health, prevent disease, evaluate symptoms, and restore health—either with or without participation by professionals.

PREVALENCE

Studies report that 80 to 95 percent of all health problems are managed at home through self-care and that most people who consult a physician have tried treating themselves before seeking medical advice. The seriousness of the health problem and the extent and type of disability, including its affect on daily activities, are the best determinants of whether an individual uses self-care practices or seeks help from a professional. In one study of older persons, J. Norburn and colleagues (1995) found that race, gender, education, place of residence, and socioeconomic status did not significantly influence the likelihood of self-care behaviors. Persons with chronic health conditions often become more knowledgeable about their conditions than the average health care professional, and they frequently participate in group or community self-care educational and support programs.

HISTORICAL DEVELOPMENT

Some authors discuss self-care as a kind of social movement and not in terms of specific health-related behaviors and activities. A major influence in the modern interest in self-care developed in the 1960s with the advent of social movements, such as the women's movement and consumerism. Such movements were concerned with issues of autonomy, self-determination, and independence in both health and illness. A shift from physician-dominated health care was catalyzed by the realization that individuals play a large role in directing their own health and therefore they should become more involved in making decisions that affect their health. During the following decades, several factors contributed to the growth in self-care, including a shift in patterns of disease from acute to chronic illnesses; a change in emphasis from cure to care; an increasing discontent with excessive technology and depersonalized medical care; a growth in lay knowledge; a desire for increased personal control in interactions with health care professionals; a need to control escalating health care costs; an increased level of education and knowledge among the general population; a broader dissemination of health-relevant information; a greater emphasis on the rights of consumers; and an increasing knowledge about the importance of lifestyles for longevity and quality of life.

Self-care now is concerned with development and use of personal health practices and coping skills, making decisions involving consulting others (including lay persons and professionals), and using one's own resources to manage health problems.

Several health care disciplines have achieved consensus on what characterizes self-care. Self-care is situation and culture specific; involves the capacity to act and make choices; is influenced by knowledge, skills, values, motivations, control, and confidence; and it focuses on aspects of health care under individual control, as opposed to aspects governed by social policy or legislation.

THEORETICAL APPROACHES TO SELF-CARE

In general, researchers have relied on existing, general theories of behavior change to explain self-care. These major theories include the social learning theory, the health belief model, the theory of reasoned action, and the transtheoretical model of behavior change. They have met with varying degrees of success in explaining self-care practices and why some people do or do not engage in these activities.

Two theories are specific to self-care: D. E. Orem's theory of self-care (1991), which is a conceptual theory and not empirically derived, is specific to managed-care environments in which nursing interventions occur; and the self-regulation model of self-care developed by E. Leventhal, H. Leventhal, and C. Robitaille.

This latter theory has been tested to a limited extent and appears to hold promise in explaining why people do or do not engage in self-care behavior. It posits that an individual's differences and motivations play a critical role in explaining decisions to initiate and sustain self-care behaviors. The following diagram illustrates the basics of this theory.

In this model, an individual's reality and the emotional reactions to this reality interact. Concurrently, action plans and procedures for managing the symptoms are generated. Finally, there is an appraisal of anticipated and actual outcomes, with this feedback possibly leading to changes in emotional reactions and perceptions of reality, which in turn lead to changes in action plans, and so forth. This theory essentially explains how people represent and manage health threats and how this changes over time in relation to experiences and the course of the health threat.

PATRICK McGOWAN

(SEE ALSO: *Alternative, Complementary, and Integrative Medicine; Behavior, Health-Related; Breast Self-Examination; Contraception; Enabling Factors; Folk Medicine; Foods and Diets; Health Belief Model; Internet; Predisposing Factors; Self-Help Groups; Theory of Reasoned Action; Transtheoretical Model of Stages of Change; Wellness Behavior*)

BIBLIOGRAPHY

Dean, K. (1986). "Lay Care in Illness." *Social Science Medicine* 22:275–284.

—— (1996). "Self-Care Behavior: Implications for Aging." In *Self-Care and Health in Old Age: Health*

Figure 1

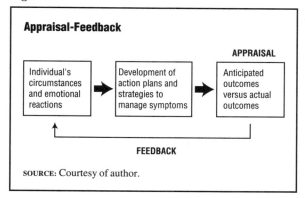

Appraisal-Feedback

APPRAISAL

Individual's circumstances and emotional reactions → Development of action plans and strategies to manage symptoms → Anticipated outcomes versus actual outcomes

FEEDBACK

SOURCE: Courtesy of author.

Behavior Implications for Policy and Practice, eds. K. Dean, T. Hickey, and B. E. Holstein. London: Croom Helm.

Gantz, S. B. (1990). "Self-Care: Perspectives from Six Disciplines." *Holistic Nursing Practice* 4(2):1–12.

Health Promotion and Programs Branch, Health Canada (1997). *Supporting Self-Care: The Contributions of Nurses and Physicians.* Ottawa: Minister of Public Works and Government Services Canada.

Leventhal, E.; Leventhal, H.; and Robitaille, C. (1998). "Enhancing Self-Care Research: Exploring the Theoretical Underpinnings of Self-Care." In *Self-Care in Later Life: Research, Program, and Policy Perspectives,* eds. M. Ory and G. DeFriese. New York: Springer.

Levin, L.; Katz, A.; and Holst, E. (1976). *Self-Care: Lay Initiatives in Health.* New York: Prodist.

Norburn, J.; Bernard, S.; Konrad, T.; Woomert, A.; DeFriese, G.; Kalsbeek, W.; Koch, G.; and Ory, M. (1995). "Self-Care Assistance from Others in Coping with Functional Status Limitations among a Sample of Older Adults." *Journal of Gerontology: Social Sciences* 50B:S101–S109.

Orem, D. E. (1991). *Nursing: Concepts of Practice.* St. Louis, MO: Mosby.

World Health Organization (1983). *Health Education in Self-care: Possibilities and Limitations.* Geneva: Author.

SELF-HELP GROUPS

The primary focus of self-help groups is to provide emotional and practical support and an exchange of information. Such groups use participatory processes to provide opportunities for people to share knowledge, common experiences, and problems. Through their participation, members help themselves and others by gaining knowledge and information, and by obtaining and providing emotional and practical support. These groups have been particularly useful in helping people with chronic health conditions and physical and mental disabilities. Traumatic life events such as death and divorce are also the basis for groups. Self-help groups are voluntary, and they are mostly led by members. Generally, groups meet on a regular basis, are open to new members, and do not cost money to join. Traditionally, self-help groups have been in-person meetings, but recently Internet self-help groups have become popular.

PATRICK McGOWAN

(SEE ALSO: *Internet; Social Networks and Social Support*)

SEMMELWEIS, IGNAZ

The Hungarian physician Ignaz Semmelweis (1818–1865) graduated in medicine from Vienna in 1844. He then worked in the obstetric wards at the Allegemeines Krankenhaus in Vienna, where he was one of a generation of young medical men trained by the anatomical pathologist Karl von Rokitansky who sought to transform traditional but ineffective treatment methods by attacking difficult clinical problems with logic and mathematical precision. Semmelweis was particularly disturbed by the appalling death rate from puerperal sepsis, or childbed fever. The germ theory of disease was gaining ascendancy at that time, and Semmelweis reasoned that the women must be acquiring the infection from their medical attendants. He observed that these attendants habitually came direct to the obstetric service from autopsies on women who had died of childbed fever—without washing their hands. He initiated a rule that required his staff to take particular care to wash their hands with soap and dip their fingers in a bowl of antiseptic solution before attending women in labor. He presented unassailable proof that observing this regimen reduced deaths from childbed fever in his wards to near zero. Many senior obstetricians, however, regarded his ideas as a personal affront, and Semmelweis's confrontational style did not help him to win the argument. The combination of his abrasive personality and the hostility of the medical establishment in Vienna proved too much for him, and in 1851 he returned to Hungary as a professor of obstetrics in Budapest, where he adopted the same successful methods to reduce the toll of childbed fever.

Semmelweis belatedly published his methods and results in 1864. But by then his intellectual powers were waning, perhaps because of mental illness, and he died of septicemia the following year. Semmelweis's method was accepted immediately in parts of Bavaria as well as in Hungary, and it was developed independently in Boston by Oliver Wendell Holmes, who encountered much the same hostility and opposition from the Boston medical establishment, despite also demonstrating beyond doubt (albeit with less convincing numerical methods) that personal cleanliness by birth attendants could prevent childbed fever.

Only in 1867, when the English surgeon Joseph Lister began using the more cumbersome method of antiseptic sprays in operating rooms (but without the hand washing, at least initially) to control postoperative infection, was the problem of childbed fever effectively controlled in the English-speaking world. Had the obstetricians of the United States, France, and Great Britain heeded the evidence offered by Ignaz Semmelweis and Oliver Wendell Holmes, a whole generation of young women need not have died. (The problem of puerperal sepsis seems to have been less serious in countries where women were not attended by doctors, but supporting facts are scarce.) Semmelweis in particular deserves to be honored as the first to offer solid scientific proof that birth attendants' personal hygiene was absolutely essential to prevent unnecessary deaths from puerperal infection.

JOHN M. LAST

BIBLIOGRAPHY

Nuland, S. B. (1981). "The Enigma of Semmelweis—An Interpretation." In *The Etiology of Childbed Fever*, trans. F. P. Murphy. Birmingham, AL: Classics of Medicine Library.

SEROLOGIC TEST FOR SYPHILIS

See VDRL Test

SEROLOGICAL MARKERS

Serology is the science that deals with the characterization of serum, the noncellular component of blood. Serum contains many valuable proteins, nucleotides, and other chemicals that aid the physiological functions of the body. Between 1900 and 1950, numerous scientific studies were performed to study the production of serum and its use in monitoring and controlling diseases. This period has been called the era of International Serology.

Serological markers are used to distinguish specific diseases in individuals. These markers are invaluable in the detection of some cancers, especially due to their potential in identifying the early stages of the disease, prior to the onset of symptoms.

CRITERIA IN ASSESSING SEROLOGICAL MARKERS

Several criteria are used to assess a serological method in a clinical laboratory, including sensitivity, specificity, and predictive value. Diagnostic sensitivity (Se) is the ability to correctly identify those who have a specific disease and is defined by the ratio of true positives over true positives and false negatives. Diagnostic specificity (Sp) is the ability of the test to correctly identify those who do not have the disease and is defined by the ratio of true negatives over true negatives and false positives. Both of these indexes measure the accuracy of assays using serological markers relative to an established and standard procedure. The predictive value (Pr) contains two components: a positive predictive value (Pp) and a negative predictive value (Pn); the former describes the likelihood that a positive test result represents a true positive and the later defines the likelihood that a negative result is truly negative. All the above definitions are described in Figure 1.

EXAMPLES OF SEROLOGICAL MARKERS

Serologic markers have been studied extensively in immunology and have also been widely used in

Figure 1

Formulas for Calculating the Indexes of Serological Markers

	Disease	No Disease
Test Positive	a	b
Test Negative	c	d

a: number of true positive, b: number of false positive,
c: number of false negative, d: number of true negative.

Diagnostic Sensitivity (Se) = a / (a + c)
Specificity (Sp) = d / (d + b)
Predictive value of a positive results (Pp) = a / (a + b)
Predictive value of a negative test results (Pn) = d / (d + c)

SOURCE: Courtesy of author.

the study, clinical diagnosis, and prognosis of cancer. Prostate-specific antigen (PSA) in serum has been studied widely and used in early detection and management of prostate cancer. Several monoclonal and polyclonal antibodies have been developed for the detection of PSA, and about 25 to 75 percent of patients with the disease have PSA in their sera. Even with the potential problem of lack of specificity of the test, PSA is the most widely used tumor-associated antigen.

The most commonly used markers for diagnosis and management of epithelial ovarian cancer is CA 125, which is an antigenic determinant, part of a glycoprotein present in the sera of approximately 80 percent of patients with epithelial ovarian cancer. It is found elevated in about 40 percent of patients with Stage I ovarian cancers and about 20 percent of patients with mucinous malignancies. In addition, approximately 60 percent of pancreatic carcinomas express CA 125, as do 25 percent of all other solid tumors. However, CA 125 is not only a marker for cancer, but is also elevated in a number of benign gynecologic conditions, including pelvic inflammatory disease, endometriosis, uterine leiomyoma, and early pregnancy. This nonspecificity has limited the use of CA 125 as a tumor maker in screening and diagnosis.

Carcinoembryonic antigen (CEA), alpha-fetoprotein (AFP), and altered carbohydrate antigen 19–9 (CA19–9) have been studied in the past decade for early diagnosis of human pancreatic adenocarcinoma and gastrointestinal malignancies. The utility of CEA as a serum marker in the detection of tumors has been limited due to the finding that CEA levels are affected by a variety of factors, including liver function, biliary obstruction, and subclinical hepatitis, and because the interlaboratory variation in CEA measurements could run as high as 36 percent.

AFP was first described as a tumor marker for hepatoma in the 1960s. It is most frequently elevated among patients with hepatoma and yolk sac (endodermal sinus) tumors. AFP-positive tumors can be found throughout the gastrointestinal tract.

CA 19–9 is frequently elevated in pancreatic cancer, but is also elevated in cancers of the biliary tract, and less frequently in colorectal and gastric cancers. Studies have shown that CA 19–9 can identify, with reasonable accuracy, the majority of patients with pancreatic cancer in a highly select patient population. The utility of other markers, such as pancreatic oncofetal antigen (POA) and tumor-associated trypsin inhibitor (TATI), is still being studied.

Serological markers have great potential to be used in clinical practice, including early detection of cancer, because these markers are differently expressed—qualitatively or quantitatively, and because they vary between either people who are healthy and those that have certain diseases. However, sensitivity and specificity issues remain the critical challenge when developing new serum markers for diagnostic and prognostic purposes. Technological advancements, standardization of the tests, and acceptance by the medical community are required to allow widespread applications of serological markers in medicine.

WENDY WANG
SUDHIR SRIVASTAVA

(SEE ALSO: *Cancer; Prostate-Specific Antigen [PSA]; Screening*)

BIBLIOGRAPHY

Benjamini, E.; Coico, R.; and Sunshine, G. (2000). *Immunology: a Short Course,* 4th edition. New York: Wiley-Liss.

Gerstman, B. B. (1998). *Epidemiology Kept Simple.* New York: Wiley-Liss.

Gohagan, J. K.; Srivastava, S.; Rossi, S. C.; and Black, W. C. (1999). "New Screening Technologies." In *Cancer Screening Theory and Practice.* eds. B. S. Kramer, J. K. Gohagan, and P. C. Prorok. New York and Basel: Marcel Dekker.

Stevens, C. D. (1996). *Clinical Immunology and Serology: A Laboratory Perspective.* Philadelphia, PA: F. A. Davis Company.

SEWAGE SYSTEM

In the year 2000, it was estimated that 70 percent of the U.S. population lived in areas where domestic wastes pass through a sewage treatment plant before being discharged back into a water source. Sewage treatment systems and chlorination of water have made major contributions to the reduction of the incidence of waterborne diseases such as cholera and typhoid fever. Sewage treatment is used to improve the quality of wastewater so that it can be released into a waterway without causing damage to aquatic species or causing waterborne diseases among humans. Several levels of sewage treatment are used.

Primary sewage treatment removes larger floating objects through screening and sedimentation. The incoming wastewater flows through one or more screens and then enters a grit chamber where it slows down enough to allow sand, gravel, and other inorganic matter to settle out. In treatment plants where only primary treatment occurs, the effluent is chlorinated and discharged into circulation in a water source. The sludge, or sedimentation of larger solids, is removed, dried, and disposed of. Primary treatment removes 50 to 65 percent of suspended solids and decreases biological oxygen demand (BOD) by 25 to 40 percent. Primary treatment alone is not considered adequate for protection of the environment or people's health.

Secondary treatment relates to processes similar to natural biological decomposition. Aerobic bacteria and other microorganisms are used to break down organic materials into inorganic carbon dioxide, water, and minerals. Trickling filters, which are made from a bed of rocks with a microbial covering, are used to absorb the organic material present in the water. Activated sludge processes can be used in place of trickling filters. The level of suspended solids and BOD in wastewater after primary and secondary treatment has been decreased by 90 to 95 percent. This level of treatment is not effective in removing viruses, heavy metals, dissolved minerals, or certain chemicals.

Tertiary treatment is an advanced level of treatment. This form of treatment can decrease the level of suspended solids and BOD to approximately 1 percent of what was present in the raw sewage prior to primary treatment. Advanced treatment processes consist of several biological, chemical, or physical mechanisms.

Sewage treatment aims to destroy pathogenic organisms. Since primary and secondary treatments do not destroy a significant number of organisms, chlorination, which is effective in killing bacteria, is used to disinfect treated effluent.

Private sewage treatment, usually a septic system, is constructed on-site and is maintained by the private homeowner. In this case, the septic tank holds the solid materials while the water goes to a leach field or absorption field. The solids undergo decomposition, and on a regular basis, generally every three years, are pumped from the holding tank. This will vary according to use and capacity.

MARK G. ROBSON

(SEE ALSO: *Biological Oxygen Demand; Sanitation; Wastewater Treatment; Water Quality*)

BIBLIOGRAPHY

Brooks, S.; Gochfeld, M.; Herzstein, J.; Schenker, M.; and Jackson, R. (1995). *Environmental Medicine.* St. Louis, MO: Mosby.

Koren, H., and Bisesi, M. (1996). *Handbook of Environmental Health and Safety,* 3rd edition, Vol. 2. Boca Raton, FL: Lewis Publishers.

Morgan, M. T. (1993). *Environmental Health.* Madison, WI: Brown & Benchmark.

SEXUALLY TRANSMITTED DISEASES

Sexually transmitted diseases (STDs) are caused by a group of infectious microorganisms that are transmitted mainly through sexual activity. These agents represent a costly, burdensome global public health problem. STDs can cause harmful, often irreversible, clinical complications, including reproductive health problems, fetal and perinatal health problems, and cancer, and they are also linked in a causal chain of events to the sexual transmission of human immunodeficiency virus (HIV) infection. Although STDs are largely preventable through behavior modification and sound primary health care, they are under-recognized and under-appreciated as a public health problem by most healthcare providers, the general public, and healthcare policy makers. In 1997, the Institute of Medicine characterized STDs as "hidden epidemics of tremendous health and economic consequence" in the United States and advocated urgent national preventive action.

An estimated 333 million curable STDs occur annually worldwide. In the United States, STDs are among the most frequently reported infectious diseases nationwide. Each year an estimated 15 million new cases of STDs occur in Americans, including nearly 4 million infections in U.S. teenagers. The annual direct and indirect costs of the principal STDs, including sexually transmitted HIV infection, and their complications are estimated at $17 billion.

More than twenty-five bacteria, viruses, protozoa, and yeasts are considered sexually transmissible. Bacterial STDs include those caused by *Chlamydia trachomatis* (chlamydia), *Neisseria gonorrhoeae* (gonorrhea), *Treponema pallidum* (syphilis), *Haemophilus ducreyi* (chancroid), and other common sexually transmitted organisms. Chlamydia and gonorrhea cause inflammatory reactions in the host. In women, these organisms can ascend into the upper reproductive tract where pelvic inflammatory disease (PID) can cause irreparable damage to the reproductive organs and result in infertility, ectopic pregnancy, and chronic pelvic pain. In its early stages, syphilis causes painless genital ulcers and other infectious lesions. Left untreated, syphilis moves through the body in stages, damaging many organs over time. Chancroid is associated with painful genital lesions. In pregnant women, acute bacterial STDs can cause potentially fatal congenital infections or perinatal complications, such as eye and lung infections in the newborn. Effective single-dose antimicrobials can cure chlamydia, gonorrhea, syphilis, and chancroid.

Viral STDs include the sexually transmitted viral infections caused by human immunodeficiency virus (HIV infection), herpes simplex virus type 2 (genital herpes), and human papillomavirus (HPV infection). Initial infections with these organisms may be asymptomatic or cause only mild symptoms. Treatable but not curable, viral STDs appear to be lifelong infections. HIV is the virus that causes acquired immunodeficiency syndrome (AIDS). Herpes causes periodic outbreaks of painful genital lesions. Some strains of HPV cause genital warts, and others are important risk factors for cervical dysplasia and invasive cervical cancer. Hepatitis B virus (HBV) is another acute viral illness that can be transmitted through sexual activity. Most persons who acquire HBV infection recover and have no complications, but it can sometimes become a chronic health problem.

Trichomonas vaginalis (trichomoniasis) is a common protozoal STD, and *Candida species* (candidiasis) are sexually transmitted yeasts. Both are frequently associated with vaginal discharge.

BIOLOGICAL FACTORS IN THE SPREAD OF STDS

STDs are behavior-linked diseases that result from unprotected sex. Nonetheless, several biological factors contribute to their spread. These include the asymptomatic nature of STDs, the long lag time between infections and complications, the higher susceptibility of women to STDs, and the way that STDs facilitate the transmission of HIV infection.

The silent nature of STDs represents their greatest public health threat. Most STDs cause some symptomatic illness, but many produce symptoms so mild or nonspecific that infected persons are not alerted to seek medical care. As many as one in three men and two in three women with chlamydia infection have no obvious signs of infection. Without treatment or other interventions, infected persons can continue to infect new sex partners. Moreover, serious complications that cause irreversible damage can occur "silently" before any symptoms are apparent. A related problem is the long interval that can elapse between acquiring an STD and recognizing a clinically significant health problem. Women can develop cervical cancer many years after infection with some strains of HPV. A woman may first suspect she had an asymptomatic infection with chlamydia or gonorrhea when she finds out later in life that she is infertile or has an ectopic pregnancy. Because the original infection was likely to have been asymptomatic, there is frequently no perceived connection between the original sexually acquired infection and the resulting health problem. The lack of awareness of this connection leads people to underestimate their risk and to forego preventive precautions.

Gender and age are also associated with increased risk for STDs. Women are at higher risk than men for most STDs, and young women are more susceptible to certain infections than older women. Due to cervical ectopy that is extremely common in adolescent females, the immature cervix of adolescent females is covered with cells that are especially susceptible to STDs such as chlamydia.

The presence of other STDs, especially those that cause genital ulcers or inflammation, influences the sexual transmission and acquisition of HIV infection. Studies have repeatedly demonstrated that people are two to five times more likely to become infected with HIV through sexual contact when other STDs are present. In addition, dually infected persons (persons who are infected with both HIV and another STD) are more likely to transmit HIV infection during sexual contact. Conversely, effective STD detection and treatment can slow the spread of HIV infection at the individual and community levels. For example, in a study in Malawi in the mid-1990s, treatment of gonorrhea in HIV-infected men returned the frequency and concentration of HIV genetic material in semen to levels comparable to levels found in HIV-infected men who were not infected with other STDs. Similarly, a community trial in Tanzania in the mid-1990s demonstrated that treatment of symptomatic STDs resulted in a 42-percent decrease in new heterosexually transmitted HIV infections.

SOCIAL FACTORS THAT AFFECT THE SPREAD OF STDS

Some social factors directly affect STD spread especially in vulnerable populations. In addition, the stigma that continues to surround STDs in the United States indirectly interferes with establishing new social norms pertaining to sex and sexuality.

When there are barriers to health care, it is difficult to detect and treat STDs early. Infected persons also miss an opportunity for behavioral change counseling. Health care access barriers keep infected persons in the community where they continue to spread STDs. In the United States, groups with the highest rates of STDs are the same groups in which access to health care services is limited or absent.

Perhaps the greatest social factor contributing to the spread of STDs, and the factor that most significantly separates the United States from industrialized countries with low STD rates, is the stigma that continues to be associated with sexually transmitted infections. Although sex and sexuality pervade many aspects of American culture, most Americans are secretive and private about their sexual behavior. Talking openly and comfortably about sex and sexuality is difficult even in intimate relationships. This secrecy about sexuality and STDs adversely affects STD prevention in the United States by thwarting sexuality and STD education programs for adolescents, hindering communication between parents and children and between sex partners, promoting unbalanced sexual messages in the media, obstructing education and counseling activities, and impeding research on sexual behaviors.

GROUPS DISPROPORTIONATELY AFFECTED BY STDS

All racial, cultural, economic, and religious groups are affected by STDs, and people in all communities and sexual networks are at risk. Nevertheless, some persons are disproportionately affected by STDs and their complications.

STDs disproportionately affect disenfranchised persons and individuals who are in social networks characterized by high-risk sexual behaviors, substance abuse, and limited access to health care. Some notable disproportionately affected groups include sex workers, homeless persons and runaways, adolescents and adults in detention, and migrant workers. Many studies document the association of substance use, especially alcohol and drug use, with STDs. The introduction of illicit substances into communities can dramatically alter sexual behavior in high-risk sexual networks leading to epidemic spread of STDs. The national U.S. syphilis epidemic of the late 1980s was fueled by the effect of increased crack cocaine use, especially in minority communities. Crack cocaine led to increases in sex exchanged for drugs and in the number of anonymous sex partners and decreased health care-seeking behavior and motivation to use barrier protection—all factors that can increase STD transmission in a community. Other substances, including alcohol, can also affect a person's cognitive and negotiating skills before and during sex, lowering the likelihood that preventive action will be taken to protect against STDs and pregnancy.

Gender disparities are an important aspect of the epidemiology of STDs. Compared to men, women suffer more frequent and serious STD complications, including PID, ectopic pregnancy, infertility, and chronic pelvic pain. Women are biologically more susceptible to infection when exposed to a sexually transmitted agent, and STDs are often more easily transmitted from a man to a woman than from a woman to a man. Given that some newly acquired STDs (and even some long-term complications) are only mildly symptomatic or completely asymptomatic in women, the combination of increased susceptibility and silent infection frequently results in delayed STD diagnosis and treatment. A further complication is that STDs are more difficult to diagnose in women due to the complex anatomy of the female reproductive tract and the frequent need for a speculum examination and diagnostic culture tests.

In pregnant women, STDs can result in serious health problems or death to a developing fetus or newborn. Sexually transmitted pathogens can be transmitted across the placenta, resulting in congenital infection, or can reach the newborn during vaginal childbirth, resulting in perinatal infection. Regardless of the route of infection, these organisms can permanently damage the fetal or newborn brain, spinal cord, eyes, auditory nerves, or immune system. Even when the organisms do not reach the fetus or newborn directly, they can cause spontaneous abortion, stillbirth, premature rupture of the membranes, and preterm delivery.

For a variety of behavioral, social, and biological reasons, STDs also disproportionately affect adolescents. In 1998, U.S. teenagers 15 to 19 years old had the highest reported rate of chlamydia and the second highest rate of gonorrhea. The herpes infection rate among white youth in the United States aged twelve to nineteen increased nearly fivefold from the late 1970s to the early 1990s. Because not all teenagers are sexually active, the actual rate of STDs among teens is even higher than the observed rates suggest. There are several contributing factors. Many teenagers are, in fact, sexually active and at risk for STDs, and they are having sex with partners from sexual networks that are already highly infected with untreated STDs. In 1999, among U.S. high school youth interviewed for the Youth Risk Behavior Surveillance System survey, half (49.9%) indicated they had had sexual intercourse during their lifetimes. Early sexual activity and multiple sexual partners were commonly reported among American high school youth; 8.3 percent of students indicated they had first had sex before age thirteen, and 16.2 percent said they had four or more sex partners during their lifetime. Despite the supposedly easy access to condoms that can lower STD transmission risk considerably, only 58 percent of sexually active students said they used a condom the last time they had intercourse. Sexually active teenagers are often reluctant to seek STD services or face serious obstacles to obtaining such services. In addition, health care providers are often uncomfortable discussing sexuality and risk reduction with young persons.

Some minority racial and ethnic groups (mainly black and Hispanic populations) in the United States have higher rates of STDs compared with rates for whites. Race and ethnicity in the United States are risk markers that correlate with other more fundamental determinants of health status such as poverty, access to quality health care, health care-seeking behavior, illicit drug use, and living in communities with high STD prevalence. Public health data may over-represent STDs among racial and ethnic groups who are more likely to receive STD services from public sector STD clinics characterized by timely and complete reporting of public health statistics. However, even when random sampling techniques are used to study health problems, higher rates of STDs are often found among African Americans and Hispanics compared with whites.

FACTORS IMPORTANT TO THE PREVENTION AND CONTROL OF STDS

The dynamics of how STDs spread in populations have been studied extensively to derive approaches to prevention and control. Three main factors predict how fast and at what level STDs will spread in a population: the nature of sexual relationships, the degree to which susceptibility to STDs can be modified, and the timeliness and completeness of treatment.

The nature of sexual relationships refers to the decisions people make about when to become and remain sexually active and whom to select as sex partners. The earlier that vaginal, oral, or anal sexual intercourse begins and the greater the number of lifetime sex partners, the more likely a person is to acquire one or more STDs in a lifetime. Behavioral interventions that help delay the initiation of intercourse and reduce the lifetime number of sex partners will have a positive effect on slowing STD transmission.

Susceptibility to STDs can be modified with vaccines or barrier contraceptives such as condoms. If uninfected persons are somehow immune to STDs, then no transmission will occur. The availability of effective vaccines against STDs could dramatically slow increases in or even eliminate some STDs. For example, there is an effective and widely available vaccine for hepatitis B, a viral STD. Current strategies to immunize all children against hepatitis B before they become sexually active could greatly reduce the societal burden of this disease. Susceptibility can also be altered each time sex occurs. The correct and consistent use of condoms can reduce the rate of STD transmission in a population. Persons who choose to engage in sexual behaviors that place them at risk of STDs should use latex or polyurethane condoms every time they have sex. A condom put on the penis before starting sex and worn until the penis is withdrawn can help protect both the male and the female partner from most STDs. When a male condom cannot be used appropriately, sex partners should consider using a female condom. However, condoms do not provide complete protection from all STDs. Sores and lesions of STDs on

infected men and women may be present in areas not covered by the condom, resulting in transmission of infection to a new person. This is common with genital warts and other genital HPV infections.

Although condom use has been on the rise in the United States over the past few decades, women who use the most effective forms of contraception (sterilization and hormonal contraception) are less likely than other women to use condoms for STD prevention. The most effective methods of contraception are not the most effective methods of STD prevention; likewise, methods that give a considerable measure of protection against STDs are considered to be good, but not the most effective, methods of pregnancy prevention. This suggests that, especially for young women who are at highest risk for unwanted pregnancy and STDs, using dual protection (condoms and hormonal contraception) will offer the best overall protection against both.

The third factor in STD prevention and control focuses on finding and treating infected persons and their sex partners. The longer someone has an untreated STD (especially if the person is asymptomatic), the longer that person can potentially infect others. If that interval can be shortened for the millions of persons who acquire STDs each year, then transmission would slow appreciably. Screening and treatment are the biomedical approaches that can be applied to this situation. For STDs that are frequently asymptomatic, screening and treatment also benefit those likely to suffer severe complications (especially women) if infections are not detected and treated early. For example, in the early 1990s, chlamydia screening in a large metropolitan managed-care organization reduced the incidence of subsequent PID in the screened group by 40 percent. Identifying and treating partners of persons with curable STDs has always been an integral part of organized control programs. Theoretically, this can break the chain of transmission in a sexual network. Early antibiotic treatment of a sex partner can interfere with an STD taking hold in a recently exposed person. Partner treatment benefits the original patient by reducing the risk of reinfection, and the partner benefits by avoiding acute infection and potential complications. Because future sex partners are protected by treating partners, this strategy also benefits the community. New screening tests (some of which can be performed on urine specimens) that facilitate STD screening in nontraditional settings are now available.

Many examples demonstrate the effectiveness of organized approaches to STD prevention and control that incorporate these strategies on a large scale. When a sustained, collaborative, multifaceted approach to STD prevention and control is undertaken, dramatic results can be achieved. One need only observe the results of sustained STD prevention efforts in many countries in Western and Northern Europe, Canada, Japan, and Australia, where STD rates are many times lower than in the United States, to conclude that STD prevention programs can work on a national scale.

ALLISON L. GREENSPAN
JOEL R. GREENSPAN

BIBLIOGRAPHY

American Social Health Association (1998). *Sexually Transmitted Diseases in America: How Many Cases and at What Cost?* Menlo Park, CA: Kaiser Family Foundation.

Anderson, J.; Brackhill, R.; and Mosher, W. (1996). "Condom Use for Disease Prevention among Unmarried U.S. Women." *Family Planning Perspectives* 28:25–28, 39.

Anderson, R. M., and May, R. M. (1991). *Infectious Diseases of Humans: Dynamics and Control.* Oxford: Oxford University Press.

Centers for Disease Control and Prevention (1998). "1998 Guidelines for Treatment of Sexually Transmitted Diseases." *Morbidity and Mortality Weekly Report* 47(RR-1):1–116.

—— (1999). *Sexually Transmitted Disease Surveillance, 1998.* Atlanta, GA: Centers for Disease Control and Prevention, 1–115.

—— (2000). "Youth Risk Behavior Surveillance: United States, 1999." *Morbidity and Mortality Weekly Report* 49(SS-5).

Cohen, M. S.; Hoffman, I. F.; Royce, R. A. et al. (1997). "Reduction of Concentration of HIV-1 in Semen after Treatment of Urethritis: Implications for Prevention of Sexual Transmission of HIV-1." *Lancet* 349:1868–1873.

Fleming, D. T.; McQuillan, G. M.; Johnson, R. E. et al. (1997). "Herpes Simplex Virus Type 2 in the United States: 1976–1994." *New England Journal of Medicine* 337:1105–1111.

Goldenberg, R. L.; Andrews, W. W.; Yuan, A. C. et al. (1997). "Sexually Transmitted Diseases and Adverse Outcomes of Pregnancy." *Clinics in Perinatology* 24(1):23–41.

Grosskurth, H.; Mosha, F.; Todd, J. et al. (1995). "Impact of Improved Treatment of Sexually Transmitted Diseases on HIV Infection in Rural Tanzania: Randomised Controlled Trial." *Lancet* 346:530–536.

Gunn, R.; Montes, J.; Tomey, K. et al. (1995). "Syphilis in San Diego County, 1983–1992: Crack Cocaine, Prostitution, and the Limitations of Partner Notification." *Sexually Transmitted Diseases* 22:60–66.

Hillis, S.; Nakashima, A.; Amsterdam, L. et al. (1995). "The Impact of a Comprehensive Chlamydia Prevention Program in Wisconsin." *Family Planning Perspectives* 27:108–111.

Holmes, K.; Mardh, P.; Sparling, P. et al., eds. (1999). *Sexually Transmitted Diseases,* 3rd edition. New York: McGraw-Hill.

Institute of Medicine. Committee on Prevention and Control of Sexually Transmitted Diseases (1997). *The Hidden Epidemic: Confronting Sexually Transmitted Diseases,* eds. T. R. Eng and W. T. Butler. Washington, DC: National Academy Press.

Scholes, D.; Stergachis, A.; Heidrich, F. et al. (1996). "Prevention of Pelvic Inflammatory Disease by Screening for Cervical Chlamydial Infection." *New England Journal of Medicine* 334:1362–1366.

St. Louis, M. E.; Wasserheit, J. N.; and Gayle, H. D. (1997). "Editorial: Janus Considers the HIV Pandemic: Harnessing Recent Advances to Enhance AIDS Prevention." *American Journal of Public Health* 87:10–12.

Tsui, A.; Wasserheit, J.; and Haaga, J. (1997). *Reproductive Health in Developing Countries: Expanding Dimensions, Building Solutions.* Washington, DC: National Academy Press.

SHAMANIC HEALING

The rise of shamanism was probably a result of the earliest human societies' efforts to make sense of and better control the world they lived in. Evidence that magic and religious ritual played a part in the life of early *Homo sapiens* can be seen in early burial practices, artifact material, and cave art, where one can see what appear to be depictions of hunting magic in the form of animals and hunters with weapons painted on the walls of caves. Injuries and illnesses would have been a common occurrence in ancient times, and a need developed for someone to explain such events, and to treat them through the application of a healing substance or by entreating a supernatural force.

Anthropologists have long studied how cultural groups living in the world today view and attempt to control their living environments. In many of these groups there are individuals who perform rituals and ceremonies to ensure a good hunt, adequate crops, good health, and whatever else is deemed important. Rites are performed to keep the community safe, healthy, and well fed, and to ensure the favor of the gods and other natural and supernatural forces. These individuals may also be called upon to diagnose and treat illnesses and disease. "Shaman" is one of many names given to those who perform rituals and healing ceremonies.

A shaman is a person who makes journeys into the spiritual world to seek wisdom for healing, divining the future, or to communicate with the spirits of the dead. They may be male or female and may have received their calling to become a shaman as a result of a near-death experience in which they were carried into the spirit world and met teachers who helped them to learn healing songs, medicines, and revelations about the future. A shaman may also be born into the role, or be trained for it after demonstrating some special aptitude for healing. Shamans are believed to possess special powers that allow them to control the weather, call game animals for a hunt, determine the best time for planting or for moving a village, and especially for curing illness and disease. A shaman often uses trance-like states to move into another dimension to seek help in diagnosing and treating a sick person. These trances may be brought on by dancing, singing, drumming, or other methods. The trance brings the shaman into the spiritual world, where a spirit teacher provides guidance on how to cure an illness or solve a problem. Shamanic healing practices include the use of gongs, rattles, finger bells, dancing rituals, purification ceremonies, physical manipulation, prayer, healing herbs, or removal of something inside a sick person, such as a stone, feather, piece of bone, or other material.

There are different types of healers involved in traditional medical practices. The vast majority of these types (i.e., curanderos, root doctors, spirit mediums, herbalists, and related types) are trained into their professions. (Sorcerers and witches may also be consulted in folk healing systems.) Often, these professions are handed down through the family when a child or young adult demonstrates an interest or aptitude for healing or is born with some peculiarity such as a vale over the face (i.e., a piece of the amniotic sac covering the face). In these cases, individuals may undergo a long period of apprenticeship in which they are trained in the healing arts. A shaman may undergo a long period of training following being called to the profession, but already have the ability to travel out of his or her body to another plane or dimension where guidance, special songs or prayers, and predictions of the future are received.

When performing a healing ritual shamans often go into such trance-like states where they leave their body and travel to a dimension where they meet a teacher or guide. Here they ask for or are given guidance and direction about the nature of the illness they are trying to cure. A shaman may use herbs and other devices in his or her healing ceremonies, but these have come from the teaching the shaman has received either in the out of body experience or from later training from another shaman. In contrast, other traditional healers do not typically travel out of body.

When considering the impact of all the healing systems outside modern medical practice, it is important to understand that an individual's cultural tradition plays a significant role in how the causes and treatments for illness and disease are perceived. For those who believe some supernatural force or an imbalance within them causes their illness, modern Western medicine may have little value and traditional medical practices provided by a shaman or other traditional healer may be the first choice for treatment. Modern medical practitioners are becoming more aware that bringing traditional healing practices into clinics and hospitals can help patients from that culture get well more quickly, or to better accept modern treatments when they are combined with traditional healing methods.

ROBERT M. HUFF

(SEE ALSO: *Black Magic and Evil Eye; Faith Healers; Folk Medicine*)

BIBLIOGRAPHY

Eliade, M. (1964). *Shamanism: Archaic Techniques of Ecstasy.* Princeton, NJ: Princeton University Press.

Huff, R. M., and Kline, M. V., eds. (1999). *Promoting Health in Multicultural Populations: A Handbook For Practitioners.* Thousand Oaks, CA: Sage Publications.

Kalweit, H. (1988). *Dreamtime and Inner Space: The World of the Shaman.* Boston: Shambhala Publications.

Kleinman, A. (1980). *Patients and Healers in the Context of Culture.* Berkeley: University of California Press.

Ripinsky-Naxon, M. (1993). *The Nature of Shamanism: Substance and Function of a Religious Metaphor.* Albany, NY: State University of New York Press.

SHATTUCK, LEMUEL

Lemuel Shattuck was born in 1793 in Ashby, Massachusetts, and he died in 1859 in Boston. Shattuck grew up in a small farming community in New Hampshire where, at the age of nineteen, a religious revival movement inspired him to dedicate his life to improving society. He came to believe that he could enhance the ability of government to respond to social ills through the collection of statistics. After relocating several times throughout New England, Shattuck settled in Concord, Massachusetts, in 1823. There, in 1835, he gained attention for writing *A History of the Town of Concord*, which included a statistical analysis based on church and municipal records. Shattuck was also responsible for Concord's new code of school regulations, which was based on a method he devised to evaluate the progress of every student in the town.

In 1835, Shattuck moved to Boston, where he became a bookseller and helped form the American Statistical Association. After being elected to the Boston City Council in 1837, Shattuck was asked to create a report analyzing Boston's vital statistics from 1810 to 1841. In addition to his findings, which were published in the *American Journal of Medical Sciences*, Shattuck outlined a method for the systematic gathering of vital statistics and a plan for analyzing that data. Based on his suggestions, Massachusetts passed the Registration Act of 1842.

Shattuck was also renowned for his 1850 survey of sanitary conditions throughout the state, the *Report of the Sanitary Conditions of Massachusetts*, which was commissioned by the state legislature. In this report, Shattuck proposed the creation of a permanent statewide public health infrastructure, and he recommended establishing health offices at the state and local levels in order to gather statistical information on public health conditions. Although the legislature did not adopt his comprehensive plan, his specific proposals became routine public health activities over the course of the twentieth century.

JENNIFER KOSLOW

(SEE ALSO: *Statistics for Public Health; Vital Statistics*)

BIBLIOGRAPHY

Cassedy, J. H. (1975). "The Roots of American Sanitary Reform 1843–1847: Seven Letters from John H. Griscom to Lemuel Shattuck." *Journal of the History of Medicine and Allied Sciences* 30(2):136–147.

—— (1984). *American Medicine and Statistical Thinking, 1800–1860.* Cambridge, MA: Harvard University Press.

Rosenkrantz, B. G. (1972). *Public Health and the State: Changing Views in Massachusetts, 1842–1936.* Cambridge, MA: Harvard University Press.

SHIGELLOSIS

Shigellosis, also known as bacillary dysentery, is a common food-borne infection that causes diarrhea with fever, toxemia, and general prostration. Blood and mucous are often mixed with the loose, watery stools, indicating severe inflammation of the intestinal lining. The causative organisms are several varieties of the genus *Shigella*. Infection is transmitted by active or convalescent cases (e.g., person to person). Food handlers working in unhygienic kitchens or restaurants sometimes become the index case for large epidemics. The incubation period is short, from one to three days, so it can be relatively easy to trace the source of an outbreak. The diarrhea and other symptoms usually run their course in a week or so, but the infectious agents can persist in feces for several weeks—which is the reason that food handlers should not be allowed to return to work, preferably for several weeks or until stool examinations for *Shigella* organisms are negative.

Control of shigella dysentery can be difficult, especially in settings such as military campaigns. Meticulous hygiene in all aspects of food handling and meal preparation are essential; everyone in the kitchen must scrupulously observe the rules for hand washing with warm water and soap after visiting the toilet and before handling food. The use of disposable plastic gloves is desirable, but these must be changed frequently. Flies must be kept out of kitchen areas.

Shigellosis is a notifiable disease in many jurisdictions, so local public health authorities will ensure that suspect premises and all persons working in such premises are inspected. Cases are treated by fluid and salt replacement, and often benefit from antibiotics.

JOHN M. LAST

(SEE ALSO: *Communicable Disease Control; Food-Borne Diseases; Regulations Affecting Restaurants*)

SHINGLES

See Chicken Pox and Shingles *and* Herpes Zoster

SICK BUILDING SYNDROME

The term "sick building syndrome" (SBS) more specifically termed "nonspecific building-related illness," describes a set of common and nonspecific symptoms that are experienced by individuals in office and other nonindustrial workplace settings but remit when the individuals are away from that environment. Symptoms typically include fatigue; cognitive complaints; headache; shortness of breath; irritation of the nose, oropharynx, and eyes; rashes; and complaints of unpleasant odor in the workplace. It is critical to distinguish SBS from building-related illness, which refers to conditions more readily diagnosable by practitioners and characterized by abnormal signs. These include carbon

monoxide poisoning, asthma, hypersensitivity pneumonitis, and upper respiratory infections. The symptoms and paucity of signs that characterize SBS overlap substantially with the symptoms of various other medically unexplained syndromes such as chronic fatigue syndrome, fibromyalgia, multiple chemical sensitivities, and even psychiatric conditions characterized by somatic symptoms. The key is that with SBS the symptoms wax and wane with exposure to a particular building environment. Sorting out their diverse causal influences is the key to prevention, and involves integration across many fields.

A number of factors have been identified in experimental and field studies which contribute to SBS, although there remains much uncertainty about specifics of exposure, dose, susceptibility, and in particular the development of chronic symptoms once an afflicted individual is removed from a building exposure. Strong observational epidemiologic data has shown relatively high rates of symptoms in office workers in a variety of countries and climates. At least 20 to 35 percent of workers report such symptoms, even in nonproblem buildings. One important clue to SBS is that rates of symptoms are strongly correlated with mechanical ventilation systems as opposed to natural ventilation. Elevated carbon dioxide levels are a marker for inadequate ventilation, but are not toxic, per se. Relative humidity below 20 percent and above 60 percent are correlated with mucous membrane discomfort or general symptoms.

It is clear from controlled exposure studies, as well as observational studies, that even relatively low levels of volatile organic compounds (VOCs) can acutely produce many of the symptoms of SBS, and that these symptoms remit once exposure is terminated. Attempts to document objective correlates of these symptoms with neuropsychological or respiratory tests have not been very successful. VOCs are emitted from many construction materials as well as office products, and while most noticeable with new buildings, many emission sources are chronic. VOCs can also be reintroduced during building maintenance and renovation, as well as normal business activities.

A number of studies document an increased rate of symptoms, independent of allergy, in buildings with moisture problems and/or documented bacterial and mold growth. Atopy (the tendency to be allergic) is a risk factor for symptoms, perhaps due to allergies to bacteria and fungi. Much work remains to be done in sorting out whether those reporting symptoms have a specific building-related illness (e.g., asthma, rhino-sinusitis, interstitial lung disease) as opposed to SBS. Reports of systemic disease and immune system damage from mycotoxins also requires further study and verification, but there is compelling preventive logic to taking steps to avoid excessive moisture in buildings and to responding promptly when it occurs to reduce microbial growth.

Workplace stress can contribute to symptoms, according to numerous studies. The mechanism and degree of interaction of SBS with physical factors needs further study. Individual psychological characteristics can certainly influence who reports symptoms and the degree of distress associated with a given level of symptoms. Nevertheless, the strong ability of environmental factors to trigger symptoms means that preventive or ameliorative strategies aimed solely at workplace stress or personal characteristics will not be satisfactory over the long run.

HOWARD M. KIPEN

(SEE ALSO: *Ambient Air Quality [Air Pollution]; Asbestos; Asthma; Environmental Determinants of Health; Occupational Disease; Residential Housing*)

BIBLIOGRAPHY

Hodgson, A. T.; Daisey, J. M.; and Grot, R. A. (1991). "Sources and Source Strengths of Volatile Organic Compounds in a New Office Building." *Journal of Air and Waste Management Association* 41(11):1461–1468.

Lynch, R. M., and Kipen, H. (1998). "Building Related Illness and Employee Lost Time Following Application of Hot Asphalt Roof: A Call for Prevention." *Journal of Toxicology and Industrial Health* 14(6): 857–868.

Mendell, M. J.; Fisk, W. J.; Deddens, J. A.; Seavey, W. G.; Smith, A. H.; Smith, D. F.; Hodgson, A. T.; Daisey, J. M.; and Goldman, L. R. (1996). "Elevated Symptom Prevalence Associated with Ventilation Type in Office Buildings." *Epidemiology* 7:583–589.

Menzies, D., and Bourbeau, J. (1997). "Building-Related Illnesses." *The New England Journal of Medicine* 337(21):1524–1531.

SICKLE CELL DISEASE

The sickle cell diseases are a group of disorders that have in common the propensity of the red blood cells to become deformed when oxygen tension in the blood is lowered, causing anemia, occlusion of blood vessels by misshapen cells, and various associated clinical consequences, including death. In sickle cell disease, a mutation of the beta-globin gene results in the substitution of valine for glutamic acid in the sixth amino acid of the chain, producing a hemoglobin, designated hemoglobin S, that has less solubility than does normal hemoglobin A. Inheriting one gene for hemoglobin S, together with a normal gene, results in the formation of red cells that contain approximately 40 percent of the abnormal hemoglobin and 60 percent of the normal hemoglobin, an essentially harmless state that is designated as sickle cell trait. But if the gene inherited together with the sickle gene is not normal, then the sickle cell disease may develop. The most common hemoglobin that interacts with sickle hemoglobin is hemoglobin C, and the ß-thalassemia (beta-thalassemia) mutation also interacts with the sickle gene by restricting the formation of normal hemoglobin.

The sickle gene, and genes that interact with it, are common in a number of different populations, but the highest gene frequencies are observed in Africa. The gene is also found in southern Europe, the Middle East, and India. A single dose of the sickle gene provides protection against malaria. Since malaria was a major cause of death in Africa, persons who carried the sickle gene had a survival advantage over those who did not. Thus, the number of persons carrying this mutation has tended to increase generation after generation in areas where malaria was a major killer. Among African Americans, approximately 7.8 percent are carriers of the sickle mutation, that is, they have sickle cell trait; while 2.3 percent have hemoglobin C trait (one copy of the hemoglobin C gene); and 0.8 percent have ß-thalassemia trait.

Although a single copy of the hemoglobin S gene is quite harmless, if a person inherits two copies of the hemoglobin S genes, he or she will have sickle cell disease. If one hemoglobin S gene and one hemoglobin C gene are inherited, the patient has hemoglobin S-C disease. Coinheritance of the beta-thalassemia and sickle hemoglobin result in sickle cell thalassemia. Patients with these three disorders have a similar clinical disease. Anemia occurs as a result of the rapid destruction of red blood cells. The red cells may have the shape of sickles, hence the term "sickle cell disease." However, the cells may assume may other forms. The misshapen red cells occlude blood vessels and cause pain and even tissue death.

In small children, one of the great problems incident to sickle cell disease is infections. If these are treated promptly, most children with sickle cell disease survive into adult life. One of the most characteristic manifestations of the disease in adults and older children is "pain crises." These occur at regular intervals, often at a time of stress, and may cause frequent hospitalizations and varying degrees of dependence upon pain-killing drugs. As patients with the sickle cell disease grow older they begin to suffer from the results of accumulated damage in small blood vessels all through the body. Dysfunction of the lungs, kidneys, and heart are common. Strokes may occur. Interruption of the blood supply to bones may result in areas of bone death, particularly in the hips.

Although sickle cell disease is a disorder that has been better understood and studied in more detail than most other disorders, treatment is still very unsatisfactory. Prenatal diagnosis can be carried out quite easily and very reliably, and parents are provided with the option of terminating the pregnancy. Antibiotics and immunization programs have drastically reduced the mortality rate among young children. Transfusion of red blood cells improves the flow properties of blood and may ameliorate the symptoms. Hydroxyurea has been administered to increase the amount of fetal hemoglobin, a hemoglobin that does not interact with sickle hemoglobin. This treatment has met with some success.

The disease is cured by bone marrow transplantation, a procedure with a relatively high risk, even in those patients in whom a match can be found. Ultimately the disease may be treated by putting a normal beta-globin gene into a stem cell of the patient, and then transplanting that patient with his or her own transduced cells, but there are many barriers to implementing such a strategy. Because stem cells do not divide often, they are relatively resistant to many gene-transfer methods. It is not enough to put a normal globin gene in the cell; the abnormal globin gene needs to be inactivated. There is also a tendency for normal human cells to shut off the function of foreign genes that are implanted in them. It is likely that these technical obstacles to gene therapy will be overcome eventually, and that the treatment of this group of diseases will give better results in the future.

ERNEST BEUTLER

(SEE ALSO: *Genes; Genetic Disorders; Hemoglobin; Hemoglobinopathies; Malaria; Medical Genetics*)

SIGMOIDOSCOPY

See Colorectal Cancer

SIGNIFICANCE TESTS

See Statistics for Public Health

SIMON, JOHN

John Simon (1816–1904), an English physician, was appointed surgeon and lecturer in pathology at St. Thomas's Hospital in London in 1847. In 1848 he became the first medical officer of health to the City of London, holding this position until 1855. His cogent, well-written reports on the health problems of the city, and the steps taken to deal with these problems, are regarded as models of preventive medicine and the administration of public health services. In 1858, Simon became medical officer to the Privy Council, a post equivalent to the modern office of chief medical officer or, in the United States, surgeon general. Simon had overall responsibility for the organization and administration of national public health services. He oversaw the passage of the Public Health Act of 1875, but resigned the following year because of disagreements about implementing policies he advocated.

Among Simon's principal achievements, two stand out. The first was his supervision of measures taken in 1866 to enhance public sanitation, including the provision of clean drinking water and safe sanitary disposal; the second was the establishment of the General Medical Council, the licensing body for medical practitioners in the United Kingdom. His work on sanitary science and public health practice made Britain the European (and world) leader in public health in the late nineteenth century. His books include two classics of public health, *Public Health Reports* (1887) and *English Sanitary Institutions* (1890). Modern readers can gain much useful insight into public health practice from either of these books. Simon was awarded a knighthood in 1897.

JOHN M. LAST

(SEE ALSO: *History of Public Health; Sanitation*)

SKIN CANCER

Skin cancer is the most common cancer in humans. There are three main types. Basal cell carcinoma is the most common, with over 1 million cases diagnosed in the United States in the year 2000. Basal cell carcinoma is locally destructive with an extremely low rate of metastasis. Squamous cell carcinoma is the second most common type of skin cancer. It is more lethal than basal cell carcinoma with an overall rate of metastasis of between 1 and 5 percent. Malignant melanoma is the most lethal form of skin cancer. With an incidence of nearly fifty thousand cases in the United States each year, melanoma results in nearly eight thousand fatalities, often striking young adults. Sun exposure is the major risk factor for the development of skin cancer. Surgical removal is the treatment of choice, and sun protection has been shown to dramatically reduce the incidence of this illness.

GREGG M. MENAKER

(SEE ALSO: *Cancer; Melanoma; Ultraviolet Radiation*)

BIBLIOGRAPHY

Koh, H. K.; Barnhill, R. L.; and Rogers, G. S. (1996). "Melanoma." In *Cutaneous Medicine and Surgery*, eds. K. A. Arndt, P. E. Leboit, J. K. Robinson, and B. U. Weintroub. Philadelphia: W. B. Saunders.

Leshin, B., and White, W. (1996). "Malignant Neoplasms of Keratinocytes." In *Cutaneous Medicine and Surgery*, eds. K. A. Arndt, P. E. Leboit, J. K. Robinson, and B. U. Weintroub. Philadelphia: W. B. Saunders.

SLUMS

See Poverty *and* Urban Sprawl

SMALLPOX

Epidemic smallpox was one of the deadliest scourges ever to afflict humankind. It killed ancient Egyptian Pharoahs, villagers in teeming Asian villages, aristocrats in Paris and St. Petersburgh, and children in colonial New England. It contributed substantially to the collapse of the Aztec empire in Mexico, where it was introduced by the Spanish conquistadors. It was an ever-present threat, always lurking, occasionally breaking out in large epidemics. Smallpox occurred in two forms, variola major and variola minor. Variola major was the fulminant, often epidemic, variety, with a mortality rate of 40 percent or more and severe complications among survivors. Variola minor was more mild, with a mortality rate of less than 5 percent.

About 1,000 years ago, Chinese physicians discovered that susceptible persons inoculated with secretions from a smallpox scab generally had only a mild attack, and thereafter were immune. This procedure, called variolation, reached Constantinople about 1700, and was reported in a letter by Lady Mary Wortley Montagu, wife of the British plenipotentiary, to a friend in England in 1717. In 1798, Edward Jenner, a Gloucestershire doctor, vaccinated a boy with secretions from a cowpox blister, and soon reported successful vaccination of over twenty others. This was the prelude to the twentieth-century eradication of smallpox in a worldwide vaccination campaign coordinated by the World Health Organization. The last naturally occurring case was a girl in Somalia in 1977 (two further laboratory cases occurred in England in 1978).

Smallpox was an acute illness with high fever, a widespread skin rash with blebs and blisters, generalized prostration, collapse, and, commonly, death. Survivors often carried disfiguring scars for the rest of their lives, and were usually blind if lesions affected their eyes. The cause was a brick-shaped virus in the orthopox virus family. Humans were its only natural host. The virus survives now only in tissue cultures in two or three high-security microbiology research institutes. Total eradication was made possible by unique epidemiological features—i.e., there is no nonhuman host and vaccination was rapidly efficacious, so those who had been exposed to a case were protected from infection if they were immediately vaccinated. This was the basis for the containment strategy that was ultimately the key to global eradication.

Smallpox has been identified as a potential biological weapon. It would wreak havoc in an unvaccinated population, and it would be difficult for a vulnerable nation to mount an effective vaccination campaign in time to prevent national devastation. However, attackers who used small-pox as a weapon would have to ensure that they were all vaccinated, and it would be difficult to conceal a vaccination program against smallpox from the world.

JOHN M. LAST

(SEE ALSO: *Communicable Disease Control; Epidemics; Immunizations; Jenner, Edward; Montagu, Lady Mary Wortley*)

SMOG (AIR POLLUTION)

"Smog" is a popular term used to describe polluted air. It was originally used as an abbreviation of the combination of coal smoke and fog that, along with sulfur dioxide vapor, characterized polluted air in London and other British cities in the 1950s. The term came into more widespread use as a summary description for the quite different pollution mixture of ozone (O_3) and other photochemical oxidants (e.g., hydrogen peroxide, hydroxgl radical peroxy acetylnitrate) that characterized the air pollution in Southern California beginning in the 1950s, and in many other urban areas in the United States in the decades that followed. In the United Kingdom, the smog was black and acidic, while the smog in California was lighter in color and more highly oxidizing.

The black smoke in Britain was heavier in the winter months, and was most closely associated with its reducing power as a chemical (i.e., antioxidant), and with excess mortality, from chronic bronchitis and respiratory symptoms. By contrast, the California mixture was worse in the summer, and was characterized in terms of its oxidizing power. It attacked rubber and chemical polymers, and was associated with eye irritation, reduced lung function, and impaired athletic performance. In both mixtures there were fine particles that caused light to scatter and reduced the range of visibility.

In the United States, United Kingdom, and other economically developed countries in the twentieth century, the black smoke components of past pollution have largely been controlled, and the residual pollution problem is most closely related to the concentrations of light-scattering fine particles and ozone that form in the atmosphere from gaseous precursors (ie, pollutant chemicals whose reaction products have low vapor pressures and condense into fine particles). Such pollution mixtures are generally referred to as smog. While generally present at lower concentrations than in the past, these mixtures are still associated with excess cardiopulmonary mortality, morbidity, and physiologic function deficits. Attribution of the effects to specific components of the pollution mixture remains controversial, and further chemical characterization and health-effects research is now underway to resolve the remaining uncertainties.

MORTON LIPPMANN

(SEE ALSO: *Airborne Particles; Air Quality Index; Ambient Air Quality [Air Pollution]; Automotive Emissions; Carbon Monoxide; Clean Air Act; Environmental Determinants of Health; Fossil Fuels; Fuel Additives; Inhalable Particles [Sulfates]*)

SMOKING BEHAVIOR

The act of smoking has been the object of extensive research, especially since the 1950s. It remains difficult, however, to know the historical influences that prompted the early use of tobacco. It is known that smoking developed social significance through tribal ceremonies and customs of the indigenous populations of North America. As industrial societies became established, mass production and corporate marketing took advantage of the stimulative and addictive properties of nicotine. The use of tobacco also took on a new social meanings as it was marketed to fulfill psychosocial needs such as a attaining independence or being part of a "cool" trend. The result was widespread and frequent usage, particularly through the smoking of cigarettes. High consumption has since produced devastating health effects. Although early opponents had to rely primarily on moral and emotional persuasion, epidemiological evidence of tobacco's impact on morbidity and mortality now provides the principal impetus to develop policies to prevent smoking.

The abundance of information that now exists on smoking necessitates the use of various frameworks, theories, and models in order to achieve a comprehensive and coherent perspective. A frame work, such as PRECEDE-PROCEED, helps depict the broad context of smoking and encourages the analysis of a comprehensive range of variables; a theoretical approach facilitates explanations as well as predictions; and modeling enhances visual representation or mathematical relations. Most of the major public health models and theories have been applied to smoking, and the literature contains support for many of these theories. This is partly due to the generality of the theoretical concepts.

Figure 1 is a graph of the prevalence of smoking across age groups in Canada. This graph shows that daily smoking largely begins and expands during the teenage years, and then peaks among young adults before decreasing. The behavior follows a sequence of experimentation, initiation, maintenance, and cessation. While the major behavioral change occurs during the teenage years, many of the predisposing factors develop at an earlier age. Beliefs, attitudes, and values begin to develop very early in life, and these influence later behavioral patterns.

DEVELOPMENT OF BEHAVIOR PATTERNS

Human beings have a long period of infant and child development, which allows children to adapt and acquire coping skills that help them survive in

Figure 1

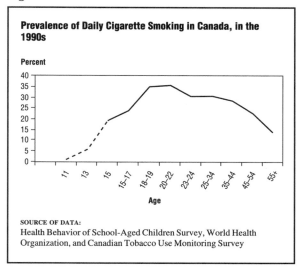

SOURCE OF DATA:
Health Behavior of School-Aged Children Survey, World Health Organization, and Canadian Tobacco Use Monitoring Survey

their environments. Due to the increasingly complex nature of society, the early socialization process needs to build capacities for communication, learning, and making decisions for healthful behavior. The initiation of smoking tends to exist among young people who report having a home environment that includes difficulty communicating with parents, lack of parental understanding, low levels of trust, and a generally unhappy home life. This type of family setting creates conditions conducive to a lifestyle that includes smoking. Such predisposing factors are also evident as social networks expand during the teenage years.

The teenage years are a time of transition. They form a bridge between the relatively sheltered environment of childhood and the roles of adulthood. Teenagers begin to confirm their own identities and emulate adult roles. There is a heightened awareness of role models and a tendency to establish boundaries through experimentation and experiencing new risks. School is obviously an important environment for teenagers and students who smoke at this age are more likely to experience difficulties in the academic setting. They experience lower grades, poor student-teacher interactions, minimal academic aspirations for the future, and often complain of unfair school rules. Teenage smokers also tend to have lower self-esteem—they are more likely to report feelings of unhappiness and loneliness, a lack of confidence, and a sense of being unhealthy.

Young people who smoke generally have a reduced capacity to implement practices that promote advancement at home and at school, and in other important settings. This can affect their ability to maintain a healthy sense of identity that includes belonging, worthiness, and hope for the future. Tobacco advertisements prey on these needs by offering an image of suave independence. The insinuation is that smoking will help an individual to achieve desirable qualities. Data are not readily available to quantify the behavioral impact of this practice. It has been shown, however, that young people are readily able to identify images and brands promoted by the tobacco industry.

Other aspects of the social environment have promoted the acceptability of smoking, such as smoking by role models in the movie industry and the widespread visibility of smoking. Studies indicate that smokers tend to overestimate the prevalence of smoking and underestimate the health hazards. All these processes and conditions are set in place during the early years of socialization, and they contribute toward a predisposition that smoking is acceptable and even desirable. Once individuals are predisposed toward the possibility of smoking, enabling factors facilitate the actual behavior.

ENABLING FACTORS

Two obvious requirements are necessary for someone to smoke: being able to acquire cigarettes and having a setting that is conductive to lighting up. Increased access to a supply of cigarettes is closely related to the expansion of a person's boundaries and social networks. Peer groups create an important source and setting for the uptake and maintenance of smoking. During their midteens, smokers tend to have a larger number of friends and spend a great deal of time with them outside of school activities. Friends and relatives often supply cigarettes to begin smoking, but commercial outlets quickly become the main source. Studies have found that young people do not have difficulty obtaining tobacco, even with recent legislation to prevent the sale of tobacco to minors.

When prices are increased, largely through taxation, additional sources become important. These include roll-your-own tobacco, illegal smuggling, tax-free sales on Indian reservations, and mail order. The inverse relationship between price and consumption may be because smoking is more prevalent among persons with a lower socioeconomic status who have a limited amount of money to spend on tobacco products. However, once smoking has begun there is a tendency toward continuance and an integration of smoking into one's lifestyle. The predisposing and enabling factors develop into patterns that reinforce the behavior, as do the addictive properties of nicotine.

REINFORCING BEHAVIOR PATTERNS

Reinforcing patterns begin with having friends who are smokers. Spending time with such friends provides ample opportunities to reinforce smoking behavior. Patterns develop to have a cigarette during breaks at work, with food and beverages, and during social events such as parties. Strong correlations exist between smoking and the consumption of caffeine, alcohol, and marijuana. These patterns move smokers away from healthy and productive lifestyles. There are thus a host of illness symptoms and premature deaths attributable directly to smoking as well as indirectly to the broader pattern of unhealthful behavior.

In 1999, The World Health Organization reported that "the joint probability of trying smoking, becoming addicted, and dying prematurely is higher than for any other addiction." Although smokers downplay the consequences of smoking, they do recognize that a risk exists, though they find it difficult to quit. Many teenagers believe they will only smoke for a short duration. Others state they can "quit anytime." Unfortunately, a significant number are in for a long struggle, and perhaps a lifetime addiction to tobacco. Most of the decline in the proportion of smokers does not occur until past the age of forty. This is partially related to successful quitters and premature deaths of smokers. More than two out of three adult smokers report a desire to quit smoking. The most common reason for successful quitting is a concern about future health. The influence of these health concerns is enhanced by a continual decline in the proportion of adult smokers subsequent to the publication of the 1964 Surgeon General's report outlining the consequences of smoking. However, during the 1990s there was a slightly upward trend in the proportion of high school students who are smoking. For young people, the subjective meaning of smoking extends beyond the concern about future health consequences.

The principal predisposing and enabling factors for smoking occur during the socialization process. Personal insecurities, problems at home, and difficulties in academic environment are all preyed upon by a tobacco industry driven by profits, and smoking cigarettes and intake of nicotine become entrenched into behavioral patterns that create a high-risk trajectory and bleak outlook for the health of individuals and the population. The underlying causes of smoking are complex and deeply rooted, and the necessary research on smoking continues to expand. Public health advocates recognize the need for comprehensive tobacco control strategies, but also admonish individuals that: If you don't smoke, don't start, and if you do smoke, quit. Social changes and changes in individual behavior are required to achieve a significant reduction in tobacco use.

RONALD A. DOVELL

(SEE ALSO: *Addiction and Habituation; Adolescent Smoking; Advertising of Unhealthy Products; Behavior, Health-Related; Counter-Marketing of Tobacco; Enforcement of Retail Sales of Tobacco; Smoking Cessation*)

BIBLIOGRAPHY

Green, L. W., and Kreuter, M. W. (1999). *Health Promotion Planning: An Educational and Ecological Approach.* Mountain View, CA: Mayfield.

Health Canada. *Tobacco Use Monitoring Survey, Wave 1 Fact Sheets.* Available at http://www.hc-sc-.gc.ca/hpb/lcdc/bc/ctums/pdf/ctums99.pdf.

Lalonde, M. (1974). *A New Perspective on the Health of Canadians: A Working Document.* Ottawa: Canadian Department of National Health and Welfare.

National Association of County and City Health Officials (2000). *Programming and Funding Guidelines for Comprehensive Local Tobacco Control Programs.* Available at http://www.naccho.org/downloadfile2.cfm/General185.pdf.

Pollay, R. W. (2000). "Targeting Youth and Concerned Smokers: Evidence from Canadian Tobacco Industry Documents." *Tobacco Control* 9:136–147.

World Health Organization (1999). "Combating the Tobacco Epidemic." In *The World Health Report 1999–Making a Difference.* Available at http://www.who.int/whr/1999/.

SMOKING CESSATION

Smoking prevalence has been declining in countries such as the United States, Australia, Canada, and the United Kingdom, but these declines are matched by increasing rates in most other countries. The *Healthy People 2010* goal in the United States is to decrease prevalence from 24 percent to 12 percent by the year 2010. This goal can only be achieved by helping current smokers to quit. Increasing the incidence of quitting is achieved through medications, counseling strategies, and public health approaches.

IMPACT OF SMOKING

In the United States smoking became increasingly popular from the early 1900s through the mid-1960s, but it then declined substantially. During the 1950s, the link between smoking and respiratory diseases and cancer became known. In 1964, the first Surgeon General's Report on smoking noted the substantial health hazards associated with smoking. Cigarette smoke contains more than 4,000 chemicals, of which forty-three are known to cause cancer. Among the more toxic chemicals in tobacco are ammonia, arsenic, carbon monoxide, and benzene. Cigarette smoking is now known to cause chronic obstructive pulmonary disease (COPD), heart disease, stroke, multiple cancers (including lung cancer), and adverse reproductive outcomes. Smoking causes about 21 percent of all deaths from heart disease, 86 percent of deaths from lung cancer, and 81 percent of all deaths from chronic lung disease.

Nicotine is highly addictive and causes persistent and compulsive smoking behavior. Most users make four to six quit attempts before they are able to remain nicotine-free. Smoking cessation produces major and immediate health benefits by reducing mortality and morbidity from heart disease, stroke, cancer, and various lung diseases.

SECONDHAND SMOKE

Secondhand smoke, or environmental tobacco smoke (ETS), causes lung cancer and cardiovascular disease in nonsmoking adults. About 43 percent of U.S. children are exposed to cigarette smoke by household members. Childhood exposure to ETS has been shown to cause asthma and to increase the number of episodes and severity of the disease. ETS exposure of very young children is also causally associated with an increased risk of bronchitis, pneumonia, and ear infections. For these reasons, the importance of smoking cessation extends beyond the health benefit of the smokers themselves.

EFFECTIVE INTERVENTIONS

In general, clinical interventions to treat tobacco use double unassisted quit rates. Effective interventions include the provision of advice to quit by a health care provider, the provision of behavioral counseling, and medications. Since the 1980s, efforts to reduce tobacco use have shifted away from an exclusive focus on clinical interventions to include a broader public health approach. This broader approach increases quitting by changing societal norms around tobacco use and increasing the motivation and support for people to attempt to quit.

CLINICAL INTERVENTIONS

Tobacco dependence is a chronic relapsing condition that often requires repeated intervention. The U.S. Public Health Service's "Treating Tobacco Use and Dependence" Clinical Practice Guideline describes the strong science base behind current treatment recommendations. Guidelines from Canada and the United Kingdom provide similar recommendations.

Brief advice to quit smoking from a health care provider increases quit rates by 30 percent. Every person who uses tobacco should be offered at least brief advice to quit smoking because failure to do so becomes a reason for smokers to assume their doctor does not consider it important to their health. More intensive counseling (individual, group, and telephone counseling) and medications are even more effective and should be provided to all tobacco users willing to use them.

Counseling. All patients should be asked at every visit to their physician whether they smoke, and this information should be recorded in the patient chart. Providers are encouraged to incorporate the five As: Ask, Advise, Assess, Assist, and Arrange into their treatment strategy. Asking if a

person smokes prompts the provider to give advice to quit. The assessment process determines whether the person is ready to quit in the near future; the clinician's message can then be tailored either to provide advice about quitting or to a motivational message to increase interest in quitting. Assistance is given by reviewing information on the quitting process, providing more intensive counseling and by encouraging the use of medications. Arranging means following up with the patient to determine the effectiveness of treatment.

Medication. Five medications have been approved by the U.S. Food and Drug Administration for treating nicotine dependence. All produce approximately a doubling of quit rates. Bupropion SR works on the nicotine receptors in the brain and seems to curb the craving for nicotine. Nicotine replacement therapy (NRT) products are produced in four forms in the United States: gum, patch, nasal spray, and inhaler. Nicotine tablets are also available in Europe. These products provide nicotine without the toxic chemicals that one inhales with smoke or absorbs through the mouth with chew or spit tobacco. Currently, the patch and gum are available in over-the-counter form; the nasal spray and inhaler are available by prescription.

HEALTH CARE SYSTEM SUPPORT FOR TREATMENT OF TOBACCO-USE

Several guidelines recommend that health care systems institutionalize the consistent identification, documentation, and treatment of every tobacco users. Another recommendation is to provide full insurance coverage for medication and counseling related to tobacco use. Data show that reducing cost barriers not only increases the use of more effective treatments but also increases the number of people who successfully quit.

Tobacco-dependence treatments are both clinically effective and highly cost-effective relative to other medical and disease prevention interventions. Treatment of tobacco use costs $2,600 per year of life saved compared with $62,000 for mammograms and $23,000 for the treatment of hypertension.

Model Clinical Treatment Programs. Group Health Cooperative (GHC) of Puget Sound, a

Seattle-based managed care organization, provides comprehensive coverage for smoking cessation. Treatment includes telephone or group behavioral counseling and medications to support the quit process. This program enrolls 8 percent of all smokers in GHC into the treatment program each year and has a 30 percent long-term quit rate. Smoking has declined at a faster rate among GHC enrollees than among the general population of Washington State. It is estimated that this program paid for itself within four years.

SPECIAL POPULATIONS

Pregnant Women. If a woman is pregnant or nursing it is especially important for her to quit smoking—to protect her own health and the health of the baby. Counseling is the primary treatment recommended for pregnant women. A pregnant woman who is a heavy smoker and unable to quit should consult her physician about the possible use of medication.

Young People. Since most tobacco use begins during adolescence, it is important to prevent onset of tobacco use and to encourage cessation at a young age. Half of adolescent smokers say they want to stop smoking cigarettes completely and about six of ten report that they seriously tried to quit in the past year. Unfortunately, adolescent tobacco users can become addicted to nicotine within the first weeks of use, and most adolescents experience symptoms of nicotine withdrawal when they try to quit. Therefore, adolescents are as likely to relapse as adults are. It is unclear which interventions will help adolescents quit. However, some adolescent prevention and cessation programs show promise in increasing quit rates.

POPULATION APPROACHES TO CESSATION

The Community Preventive Services Task Force reviewed the effect on cessation of population approaches, including media campaigns, cigarette tax increases, and clean indoor air laws, and found that media campaigns and price increases promoted cessation. Clean indoor air policies decrease the number of cigarettes smoked per day; though the impact on cessation is less clear.

CESSATION ACTIVITIES IN THE UNITED STATES

California and Massachusetts have developed comprehensive programs that include media campaigns, community interventions, and state-sponsored telephone quit lines. These programs have been successful in increasing smoking cessation. Oregon has collaborated with managed care organizations to improve treatment and also provides telephone counseling and medication to Medicaid clients. Florida has developed a very successful media campaign and community intervention that reduced smoking by young people.

Comprehensive programs directed at both young people and adults that focus on decreasing initiation, increasing cessation, and decreasing exposure to ETS have proven effective. In California, comprehensive tobacco-control programs and policies have been associated with accelerated declines in cardiovascular disease and deaths from lung cancer compared to the rest of the nation.

State Roles. The Center for Disease Control and Prevention's 1999 *Best Practices for Comprehensive Tobacco Control Programs* suggests that comprehensive state programs include the following (1999):

- Community programs to reduce tobacco use.

- Chronic disease programs to reduce the burden of tobacco related disease.

- School programs to reduce tobacco use by young people.

- Enforcement of clean indoor air and minors' access laws.

- Statewide programs.

- Counter-marketing campaigns.

- Cessation programs.

- Surveillance and evaluation.

- Administration and management.

Combining individual, systems, and population-based approaches that increase cessation offers the best opportunity to reduce morbidity and mortality from tobacco use, which is the leading preventable cause of death in the United States.

The clinician's role is to assess every patient's tobacco use and interest in quitting, advise those who smoke to stop, offer individual, group, or telephone counseling, and encourage patients to use effective medications. The role of the health care system is to implement system changes to support routine tobacco treatment by clinicians and to monitor the effect of treatment through quality performance measures.

Employers also play a role, which consists of providing insurance coverage for cessation services, providing treatment services at the worksite, and establishing smoke-free buildings or campuses. Finally the role of the government is to increase the price of tobacco products, implement media campaigns, enact clean indoor air policies and laws, regulate tobacco products, and ensure insurance coverage of tobacco use treatment.

CORINNE G. HUSTEN
ABBY C. ROSENTHAL
MICAH H. MILTON

(SEE ALSO: *Addicition and Habituation; Adolescent Smoking; Advertising of Unhealthy Products; Media Advocacy; Office on Smoking and Health; Tobacco Control*)

BIBLIOGRAPHY

Canadian Task Force on the Periodic Health Examination (1994). *Canadian Guide to Clinical Prevention Health Care,* 2nd edition. Ottawa: Canada Communication Group.

Centers for Disease Control and Prevention (1999). *Best Practices for Comprehensive Tobacco Control Programs–August 1999*. Atlanta, GA: Author.

Corrao, M. A.; Guindon, G. E.; Sharma, N.; and Shokoohi, D. F., eds. (2000). *Tobacco Control: Country Profiles*. Atlanta, GA: American Cancer Society.

Cromwell, J.; Bartosch, W. J.; Fiore, M. C.; Hasselblad, V.; and Baker, T. (1997). "Cost-Effectiveness of the Clinical Practice Recommendation in the AHCPR Guideline for Smoking Cessation." *Journal of the American Medical Association* 278(21):1759–1766.

DiFranza, J. R.; Rigotti, N. A.; McNeill, A. D.; Ockene, J. K.; Savageau, J. A.; St. Cyr, D.; and Coleman, M. (2000). "Initial Symptoms of Nicotine Dependence in Adolescents." *Tobacco Control* 9:313–319.

Fichtenberg, C. M., and Glanz, S. A. (2000). "Association of the California Tobacco Control Program with Declines in Cigarette Consumption and Mortality from Heart Disease." *New England Journal of Medicine* 343:1772–1777.

Fiore, M. C.; Bailey, W. C.; Cohen, S. J. et al. (2000). *Treating Tobacco Use and Dependence. Clinical Practice Guideline*. Rockville, MD: U.S. Public Health Service.

McAffee, T.; Wilson, J.; Dacey, S.; Sofian, N.; Curry, S.; and Wagener, B. (1995). "Awakening the Sleeping Giant: Mainstreaming Efforts to Decrease Tobacco Use in an HMO." *HMO Practice* 9(3):138–142.

National Cancer Institute (1999). *Health Effects of Exposure to Environmental Tobacco Smoke: The Report of the California Environmental Protection Agency*. Smoking and Tobacco Control Monograph No. 10. Bethesda, MD: Author.

Raw, M.; McNeill, A.; and West, R. (1998). "Smoking Cessation Guidelines for Health Professionals. A Guide to Effective Smoking Cessation Interventions for the Health Care System." *Thorax* 53(1):S1–S19.

Silagy, C., and Ketteridge, S. (1998). "The Effectiveness of Physician Advice to Aid Smoking Cessation. Database of Abstracts of Reviews of Effectiveness." In *The Cochrane Library, Issue 2*. Oxford: Update Software.

Task Force on Community Preventive Services (2001). "Recommendations Regarding Interventions to Reduce Tobacco Use and Exposure to Environmental Tobacco Smoke." *American Journal of Preventive Medicine* 20(2S).

U.S. Department of Health and Human Services (1989). *Reducing the Consequences of Smoking: 25 Years of Progress. A Report of the Surgeon General*. Atlanta, GA: CDC, Office on Smoking and Health.

—— (1990). *The Health Benefits of Smoking Cessation: A Report of the Surgeon General*. Atlanta, GA: CDC, Office on Smoking and Health.

—— (1994). *Preventing Tobacco Use Among Young People: A Report of the Surgeon General*. Atlanta, GA: CDC, Office on Smoking and Health.

—— (2000). *Reducing Tobacco Use: A Report of the Surgeon General*. Atlanta, GA: CDC, Office on Smoking and Health.

U.S. Department of Health, Education, and Welfare (1964). *Smoking and Health: Report of the Advisory Committee to the Surgeon General of the Public Health Service*. Washington, DC: U.S. Public Health Service, Centers for Disease Control and Prevention.

Wagner, E. H.; Curry, S. J.; Grothaus, L.; Saunders, K. W.; and McBride, C. M. (1995). "The Impact of Smoking and Quitting on Health Care Use." *Archives of Internal Medicine* 155:1789–1795.

SMOKING: INDOOR RESTRICTIONS

In the mid-1970s, the nonsmokers' rights movement began to press for the adoption of laws to control exposure to environmental tobacco smoke (ETS)—also know as second-hand smoke. In 1973, Arizona became the first U.S. state to restrict smoking in public places for health reasons. In 1975, Minnesota passed a comprehensive state-wide law.

Although a 1972 U.S. Surgeon General's Report raised the issue of ETS, it was in the 1980s that the scientific understanding of the health effects of ETS increased notably. In 1986, the Surgeon General concluded that "involuntary smoking is a cause of disease, including lung cancer, in healthy nonsmokers." In 1997, the California Environmental Protection Agency concluded that ETS caused 3,000 lung cancer deaths and 35,000 to 62,000 heart disease deaths in the United States each year. Among children, ETS causes bronchitis, pneumonia, and middle ear infections, and induces asthma attacks. ETS has also been linked to new cases of asthma, and to sudden infant death syndrome.

As knowledge of the health effects of ETS has increased, so has the strength of restrictions. The hazards of ETS are entirely preventable, and ETS restrictions protect both workers and the public. Apart from the serious health hazards, most nonsmokers are annoyed by ETS exposure.

The World Health Assembly, parent body of the World Health Organization, has adopted a number of resolutions referring to ETS, including urging member countries in 1978 "to protect the rights of nonsmokers to enjoy an atmosphere unpolluted by tobacco smoke." North America, along with Australia and New Zealand, have been further ahead than most countries in restricting smoking in workplaces and public places, although particular progress has been made in places such as Singapore, South Africa, and Scandinavia.

As of 2000, at least 930 municipal ordinances restricting ETS in varying degrees were in force in the United States, and at least 300 in Canada. Forty-five U.S. states, the District of Columbia, and seven Canadian provinces had laws restricting ETS in 2000.

In 1985, Aspen, Colorado, became the first North American municipality to require smoke-free restaurants. As of 2000, at least 280 U.S. municipalities and twenty-five Canadian municipalities had local laws in force requiring smoke-free restaurants. Utah (1993), California (1995), Vermont (1995), and Maine (1999) have passed state-wide laws requiring smoke-free restaurants. Numerous studies have demonstrated that such laws do not adversely impact restaurant sector sales. As of 2000, at least thirty municipalities in the United States and fifteen in Canada require smoke-free bars.

In 1987, Canada (and the United States in 1988) prohibited smoking on domestic airline flights of two hours or less. Canada banned smoking on all domestic flights of Canadian airlines in 1989, and all international flight in 1994. The United States prohibited smoking on all domestic flights of six hours or less in 1990. Worldwide, smoke-free flights have become the norm, with the support of the International Civil Aviation Organization.

There have been a number of legal initiatives by nonsmokers to pursue smoke-free environments, including labor arbitrations, claims under workplace safety and worker compensation laws, and claims under the Americans with Disabilities Act. In 1997, the Broin class action lawsuit against tobacco manufactures by flight attendants exposed to ETS resulted in a $349 million out-of-court settlement.

Smoking laws are generally respected and easy to enforce, especially after an initial implementation period. Measures that facilitate enforcement include posting of "no smoking" signs; requiring employers/proprietors to not permit illegal smoking; and prohibiting ashtrays where smoking is banned. Public support for smoking laws is generally high and often increases after implementation.

Smoke-free workplaces may benefit employers through increased productivity among non-smokers, and through reduced costs due to cleaning, maintenance, property damage, fire risk and insurance, absenteeism, sick pay, and worker's compensation.

Apart from protecting nonsmokers, smoking restriction laws have a major impact in reducing smoking overall; such laws motivate smokers to quit or cut back, reduce smoking's social acceptability, and reduce visible role modeling. Numerous studies have found that workplace smoking restrictions reduce cigarette consumption. In a Philip Morris document, workplace smoking bans were said to result in a 20 percent quit rate.

Recognizing the impact on sales volumes, the tobacco industry has actively opposed ETS restrictions. This has been done by conducting large-scale public relations campaigns denying that ETS is a proven harm, funding studies that cast doubt over whether ETS is harmful, lobbying against laws, funding other organizations or new "front" groups to lobby against laws, and supporting state laws that prevent municipalities from adopting ordinances. The tobacco industry has argued that public smoking restrictions cause economic harm, and that the marketplace should allow proprietors to determine whether or not to restrict smoking.

ROB CUNNINGHAM

(SEE ALSO: *Environmental Tobacco Smoke; Tobacco Control*)

BIBLIOGRAPHY

Barnes, D. E.; Hanauer, P.; Slade, J.; Bero, L. A.; and Glantz, S. A. (1995). "Environmental Tobacco Smoke: The Brown and Williamson Documents." *Journal of the American Medical Association* 274(3):248–253.

California Environmental Protection Agency (1997). *Health Effects of Exposure to Environmental Tobacco Smoke: Final Report.* Sacramento, CA: CEPA Office of Environmental Health Hazard Assessment. Available at http://www.oehha.ca.gov.

U.S. Department of Health and Human Services (1986). *The Health Consequences of Involuntary Smoking: A Report of the U.S. Surgeon General.* Washington, DC: USDHHS.

—— (2000). *Reducing Tobacco Use: A Report of the Surgeon General.* Washington, DC: USDHHS.

U.S. Environmental Protection Agency (1992). *Respiratory Health Effects of Passive Smoking: Lung Cancer and Other Disorders.* Washington, DC: EPA.

SMUGGLING TOBACCO

Smuggling tobacco is the illegal movement of tobacco products across domestic or international borders. It reduces tax revenues, thereby weakening the effectiveness of tobacco control laws. Weakened regulation results in increased access to tobacco by minors, limits enforcement of state and federal laws, and hinders surveillance efforts to track tobacco sales and consumption.

Interstate tobacco smuggling evades state or provincial tobacco taxes. It involves legal purchases of tobacco products in states with lower taxes and shipment of these products to states with higher taxes for illegal sale. Federal taxes are not affected because they are levied at the time of initial purchase.

International tobacco smuggling evades federal, state or provincial, and local taxes, and import/export duties. It involves either tobacco made abroad and smuggled into the United States or into another country, or the introduction of tobacco products into the producing country's black market.

LAWRENCE W. GREEN

(SEE ALSO: *Enforcement of Retail Sales on Tobacco; Taxation on Tobacco; Tobacco Control; Tobacco Sales to Youth, Regulation of*)

SNOW, JOHN

John Snow (1813–1858) was a London physician and a founding father of modern epidemiology. He was a pioneer anesthetist who invented a new kind of mask to administer chloroform, which he used on Queen Victoria to assist at the births of her two youngest children. He was an astute clinician and kept meticulously detailed notes about his patients and their diseases. His work on cholera was of lasting value because it demonstrated several fundamental intellectual steps that must be part of every epidemiologic investigation. He began with a logical analysis of the then available facts, which demonstrated that cholera could not be due to a "miasma," a theory that was then popular. It could only be caused, Snow determined, by a transmissible agent, most probably in drinking water.

Having arrived at this logical conclusion, Snow conducted two epoch-making epidemiological investigations in the great cholera epidemic of 1853 to 1854. One was a study of a severe, localized epidemic in Soho, using analysis of descriptive epidemiologic data and spot maps to demonstrate that the cause was polluted water from a pump in Broad Street. His investigation of the more widespread epidemic in South London involved him in an inquiry into the source of drinking water used in some seven hundred households. Snow compared the water source in houses where cholera had occurred with that in houses where it had not. His analysis showed beyond doubt that the cause of the epidemic was water that was being supplied to houses by the Southwark and Vauxhall water company, which drew its water from the Thames downriver, from London, where many effluent discharges polluted the water. Snow found that very few cases occurred in households supplied with water by the Lambeth company, which collected water upstream from London, where there was little or no pollution. Snow's work was remarkable in that it was completed thirty years before Robert Koch identified the cholera bacillus. Snow published his work in a monograph, *On the Mode of Communication of Cholera* (1855). This classic book has been reprinted in several modern editions and is still used as a teaching text in courses of epidemiology.

JOHN M. LAST

(SEE ALSO: *Filth Diseases; Miasma Theory*)

BIBLIOGRAPHY

Snow, J. (1855). *On the Mode of Communication of Cholera.* Reprint. New York: Haffner, 1965.

SOCIAL AND BEHAVIORAL SCIENCES

While it is undoubtedly true that a biomedical perspective dominated public health in the first half of the twentieth century, there has emerged, largely since World War II, a social science perspective in public health. This perspective has developed in departments of social and community medicine in Europe and in schools of public health in the United States, and it is reflected in the growth of the behavioral and social sciences in the curricula for public health professional and research degrees. This perspective is also evident in the establishment of departments of social and behavioral sciences in universities.

Many social and behavioral science disciplines are relevant to the understanding and articulation of the mission of public health. It would be impossible to document here all the various discipline areas; these include disciplines as diverse as psychology, economics, history, and anthropology. The focus here will be on those disciplines that most directly attempt to describe, understand, predict, and change the public's health.

SOCIAL AND BEHAVIORAL SCIENCES LITERATURE

A considerable literature on individual behavior and public health has developed in the second half of the twentieth century. The general failure of public health to pick up and nurture the more macro social science perspectives to the same degree has limited the full potential of the impact of the social and behavioral sciences on public health, particularly because the historical roots of public health in the latter half of the nineteenth century included a strong social structural viewpoint. Since that time, the theoretical development of economics, political science, sociology, and anthropology has accelerated, but it was often not brought to bear on contemporary public health issues because these issues were often defined in terms of the characteristics of individuals rather than as characteristics of social structure. The argument is, then, that public health picked up the wrong end of the social science stick—the individual (micro) end rather than the sociocultural (macro) end. This assertion is supported by any perusal of public health journals or literature on social and behavioral science in public health in the second half of the twentieth century. Nonetheless, as the end of the twentieth century in public health witnessed increasing concern with social concepts such as social inequity, inequality, and community interventions, the disciplines of sociology, anthropology, economics, and political science had a more important role in public health, for the determinants of health were being defined in terms of a social and behavioral perspective. For example, many individual behaviors were recognized as risk factors for poor health, but were also seen as embedded in a wider social context. In addition, a social science–informed healthful public policy was seen by many as a key to the development of public health strategies to improve health.

THE SCIENTIFIC DISCIPLINES AND PUBLIC HEALTH

As noted previously, there are several social and behavioral science disciplines applied to public health. What follows is a brief summary of each of the key disciplines, with attention given to the theory and work of each discipline relevant to public health. In some of the social science disciplines there are large subdisciplinary areas devoted to medicine. For example, there are large subdisciplinary fields such as history of medicine, medical sociology, medical anthropology, health psychology, and medical geography. Most of these subdisciplines have university departments, dedicated journals, and professional organizations. However, most of these subdisciplines are concerned with medicine in the very broadest interpretation, including health promotion, clinical care, disease prevention, and biomedical research. Only a part of a subdiscipline such as medical sociology is concerned with public health. Similarly, most of the subdiscipline of history of medicine is concerned with the development and evolution of clinical medicine rather than public health. Thus, the interpretation of the role of the social and behavioral sciences in public health is very much tied to one's definition of public health.

THE SOCIAL AND BEHAVIORAL SCIENCE DISCIPLINES

The social sciences are concerned with the study of human society and with the relationship of individuals in, and to, society. The chief academic disciplines of the social sciences are anthropology, economics, history, political science, and sociology. The behavioral sciences, particularly psychology, are concerned with the study of the actions of humans and animals. The key effort of the behavioral sciences is to understand, predict, and influence behavior. The chief academic disciplines of the behavioral sciences are anthropology, psychology, and sociology, with the distinction between social and behavioral science often blurred when these disciplines are applied in public health research and practice, particularly in schools of public health and governmental agencies. Many, if not most, public health approaches are problem focused and lead to a multidiscipline solution encompassing several social and behavioral science disciplines and combinations of them (such

as social psychology), in addition to other public health disciplines such as epidemiology and biostatistics.

Anthropology. Anthropology is a broad social science concerned with the study of humans from a social, biological and cultural perspective. Historically it is a Western-based social science with roots in Europe and North America. It includes two broad areas of physical and sociocultural anthropology; both are relevant to public health. Physical anthropology divides into two areas, one related to tracing human evolution and the study of primates, and the other concerned with contemporary human characteristics stemming from the mixture of genetic adaptations and culture. Medical anthropologists with this perspective are often concerned with the relationships between culture, illness, health, and nutrition. Sociocultural anthropology is concerned with broad aspects of the adaptation of humans to their cultures—with social organization, language, ethnographic details, and, in general, the understanding of culturally mitigated patterns of behavior. In recent decades this perspective has taken a more ecologically focused view of the human species. From a public health perspective, this approach to anthropology is probably most salient in terms of the methodological approaches used by anthropologists. They have a critical concern with understanding communities through participant observation. Indeed, participation is probably the key concept linking modern-day anthropological approaches to twentieth-century concepts of public health community interventions. Although the methodology of rapport-based structured interviews and observation is a highly developed methodology among anthropologists, it has had limited application in public health. More recent efforts in public health to address issues of inequity at the community level have created more attention to anthropological approaches.

Economics. Economics is perhaps the oldest of the social sciences, with its concern with wealth and poverty, trade and industry. However, current economic thinking generally dates from the last three centuries and is associated with the great names in economic thinking, such as Adam Smith, Robert Malthus, David Ricardo, John Stuart Mill, and Karl Marx. Present-day economics is an advanced study of production, employment, exchange, and consumption driven by sophisticated mathematical models. Basically, the field breaks into two distinctive areas: microeconomics and macroeconomics. Microeconomics is largely concerned with issues such as competitive markets, wage rates, and profit margins. Macroeconomics deals with broader issues, such as national income, employment, and economic systems. The relationship between economics and health is obvious because in developed countries the percentage of gross national product consumed by the health care industry is significant, generally ranging from 5 to 15 percent of the gross national product. In the poorer countries, the cost of disease to the overall economy can prohibit the sound economic development of the country. In recent years there has been a concern with both the global economic burden of disease as well as with investment in health. That poverty is highly related to poor public health is a widely accepted tenet of modern-day thinking in public health. However, economic systems ranging from free enterprise through liberal socialism and communism offer quite differing alternatives to the reduction of poverty and the distribution of economic resources.

Psychology. Psychology is probably the most common disciplinary background found in the application of the social and behavioral sciences to public health. Modern psychology is a large field that encompasses physiological psychology, concerned with the nervous and circulatory systems, as well as social psychology, and concerned with the behavior of individuals as influenced by social stimuli. In general, psychology is concerned with the relationship of living organisms to their environment. In addition to studies focused on physiological mechanisms, psychology is concerned with the broad area of human cognition, including learning, memory, and concept formation. The subfield of abnormal psychology is concerned with mental disorders, ranging from psychoses to neuroses. The subfield of clinical psychology offers direct patient-care mechanisms to treat mental problems in individuals. Thus the application of psychological approaches to health is quite apparent.

However, the most salient branch of psychology for public health practice, and particularly for the task of understanding the determinants of health, is probably social psychology. A major focus of social psychology is on attitudes, opinions, and behaviors. Thus, there is an emphasis on

understanding how groups and individuals interact with one another. The degree to which many interactions are easy or difficult can play a major role in determining the stability of groups and individuals. Therefore, broad concepts such as stress, social cohesion, peer influence, civic trust, and others derive strong theoretical and research support from social psychology.

Sociology. Sociology is perhaps the broadest of the social science fields applied to public health. It is also characterized by being eclectic in its borrowing from the other social sciences. Thus, sociology is also concerned with organizations, economics, and political issues, as well as individual behaviors in relation to the broader social milieu. A key concept in sociology, however, is an emphasis on society rather than the individual. The individual is viewed as an actor within a larger social process. This distinguishes the field from psychology. Thus the emphasis is on units of analysis at the collective level such as the family, the group, the neighborhood, the city, the organization, the state, and the world. Sociology is concerned with how the social fabric or social structure is maintained, and how social processes, such as conflict and resolution, relate to the maintenance and change of social structures. A sociologist studies processes that create, maintain, and sustain a social system, such as a health care system in a country. The scientific component of this study would be the concern with the processes regulating and shaping the health care system. Sociology assumes that social structure and social processes are very complex.

THE SOCIAL AND BEHAVIORAL SCIENCES WORKING TOGETHER

Many social and behavioral scientists who work in public health have strong, disciplinary-based, undergraduate and graduate training in one of the social sciences. However, the practice of academic and governmental public health involves disciplinary bases that are seldom as narrow as they would be in traditional, university-based academic departments. Indeed, in many government institutions of public health such discipline-trained social scientists may be simply referred to as health scientists or even as social epidemiologists. Public health practice is largely problem-focused, and whatever disciplinary base is appropriate to the problem will be used. Thus, it would not be uncommon for a person trained as a psychologist to be involved with a program addressed at community change or for an anthropologist to be involved with individual behavioral change. Nonetheless, all of the social and behavioral sciences share a commonality in approach to public health that differs from that of the biomedical approach. Disease is usually seen as a distal outcome, the focus being on those social and behavioral processes that prevent and reduce disease in people. Generally, the social sciences take a view that health and sickness are only one part of people's lifestyle.

The social and behavioral sciences have varied and broad-based methodologies. Discussions of methodological approaches to knowledge attainment are at the heart of many discipline-based discussions. Perhaps the greatest ongoing debate is that over the role of qualitative and quantitative approaches to understanding. Many researchers and practitioners in public health consider data to be the sine qua non of public health. Often data are perceived as being quantitative and numerate. The social and behavioral sciences take a much broader view of what data is. Data can be personal accounts and stories as well as statistical presentations. Nonetheless, the rigor underpinning the appropriate collection of good data applies to both the quantitative and qualitative approaches. There is a strong appreciation that many quasi-scientific cognitive ideas, such as race, poverty, or trust, cannot simply be quantified and understood numerically, yet still play a key role in determining health outcomes.

THE DETERMINANTS OF HEALTH

In discussing the determinants of health it is useful to distinguish between the health of individuals and populations. The determinants of health for any individual relate highly to the unique characteristics of that individual. In the first instance, these characteristics are highly determined by biology—the gender, age, and genetic background of the individual. These characteristics play a primary determining role and are usually not modifiable. For example, it is obvious that a man cannot die from ovarian cancer, or a woman from testicular cancer. Generally, only an older person will suffer from Alzheimer's disease; only a person

with a genetic deficit will suffer from Down syndrome. Medical science and public health can do little to change these powerful determinants of health in the individual. However, it is also anticipated that most individuals born in the Western world of the twenty-first century are biologically equipped to have a life expectancy of some seventy to eighty years.

The health of populations is a different concept from that of the health of individuals, and the determinants of the health of populations may be conceptualized very broadly. The following is just a short list of some of the hypothesized determinants of population health: health care services, sewers and drains, potable water, sanitation, adequate nutrition, shelter, transportation networks, supportive social environments, healthful public policy, stable child-rearing environments, healthful work environments, and peace and tranquility. What is apparent in such a broad list is that most of the hypothesized determinants are outside of the traditional medical care sector of clinics and hospitals. Many determinants of population health are determined by human conditions at the broadest level of political interaction, such as the protection from the ravages of poverty, war, and refugee status. Most important, the individual has relatively little direct control over these determinants. Even in those arenas where the individual believes he or she has control, such as in pursuit of education, occupation, and income through the life span, the reality remains that access to education, occupation, and income is socially determined.

People suffer disease and illness due to social processes that are only remotely related to personal health care. As public health moves away from personal health care as the major determinant of public health to a position where it is merely one of many determinants of public health, the role of the social and behavioral sciences becomes more important in understanding population health. The World Health Organization European Office lists ten social determinants of health that are supported by strong research evidence: (1) the social gradient (people's relative social and economic status and circumstances strongly affect their health throughout life); (2) stress (stress harms health); (3) early life (the effects of early development last a lifetime); (4) social exclusion (social exclusion creates misery and costs lives); (5) work (stress in the workplace increases the risk of disease); (6) unemployment (job security increases health, well-being, and job satisfaction); (7) social support (friendship, good social relations, and strong supportive networks improve health at home, at work, and in the community); (8) addiction (individuals turn to alcohol, drugs, and tobacco and suffer from their use, but use is influenced by the wider social setting); (9) food (healthful food is a political issue); and (10) transport (healthful transport means reducing driving and encouraging more walking and cycling, backed up by better public transport).

THE ROLE OF THE SOCIAL AND BEHAVIORAL SCIENCES

In contributing to the understanding of the determinants of health, there are two chief challenges for the social and behavioral sciences. The first is to continue to build in greater depth the knowledge and evidence base for the role of socioeconomic factors in health. The second is to develop appropriate best practices for addressing the role of socioeconomic factors in order to improve the health of the public. These are related challenges, but the first is perhaps more of a challenge for the academic world, and the second for the world of public health practice. Despite the enormous complexity inherent in these challenges, there is a large and growing literature to address both of them. There is a very large literature in Western languages addressing the role of socioeconomic status (SES) and its relationship to mortality and morbidity in infants, children, adolescents, and young and old adults. In general the available evidence is more extensive for working-aged adults, where multiple studies from many countries show powerful evidence linking low SES to increased chronic disease mortality and morbidity among males and a consistent gradient of the association between levels of SES and levels of health.

Conceptually, this is a very complex and extensive area for research because of the large number of variable combinations in any research approach. Thus, if one takes SES as the determinant of interest, it needs to be studied for its impact on every age group, gender, and ethnic or racial group, in relation to many possible outcomes, including chronic disease morbidity and mortality

and risk factors for each disease. The resulting matrix of variable combinations is indeed exceedingly complex. Even though research has looked at many of the relationships possible, they clearly have not all been explored in the detail to bring surety in conclusions. That is why the research challenge is so great—there is much more basic research that needs to be undertaken to fully understand the complexities associated with the social determinants of health.

The second challenge is even more critical and is at the heart of public health ideology. Public health is predicated on the idea that one wants to take action to prevent or control disease; at the same time public health is also concerned with promoting health and preventing disease at the population level. Thus, the ideal strategies for public health practice call for action at the population level. It is, however, one thing to understand the complex mechanisms that link social determinants to health, it is quite another to try and alter them. At first glance it would appear that the solution is simple. If poverty causes poor health, then elimination of poverty should increase the overall population health. Few could disagree; nonetheless poverty itself is the result of many contributing factors. Furthermore, many in public health might well argue that large-scale programs to eliminate poverty, such as equal income distribution policies, are well beyond the scope of public health practice and carry with them political risks and an adverse impact on economic aspects of a society.

One social-science approach is to look at the scope and characteristics of the problem and then determine what is a feasible course of action to maximize benefits within the restraints of a given social system—an approach that is based on the realities within any given country's sociopolitical system. Such an approach recognizes the diversity and variability both within and between sovereign countries, but at the same time recognizes the global interdependence of all countries. Nonetheless, when public health researchers and agencies within countries have addressed the socioeconomic determinants of health from the standpoint of interventions, several common themes emerge.

First, there is the recognition of the need to pursue macro-level economic and social policies that create investment in the physical and social determinants of health. In general, this means an effort to address broad issues to improve health care infrastructure, education, transportation systems, and housing, as well as participation in a just society. It also means addressing inequities and issues of poverty. Such approaches are made explicit in documents such as *Healthy People 2010*.

Second, there is a strong attention to the community as the setting for public health interventions. That is, the everyday living and working conditions must be improved, particularly when these are accompanied by poverty and the plight of disadvantaged groups. Increasing control of the environment by those within it is a strong component of a participation-based intervention approach.

Third, behavioral risk factors remain a critical component of interventions to address the social determinants of health. Although the social setting and milieu may produce many barriers to behavior change, there remains considerable latitude at the individual level for change. Particularly in the addictive behaviors, the role of the individual remains powerful and inescapable. Evidence-based interventions need to combine the knowledge of the social and behavioral science disciplines to address the complexity of behavioral change.

Fourth, the personal health care system is seen as a critical component of the determinants of health and is the system closest to the professions of most of those who labor in the field of public health. The critical issue for the personal health care system is to address the inequities in access to quality care. These inequities stem from many determinants, including poverty and prejudice. Sociodemographic factors such as geography and urbanization also play a key role. Adequate and equitable distribution of health care resources remains a challenge for the entire globe, as does humane treatment and attention to social and psychological factors in the overall well-being of patients and families seen in these settings.

DAVID V. McQUEEN

(SEE ALSO: *Cultural Anthropology; Cultural Factors; Diffusion Theory; Economics of Health; Environmental Determinants of Health; Ethnicity and Health; Health Promotion and Education; Inequalities in Health; Lifestyle; Medical Sociology; Psychology; Psychology, Health; Social Class; Social Determinants; Sociology in Public Health*)

BIBLIOGRAPHY

Auerbach, J. A., and Krimgold, B. K., eds. (2001). *Income, Socioeconomic Status and Health: Exploring the Relationships*. Washington, DC: National Policy Association, Academy for Health Services Research.

Coleman, J. S. (1994). *Foundations of Social Theory*. Cambridge, MA: Belknap Press of Harvard University.

Evans, R. G.; Barer, M. L.; and Marmor, T. R., eds. (1994). *Why Are Some People Healthy and Others Not? The Determinants of Health of Populations*. New York: Aldine de Gruyter.

Kahn, R. S.; Wise, P. H.; Kennedy, B. P.; and Kawachi, I. (2000). "State Income Inequality, Household Income, and Maternal Mental and Physical Health: Cross Sectional National Survey." *British Medical Journal* 321:1311–1315.

Smith, G. D.; Hart, C.; Blane, D.; Gillis, C.; and Hawthorne, V. (1997). "Lifetime Socioeconomic Position and Mortality: Prospective Observational Study." *British Medical Journal* 314:547–552.

U.S. Department of Health and Human Services (2000). *Healthy People 2010*. Washington, DC: U.S. Government Printing Office.

Wilkinson, R. G. (1996). *Unhealthy Societies: The Afflictions of Inequality*. London: Routledge.

Wilkinson, R., and Marmot, M., eds. (1998). *Social Determinants of Health: The Solid Facts*. Copenhagen: World Health Organization, Regional Office for Europe.

SOCIAL ASSESSMENT IN HEALTH PROMOTION PLANNING

Within the context of health promotion, social assessment refers to a process in which objective and subjective information are used to identify high-priority problems, or assets, that affect the common good. Ideally, this process will use a variety of social, economic, and quality-of-life indicators, including the perceptions and concerns of representatives from the area or community being assessed.

There are strong connections between major health problems (e.g., violence, chronic disease, teen pregnancy) and their social determinants (e.g., cultural differences, variability in levels of income, social support, housing, and education). While these factors tend to cluster within neighborhoods or communities, they vary considerably between communities. Any social assessment should be designed to take these realities into account. Armed with the information generated from a social assessment, planners will be in a better position to tailor interventions to meet the unique needs of a given community.

MULTIPLE INDICATORS

There are different ways of knowing, and different interpretations of reality. An epidemiologist, an anthropologist, a health educator, and a layperson are all likely to view a given problem through different lenses. More importantly, each is quite likely to detect a glimpse of reality that the others may miss. The social assessment process will be productive to the extent that: (1) it serves as a first step in a planning process, (2) it reflects a spirit of inclusion, (3) time is dedicated to allow all stakeholders to discuss and interpret information gained in the process, and (4) those discussions are carried out in an atmosphere of mutual respect and trust.

The literature describing methods and instruments to assess quality-of-life and social indicators is extensive and growing. Included among the objective and subjective indicators that may be used as a part of social assessment include perceptions of quality of life; sense of community; perceived functional capacity; employment rates; differences in levels of income; access to transportation and transportation services; alcohol-related auto crashes; housing density; crime; trust or distrust in government; air and water quality; access to health, mental health, and social services; and education.

A wide range of methods have been used to collect data for social assessments. These include, but are not limited to, interviewing those who have a stake in the outcomes of a relevant program or project, community town meetings, focus groups, community polls and surveys, archival research, reviews of income, housing status, access to health services and other relevant social indicators, and synthetic estimates from national data interpolated to the local level. As a means to save limited resources, some planners retrieve existing information whenever possible, rather than generate new data. Federal, state, and local offices of housing and urban planning keep reasonably up-to-date summary records. Most of these data are in the public domain and are easily accessible, though a meaningful social assessment will inevitably require the allocation of resources to gather new information perceived as relevant to the population being studied.

ASSETS

As implied in the definition, a social assessment in health promotion should involve an accounting of community and individual assets as well as identification of problems or concerns. John McKnight and John Kretzmann describe a process of community asset mapping, wherein relevant skills and capacities of individuals, as well as other assets that may exist in a given community, are documented. These assets are classified into three tiers of primary, secondary, and potential building blocks. Primary building blocks are those that exist and are controlled within a given community (e.g., a local health agency, or a local teacher); they are also the assets that are most accessible. Secondary building blocks are those that exist within a community but are controlled from outside the community (e.g., a health clinic which is a satellite of a regional or corporate medical system). Potential building blocks are those located and controlled outside of the community (e.g., federal grant programs or national campaigns). An analysis of this kind will help planners keep a realistic perspective on the comparative difficulty of accessing the assets they have identified.

Another example of using positive indicators is found in Peter Benson's work on the developmental assets that influence children and adolescents. Benson describes forty developmental assets, which are classified equally into two categories: (1) internal assets related to the personal qualities of children (e.g., self esteem, achievement motivation) and (2) external assets (e.g., family and adult support, safety, programs and services). Analysis of developmental assets reveals a consistent pattern where, among youth, developmental assets are inversely related to high-risk health behaviors— the more developmental assets children have, the less likely they are to engage in behavior that puts them at health risk. High levels of developmental assets are associated with success in school and valuing diversity.

RESPECT

Lawrence Green and others have made the point that health is an instrumental value, that is, a value that facilitates the striving for, or attainment of, higher order, or ultimate values. For example, a company may value a commitment to physical fitness and nutrition to the extent that it influences employee performance and satisfaction. The implication is that health has value to the extent that it either supports or enables higher order values, which may include social benefits, overall quality of life, the capacity to function, or even an organization's bottom line. This point is relevant to social assessment because information gleaned from the process can be used to illustrate how the effective application of health-promotion programs contributes to the improvement of social benefits beyond improvements in health.

In a study designed to improve the immunization rates among children 0 to 2 years of age and born to low-income mothers in an urban setting, researchers found that marked increases in immunization coverage were attributable to tailored messages created from assessments that took into account the family characteristics, social and environmental conditions, and selected cultural factors unique to the participants. Irrespective of the methods, indicators, or instruments used in the social assessment process, a commitment to engaging the people of a community in identifying and assessing their own perceived problems and aspirations is essential. Not only does such a commitment assure that a critical view of reality will not be left out of the health-promotion program planning process, it signals a tangible sign of respect toward the members of a community.

MARSHALL KREUTER
BRICK LANCASTER

(SEE ALSO: *Assessment of Health Status; Community Health; Community Organization; Health Promotion and Education; Healthy Communities; Mobilizing for Action through Planning; Sociology in Public Health*)

BIBLIOGRAPHY

Bauer, R. A., ed. (1966). *Social Indicators.* Cambridge, MA: MIT Press.

Benson, P. L. (1997). *All Our Kids Are Our Kids.* San Francisco, CA: Jossey Bass Publishers.

Green, L. W, and Kreuter, M. W. (1999). *Health Promotion Planning: An Educational and Ecological Approach.* Mountain View, CA: Mayfield Publishing Company.

Kreuter, M. W.; Vehige, E.; and McGuire, A. G. (1996). "Using Computer-Tailored Calendars to Promote Childhood Immunization: A Pilot Study." *Public Health Reports* 111:176–178.

McKnight, J. L., and Kretzmann, J. P. (1977). "Mapping Community Capacity." In *Community Organizing and Community Building for Health.*, ed. M. Minkler. New Brunswick, NJ: Rutgers University Press.

Mootz, M. (1988). "Health (Promotion) Indicators: Realistic and Unrealistic Expectations." *Health Promotion* 3:79–84.

Noack, H., and McQueen, D. (1988). "Towards Health Promotion Indicators." *Health Promotion* 3:73–78:

Patrick, D., and Erickson, P. (1987). *Assessing Health-Related Quality of Life in General Population Surveys: Issues and Recommendations.* Washington, DC: National Center for Health Statistics.

Wilson, R. (1981). "Do Health Indicators Indicate Health." *American Journal of Public Health* 71:461.

SOCIAL CLASS

Since prehistory, all societies have perceived hierarchy among their members. Leaders and followers, strong and weak, rich and poor: social classifications are universal. Humans have invented numerous ways to classify people—by wealth, power, or prestige; by ability, education, or occupation; even by where they live. The term "social class" originally referred to groups of people holding similar roles in the economic processes of production and exchange, such as landowner or tenant, employer or employee. Such positions correspond to different levels of status, prestige, and access to political power, but social class eventually took on a more generic meaning and came to refer to all aspects of a person's rank in the social hierarchy.

Belonging to a social class is not merely an objective fact, but is generally accompanied by a perception of class identity. In this sense, social class is not merely a personal attribute, but also a contextual variable that characterizes a group of people. The shared culture of a particular class influences, and is influenced by, people's attitudes and lifestyle. Social class, therefore, influences health. Centuries of observations have linked social class to patterns of disease (see Krieger, Williams, and Moss, 1997). Accordingly, epidemiologists frequently present statistics on mortality and morbidity tabulated by social class, as shown in Figures 1 and 2. However, social class is an abstract and complex concept whose influence is blended with many others in predicting disease. Both Figures 1 and 2, for example, show how the effects of social class (here, indicated by family income and educational level) interact with racial or ethnic factors. However, classifications by age, religion, race, or sex lack the implication of hierarchy and are not normally considered under the heading of social class.

Social class may be ascribed at birth, as with royalty or nobility, or with castes in Hindu societies. More commonly, however, a person's position at birth is modified by his or her achievements, typically through education, occupation, or income. Class cannot be measured directly. Instead, indicators of socioeconomic status, typically based on educational attainment, income, wealth, or occupation, are used. While few would consider these to be ideal indicators of social class, they nonetheless show consistent associations with health status, such that poorer or less educated people die younger and experience more illness and disability than richer or more educated people. These indicators each have strengths and shortcomings.

A simple occupational classification has been used in Britain throughout the twentieth century for analyses linking social class and health. The British Registrar General for Births and Deaths ranks occupations in six broad categories that reflect a judgment of the skill level and social prestige of each occupation. This has been followed by other, more complex classifications, such as the 100-point occupational scale of Tremain. This applies internationally and allows comparisons between developing and industrial countries. These categories have the advantage of capturing the notion of shared culture implicit in social class,

Figure 1

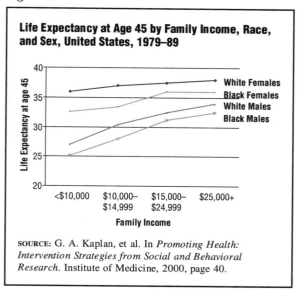

Life Expectancy at Age 45 by Family Income, Race, and Sex, United States, 1979–89

SOURCE: G. A. Kaplan, et al. In *Promoting Health: Intervention Strategies from Social and Behavioral Research.* Institute of Medicine, 2000, page 40.

but they are limited because there is no adequate way to classify people who are not in the labor force, such as retired people, housewives, or students. Furthermore, the status of occupations changes with economic development, complicating comparisons across times and across cultures. Finally, occupation shares a limitation with income, in that reverse causality may occur whereby occupational status (or income) may be influenced by the level of health.

The advantages of education as an indicator of social status include simplicity and universality: educational level can be recorded for all adults, whether working or not, and it is less likely than occupation or income to be influenced by health. But education is generally finished in early adulthood, and may no longer reflect a person's status in later years. Care must also be taken when drawing comparisons of educational levels across generations, since educational attainment changes from generation to generation.

Income or wealth are also frequently used as indicators of social class, and hold the advantage of sensitivity to variations in a person's status over time. Wealth is not simple to record, however; data on income must be supplemented by information on the number of people supported by the income, and on other assets such as savings and property. Because of shortcomings in each of

Figure 2

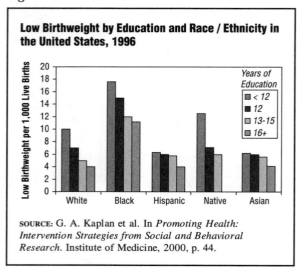

Low Birthweight by Education and Race / Ethnicity in the United States, 1996

SOURCE: G. A. Kaplan et al. In *Promoting Health: Intervention Strategies from Social and Behavioral Research.* Institute of Medicine, 2000, p. 44.

these indicators, several authors have used indicators that combine education, occupation, and income.

While socioeconomic status is generally considered a characteristic of individuals, contextual measures of social class may also be relevant in explaining patterns of health. Thus, for a population we may record not only the average level of income or wealth, but also the extent of income disparities, or class divergence, in the society. Such indicators can indicate social class characteristics of the society, rather than summarizing patterns in the society.

Contemporary epidemiologic analyses assume that it is not so much social class per se that influences health, but characteristics associated with class. There are several channels through which class or socioeconomic position may influence health:

- Certain health hazards may be directly associated with social position, such as exposure to hazardous substances or processes in the workplace.

- Alternatively, social class may influence health via behaviors that follow social patterns, such as diet, cigarette smoking, or leisure-time physical activity.

- Wealth can influence health directly, by providing access to safe and healthy housing, adequate food, and medical care and supplies when needed. Wealth also enhances educational attainment in a person's children, and so influences their subsequent earning capacity; in this manner the association between poverty and health tends to perpetuate itself across generations.

- Education also facilitates access to information that can benefit health. More educated people are better able to communicate with their physicians and interact with the health care system, and make informed choices among treatment options.

- Higher social status is associated with attitudes, such as positive self-esteem or a sense of being in control of one's life, that are positively associated with a range of indicators of health (especially mental health). Such feelings are difficult to maintain when a person is unemployed.

Contemporary analyses of social class in health research have evolved from using it as a simple classification toward using class as a starting point for a more complete analysis of possible channels of influence. The next stage, perhaps, will be to incorporate an understanding of social class dynamics into designing approaches to prevention and health promotion.

IAN MCDOWELL

(SEE ALSO: *Cultural Factors; Economics of Health; Ethnicity and Health; Inequalities in Health; Social Determinants*)

BIBLIOGRAPHY

Berkman, L. F., and Macintyre, S. (1997). "The Measurement of Social Class in Health Studies: Old Measures and New Formulations." In *Social Inequalities and Cancer.* eds. M. Kogevinas, N. Pearce, M. Susser, and P. Boffetta. Lyon: International Agency for Research on Cancer.

Krieger, N.; Williams, D. R.; and Moss, N. E. (1997). "Measuring Social Class in U.S. Public Health; Research: Concepts, Methodologies, and Guidelines." *Annual Review of Public Health* 18:341–378.

Smedley, B. D., and Syme, L. S., eds. (2000). *Promoting Health: Strategies from Social and Behavioral Research.*

Washington, DC: National Academy Press. Available at http://books.nap.edu.

Szretzer, R. S. (1984). "The Genesis of the Registrar General's Social Classification of Occupations." *British Journal of Sociology* 35:522–546.

Tremain, D. J. (1977). *Occupational Prestige in Comparative Perspective.* New York: Academic Press.

Wilkinson, R. G. (1996). *Unhealthy Societies: The Afflictions of Inequality.* London: Routledge.

SOCIAL COGNITIVE THEORY

The self-management of health requires development of self-regulatory skills. This is achieved through self-regulatory subfunctions that provide guides and motivators for self-directed change. People have to keep track of their health habits. Self-monitoring provides the information needed for setting realistic goals and for evaluating one's progress toward them. People motivate themselves and guide their behavior by the goals and challenges they set for themselves. Goals motivate by enlisting self-evaluative involvement in the activity. The evaluative self-reactions provide the means by which personal standards regulate courses of action.

PERSONAL EFFICACY

The self-management system operating through self-monitoring, goal setting, and self-reactive influence is rooted in beliefs of personal efficacy. This core belief system is the foundation of human motivation and action. Unless people believe they can produce desired effects by their actions, they have little incentive to act or to persevere in the face of difficulties.

In social cognitive theory, perceived efficacy is a key determinant because it affects lifestyle habits both directly and by its influence on other determinants. The stronger the perceived efficacy, the higher the goals people set for themselves, the more they expect their efforts to produce desired outcomes, and the more they view obstacles and impediments to personal change as surmountable.

Development of self-regulatory capabilities requires instilling a resilient sense of efficacy as well as imparting skills. Experiences in exercising control over troublesome situations serve as efficacy builders. If people are not convinced of their personal efficacy, they rapidly abandon the skills they have been taught when they fail to get quick results or suffer reverses. Efficacy beliefs affect every phase of personal change: whether people even consider changing their health habits; whether they enlist the motivation and perseverance needed to succeed; their facility to recover from setbacks; and how well they maintain the habit changes they have achieved. The self-efficacy belief system operates as a common mechanism through which psychosocial treatments affect different types of health outcomes.

PUBLIC HEALTH APPLICATIONS

People see little point in even trying if they believe they do not have what it takes to succeed. In community-wide health campaigns, people's preexisting efficacy beliefs and the efficacy beliefs instilled by the campaign contribute to adoption of health promoting habits. This calls for a change in emphasis from trying to scare people into health to enabling them to achieve self-directed change.

Effective self-management models inform people of the health risks and benefits of different lifestyles habits; create the self-regulatory skills needed to translate informed concerns into health promotive actions; build a resilient sense of efficacy to support control in the face of difficulties; and enlist social supports for desired personal changes. The guiding principles, implementative practices, and empirical documentation of effectiveness are reviewed in some detail in *Self-Efficacy: The Exercise of Control* (Bandura, 1997). By combining the high individualization of the clinical approach with the large-scale applicability of the public health approach, health self-management systems ensure high social utility.

It is easier to prevent detrimental health habits than to try to change them after they have become deeply entrenched as part of a lifestyle. The social cognitive model provides a valuable public health tool for societal efforts to promote the health of its youth. Preventive programs often produce weak results because they are heavy on didactics but meager on personal enablement. Health knowledge can be conveyed readily, but changes in values, attitudes, and health habits require greater effort. Health promotion programs that encompass the essential elements of the self-regulatory model achieve greater success.

The quality of health of a nation is a social matter, not just a personal one. It requires changing the practices of social systems that impair health rather than just changing the habits of individuals. People's beliefs in their collective efficacy to accomplish social change by perseverant group action play a key role in the policy and public health approach to health promotion. Given that health is heavily influenced by behavioral, environmental, and economic factors, health promotion requires emphasis on the development and enlistment of collective efficacy for socially oriented initiatives.

ALBERT BANDURA

(SEE ALSO: *Behavior, Health-Related; Behavior Change; Communication for Health; Enabling Factors; Health Promotion and Education; Mass Media; Predisposing Factors; Psychology, Health; Social and Behavioral Sciences*)

BIBLIOGRAPHY

Bandura, A. (1986). *Social Foundations of Thought and Action: A Social Cognitive Theory.* Englewood Cliffs, NJ: Prentice-Hall.

—— (1997). *Self-Efficacy: The Exercise of Control.* New York: Freeman.

Holden, G. (1991). "The Relationship of Self-Efficacy Appraisals to Subsequent Health Related Outcomes: A Meta-Analysis." *Social Work in Health Care* 16:53–93.

Maibach, E.; Flora, J.; and Nass, C. (1991). "Changes in Self-Efficacy and Health Behavior in Response to a Minimal Contact Community Health Campaign." *Health Communication* 3:1–15.

SOCIAL DETERMINANTS

Any case of a disease results from a long and complex chain of characteristics, circumstances, and events. The terms used to refer to the stages in this causal chain are not well agreed upon, however. Causal factors are loosely grouped into precipitating causes, which refer to agent factors, such as a virus, and some aspects of the host, such as inadequate nutrition which increases susceptibility. The events and environmental factors that give rise to the immediate causal factors are often termed "determinants." These include biological, physical, and social circumstances. Determinants account, in some measure, for the underlying rates of disease in a population, while variations in these rates are explained by risk factors. The social determinants of health include socioeconomic circumstances, social structure and function, and cultural factors. Social determinants refer to broad patterns and not to individual details—the state of being married would constitute a risk factor for some conditions, while the cultural and economic circumstances that lead to high divorce rates might form a social determinant of mental health in a particular population.

The use of the term "determinants" deserves some clarification. In most instances it does not imply a deterministic relationship, as might hold in chemistry, for example. Nor does it imply the absence of free will. Instead, determinants refer to macrosocial influences that affect health, such as poverty or social strife, and that would prove very difficult for an individual to alter.

Perhaps the broadest social determinant of health is a country's level of social and economic development. This is related to patterns of longevity, health, and disease, but the relationship is dynamic and far from simple, and economic development and health status influence one another. Patterns of disease shift as a country's economy grows, producing the epidemiologic transition from a pattern of short life expectancy and high mortality due to infectious disease, to a pattern of long life expectancy and deaths due mainly to noninfectious chronic diseases that are typical of industrial countries. Social determinants influence health through many intervening factors, such as the quality of sanitation, medical care, or food distribution systems. Examples are provided by the twentieth-century adverse impact on health seen in Eastern European countries in the former Soviet bloc.

While social determinants undoubtedly exert much of their influence through individual behaviors that promote or prevent disease, it is also clear that disease patterns cannot be fully explained in terms of individual behaviors. Health behaviors form the tip of an iceberg of social forces that also include contextual variables such as social mores, urbanization, and political changes, which seem to exert direct effects on health.

Our understanding of the social determinants of health remains in its infancy; there is little understanding of many details relating to how health is determined. Social epidemiology is still looking for its Pasteur to explain the processes involved. Current explanations are akin to stating that a car works when you put gasoline in and turn the key.

IAN MCDOWELL

(SEE ALSO: *Cultural Factors; Economics of Health; Epidemiologic Transition: Inequalities in Health; Social Class*)

BIBLIOGRAPHY

Pearl, J. (2000). *Casuality: Models, Reasoning, and Inference.* Cambridge: Cambridge University Press.

Robert, S. A. (1999). "Socioeconomic Position and Health: The Independent Contribution of Community Socioeconomic Context." *Annual Review of Sociology* 25:489–516.

Rothman, K. J., ed. (1988). *Casual Inference.* Chestnut Hill, MA: Epidemiology Resources, Inc.

SOCIAL HEALTH

The concept of social health is less intuitively familiar than that of physical or mental health, and yet, along with physical and mental health, it forms one of the three pillars of most definitions of health. This is partly because social health can refer both to a characteristic of a society, and of individuals. "A society is healthy when there is equal opportunity for all and access by all to the goods and services essential to full functioning as a citizen" (Russell 1973, p. 75). Indicators of the health of a society might include the existence of the rule of law, equality in the distribution of wealth, public accessibility of the decision-making process, and the level of social capital.

The social health of individuals refers to "that dimension of an individual's well-being that concerns how he gets along with other people, how other people react to him, and how he interacts with social institutions and societal mores" (Russell 1973, p. 75). This definition is broad—it incorporates elements of personality and social skills, reflects social norms, and bears a close relationship to concepts such as "well-being," "adjustment," and "social functioning."

Formal consideration of social health was stimulated in 1947 by its inclusion in the World Health Organization's definition of health, and by the resulting emphasis on treating patients as social beings who live in a complex social context. Social health has also become relevant with the increasing evidence that those who are well integrated into their communities tend to live longer and recover faster from disease. Conversely, social isolation has been shown to be a risk factor for illness. Hence, social health may be defined in terms of social adjustment and social support—or the ability to perform normal roles in society.

Definitions of social health in terms of adjustment derive from sociology and psychiatry. Poor social adjustment forms a common indicator of neurotic illness, and adjustment may be used to record the outcome of care, especially for psychotherapy. Adjustment may be rated subjectively, or it may be judged in terms of a person's fulfillment of social roles—how adequately a person is functioning compared to normal social expectations. Role performance can also indicate the impact of disability, bringing the concept of social health close to that of handicap, which refers to the social disadvantage resulting from impairments or disabilities (World Health Organization, 1980). As norms vary greatly between cultures, however, a challenge lies in selecting an appropriate standard against which to evaluate roles.

Mutual social support is also commonly viewed as an aspect of social health. Support attenuates the effects of stress and reduces the incidence of disease. Social support also contributes to positive adjustment in children and adults, and encourages personal growth. The concept of support underlines the theme of social health as an attribute of a society: a sense of community—or the currently fashionable concept of social capital, which refers to the extent to which there is a feeling of mutual trust and reciprocity in a community—is an important indicator of social health.

IAN MCDOWELL

(SEE ALSO: *Assessment of Health Status; Community Health; Health; Social Assessment in Health Promotion Planning; Social Determinants; Social Networks and Social Support*)

BIBLIOGRAPHY

Hawe, P., and Shiell, A. (2000). "Social Capital and Health Promotion: A Review." *Social Science and Medicine* 51:871–885.

Russell, R. D. (1973). "Social Health: An Attempt to Clarify This Dimension of Well-Being." *International Journal of Health Education* 16:74–82.

World Health Organization (1980). *International Classification of Impairments, Disabilities, and Handicaps.* Geneva: Author.

SOCIAL MARKETING

Toward the end of the twentieth century, public health professionals embraced a new strategy for promoting healthful behaviors and increasing the utilization of health services. The Centers for Disease Control and Prevention (CDC), the United States Department of Health and Human Services (USDHHS), the United States Department of Agriculture (USDA), and other federal and state agencies began using social marketing practices to promote protective and preventive health behaviors—such as fruit and vegetable consumption, physical exercise, and breastfeeding—and to increase utilization of programs and services like the Supplemental Food and Nutrition Program for Women, Infants and Children (WIC), prenatal care, and family planning.

Within the last thirty years, social marketing's application to public health problems has grown rapidly. Today, a wide range of public health and social service organizations in the United States are using social marketing, including the Centers for Disease Control and Prevention (CDC), the National Cancer Institute (NCI), the United States Department of Agriculture (USDA), the United States Department of Health and Human Services (USDHHS), and the American Association of Retired Persons (AARP). Public health administrators and health educators at the state and local level have also begun using social marketing as an approach for developing programs to bring about behavior change. Social marketing organizations have emerged to meet the growing demand for technical assistance with consumer research, strategic planning, communications, media advocacy, and other components in the social marketing process. Although formal degrees and credentialing are not awarded at this time, social marketing courses are now offered in many colleges of public health and business schools.

THE SOCIAL MARKETING APPROACH

The term "social marketing" was coined in 1971 by Kotler and Zaltman in their seminal article "Social Marketing: An Approach to Planned Social Change." It is defined as "the application of commercial marketing technologies to the analysis, planning, execution, and evaluation of programs designed to influence voluntary behavior of target audiences in order to improve their personal welfare and that of their society" (Andreasen, 1995. p. 7). Social marketing is distinguished from other management approaches by six basic principles: (1) the marketing conceptual framework is used to design behavior change interventions; (2) there is recognition of competition; (3) there is a consumer orientation; (4) formative research is used to understand consumers' desires and needs; (5) there is a segmentation of populations and careful selection of target audiences; and (6) continuous monitoring and revision of program tactics help to achieve desired outcomes.

MARKETING'S CONCEPTUAL FRAMEWORK

Social marketing relies on commercial marketing's conceptual framework to guide program development and implementation. This framework places consumers at the center of an exchange process in which they act primarily out of self-interest—attempting to maximize the ability to satisfy wants and needs and minimize the cost to do so. Social marketing identifies consumer wants and needs and then develops ways to satisfy them. Marketing's framework, or the marketing mix, includes five components involved in the exchange process: the product (in social marketing, the product is the health behavior or service being promoted); its competition (the risk behavior currently practiced); the price (social, emotional, and monetary costs exchanged for the product's benefits); place (where the exchange takes place, or the target behavior is practiced); and promotion (activities used to facilitate the exchange).

Social marketing may be used to get people to adopt new protective behaviors such as healthful diets or exercise, or to stop practicing risky behaviors such as smoking. The product may also be a service such as prenatal care or immunization, with the objective being to increase people's utilization of the service. A commodity, such as a condom, may also be promoted, but again the focus is on the behavior associated with the commodity.

The behavior being promoted must provide benefits relevant to consumers. For this reason, marketers are interested in people's aspirations and desires, as well as their social or medical needs.

The marketing model also considers the competition posed by unhealthful or risky behaviors. Often, people must make a choice between protective or healthful behaviors and risky alternatives.

In marketing terms, the price of adopting a healthful behavior is also considered from the consumer's perspective. What will the consumer exchange in order to obtain the product's benefits? Some health behaviors require consumers to exchange money for the product, such as the cost of an exercise or weight loss program. Other public health products, such as the WIC program, may appear to be free. Closer examination reveals indirect monetary costs, such as lost wages, bus fares, or childcare fees that accompany the utilization of WIC services. Often costs are nonmonetary, including time, effort, embarrassment, and the perceived loss of pride and dignity associated with participation in government assistance programs or adopting certain behaviors.

To make the exchange more attractive to consumers, social marketing seeks to lower costs and to maximize benefits. Unfortunately, many protective health behaviors come with costs that are difficult to control. For some people, safe sex practices are not as pleasurable as the riskier competition. Many people have a hard time sacrificing the taste, satiety, and perceived pleasure of a high-fat diet. Nevertheless, social marketers work to create an acceptable cost-benefit ratio.

The third "P" in marketing's framework is place—the location where services are provided, where tangible products are distributed, or where consumers receive information about new products or behaviors. Research is conducted to identify "life path points"—places that consumer's frequent—so that products and information can be placed there. Social marketing also identifies when and where a target audience will be most receptive to promotional messages.

The fourth "P" is promotion. Social marketing relies on health communications to inform and educate consumers. However, education and public information are only a part of a carefully planned set of activities designed to bring about change. In fact, an effective promotional strategy may include several communication elements, including objectives for each target audience; guidelines for designing attention-getting and effective messages; designation of appropriate communication channels; and credible, trustworthy spokespersons. Some large-scale, multifaceted projects rely on mass communications, public information, public relations, consumer education, lotteries, direct mail, and other means. Projects with more limited communications components may rely solely on personal counseling and print materials. Finally, to be effective, promotional strategies must be carefully coordinated with other components of the marketing mix. Promotional efforts cannot succeed if the product's benefits, price, and placement are not also in line with the people's wants and needs.

CONSUMER ORIENTATION

A central principle in the social marketing mindset is a commitment to understand the consumer and to design products to satisfy consumers' wants and needs. Those applying social marketing methods need to know about the people whose behavior they want to change—their aspirations and values; their relevant beliefs and attitudes; and their current behavioral patterns. They also look at the broader social and cultural factors that influence consumer behavior, recognizing that behavioral change is influenced by a combination of environmental as well as personal and interpersonal factors.

Unfortunately, many people still incorrectly equate marketing with sales and advertising. Marketing's consumer orientation is actually the antithesis of a sales orientation. In contrast to the belief that sales-stimulating devices are needed to bring results, a consumer orientation requires program planners to understand and respond to consumers' desires and needs. The social marketing approach seeks ways to design services and develop behavioral recommendations that are compatible with consumers' values and beliefs. In contrast to top-down, expert-driven approaches, social marketing attempts to create interventions that enable the target audience to solve problems and realize the dreams that people consider important.

Social marketers believe that the behaviors being promoted should contribute to the consumers' and society's well-being. However, people may have aspirations and desires that work against society's interests or conflict with their own health and well-being. There is a responsibility inherent in health promotion and education to design and deliver offerings that preserve and enhance social health, and marketing techniques do not abrogate this responsibility—they are tools that may help public health professionals reach those they need to reach.

CONSUMER RESEARCH

A consumer orientation requires an examination of consumer perceptions of product benefits, product price, the competition's benefits and costs, and other factors that influence consumer behavior. Marketing healthful behaviors relies on the social and behavioral sciences to guide formative research and subsequent program design.

Program planners use consumer research findings to identify the factors to address in promoting behavior change to the people they hope to reach. Drawing on a theoretical framework that combines elements from the Health Belief Model, Social Cognitive Theory, the Theory of Reasoned Action, and the Trans-theoretical Model of Behavior Change, research is designed to identify the mix of internal and external factors that have the greatest impact on people's health behavior. The behavioral orientation helps keep program planners on track by setting behavioral objectives for program interventions, and designing strategies that address the critical factors that determine a specific audience segment's adoption of the desired behavior. Research also helps program planners determine the specified behavioral recommendations that are most likely to be adopted by specific segments in the target population. Consumer research conducted to develop the *Loving Support Makes Breastfeeding Work* program for the National WIC Breastfeeding Promotion project

revealed that families place a strong value on establishing a close, loving bond with their babies. While health concerns are also important, the emotional benefits associated with breastfeeding are paramount for pregnant women and their relatives. This knowledge helped program planners avoid the common mistake of promoting breastfeeding as a wise medical choice instead of a way to realize parents' dreams of creating of strong family bonds. Research also learned that recommendations to breastfeed for thirteen months or longer was not viewed as realistic by many WIC participants. Program planners were careful to avoid recommending a specific time period in an effort to motivate mothers who doubted their ability to breastfeed for more than a few months. This approach helped foster successful lactation initiation, which subsequently helps instill as sense of pride efficacy to breastfeed for even short periods of time.

AUDIENCE SEGMENTATION

Another distinguishing feature of social marketing is audience segmentation. Audience segmentation is the process of dividing a population into distinct groups based on characteristics that influence their responsiveness to interventions. Segmentation may be used to identify subgroups they can realistically be reached with available resources or to determine the best way to reach particular groups. Segments may differ in terms of the benefits they find most attractive, the price they are willing to pay, the best place to communicate with them or to locate services, or their differential responsiveness to promotional tactics.

CONTINUOUS MONITORING AND REVISION

Social marketing also relies on continuous program monitoring to assess program efficacy in encouraging the desired behavior changes. Monitoring also aids in identifying activities that are effective and those that are not, and in making midcourse corrections in program interventions. Many public health programs rely on process and impact evaluations to identify components that are working and those that should be discontinued, and social marketing devotes considerable resources to this activity. There are constant checks with target audiences to gauge their responses to all aspects of an intervention, from the broad marketing strategy to specific messages and materials.

CAROL A. BRYANT
JAMES H. LINDENBERGER

(SEE ALSO: *Behavioral Change; Communication for Health; Communication Theory; Health Goals; Health Promotion and Education; Health Risk Appraisal*)

BIBLIOGRAPHY

Andreasen, A. (1995). *Marketing Social Change: Changing Behavior to Promote Health, Social Development, and the Environment.* San Francisco: Jossey-Bass.

Bryant, C.A.; Coreil, J.; D'Angelo, S.; Bailey, D.; and Lazarov, M. (1992). "A New Strategy for Promoting Breastfeeding Among Economically Disadvantaged Women and Adolescents." *NAACOG's Clinical Issues in Perinatal and Women's Health Issues: Breastfeeding* 3(4):723–730.

Cooper, P. D. (1994). *Health Care Marketing. A Foundation for Managed Quality,* 3rd edition. Gaithersburg, MD: Aspen Publishers.

Duncan, W. J.; Ginter, P. M.; and Swayne, L. E. (1998). *Handbook of Health Care Management.* Malden, MA: Blackwell Business.

Furse, D. H.; Burcham, M. R.; Rose, R. L.; and Oliver, R. W. (1994). "Leveraging the Value of Customer Satisfaction Information." *Journal of Health Care Marketing* 14(3):16–20.

Kotler P. (1999). *On Marketing.* New York: The Free Press.

Kotler, P., and Andreasen, A. (1991). *Strategic Marketing for NonProfit Organizations,* 4th edition. Englewood Cliffs, NJ: Prentice-Hall.

Kotler, P., and Armstrong, G. (1996). *Principles of Marketing,* 7th edition. Englewood Cliffs, NJ: Prentice Hall.

Kotler P., and Clarke, R. N. (1987). *Marketing for Health Care Organizations.* Englewood Cliffs, NJ: Prentice-Hall.

Kotler, P., and Zaltman, G. (1971). "Social Marketing: An Approach to Planned Social Change." *Journal of Marketing* 35:3–12.

Fishbein, M.; Guenther-Grey, C.; Johnson, W.; Wolitski, R. J.; McAlister, A.; Rietmeyer, C. A; and O'Reilly, K. (1997). "Using Theory-Based Community Intervention to Reduce AIDS Risk Behaviors: The CDC's AIDS Community Demonstration Project." In *Social Marketing: Theoretical and Practical Perspectives.* eds. M. E. Goldberg, M. Fishbein, and S. E. Middlestadt. Mahwah, NJ: Erlbaum.

Lefebvre, R. C.; Doner, L.; Johnston, C.; Loughrey, K.; Balch, G. I.; and Sutton, S. M. (1995). "Use of Database Marketing and Consumer-Based Health Communication in Message Design: An Example from the Office of Cancer Communications' '5 a Day for Better Health' Program." In *Designing Health Messages: Approaches from Communication Theory and Public Health Practice.* eds. E. Maibach and R. Parrot. Thousand Oaks, CA: Sage.

Lefebvre, C., and Flora, J. A. (1998). "Social Marketing and Public Health Intervention." *Health Education Quarterly* 15(3):299–315.

Lindenberger, J. H., and Bryant, C. A. (2000). "Promoting Breastfeeding in the WIC Program: A Social Marketing Case Study." *American Journal of Health Behavior* 24(1):53–60.

McCormack-Brown, K.; Bryant, C. A.; Forthofer, M.; Perrin, K.; Guinn, Q.; Wolper, M.; and Lindenberger, J. (2000). "Florida Cares for Women Social Marketing Campaign: A Case Study." *American Journal of Health Behavior* 24(1):44–52.

Middlestadt, S. E.; Schechter, C.; Peyton, J.; and Tjugum, B. (1997). "Community Involvement in Health Planning: Lessons Learned from Practicing Social Marketing in a Context of Community Control, Participation & Ownership." In *Social Marketing: Theoretical and Practical Perspectives.* eds. M. E. Goldbert, M. Fishbein, and S. E. Middlestadt. Mahwah, NJ: Lawrence Erlbaum.

Nitse, P. S., and Rushing, V. (1996). "Patient Satisfaction: The New Area of Focus for the Physician's Office." *Health Marketing Quarterly* 14(2):73–84.

Smith, W. A., and Middlestadt, S. E. (1993). "The Applied Behavior Change Framework." In *The World Against AIDS: Communication for Behavior Change.* Washington, DC: The Academy for Educational Development.

Wheatley, E. W. (1997). "Patient Expectations and Marketing Programming for OB/GYN Services." *Health Marketing Quarterly* 14(3):35–51.

SOCIAL MEDICINE

The concept of social medicine developed in the wake of the Industrial Revolution and its attendant social and health problems. Poor working conditions, periodic economic slumps, unemployment, lack of housing, and poverty and destitution all created an environment that had a significant impact upon people's health. Quantitative studies of mortality in England show that, for example, the average age of death in Liverpool in 1840 was 35 for gentry and professional persons and their families, 24 for tradesmen and their families, and 15 for laborers, mechanics, servants, and their families. In Manchester, the corresponding ages were 38, 20, and 17; and in Leeds they were 44, 27, and 19.

In France, Louis-René Villerme (1782–1863) studied mortality rates in the districts of Paris. During the years 1817 to 1821, the average annual mortality rate ranged from 22 deaths per 1000 inhabitants in the richest district to 42 deaths per 1000 inhabitants in the poorest.

Findings such as these led the great pathologist Rudolf Virchow (1821–1902), together with his colleagues in the German Medical Reform movement of 1848, to enunciate the basic principles of social medicine:

1. The health of the people is a matter of direct social concern.

2. Social and economic conditions have an important effect on health and disease, and these relations must be subjected to scientific investigation.

3. Steps must be taken to promote health and to combat disease, and the measures involved in such action must be social as well as medical.

These basic concepts of social medicine were extensively developed in the first half of the twentieth century in continental Europe. After World War II, a strong movement for social medicine developed in the United Kingdom. In the United States, a broad concept of social medicine was developed by the economist and public health statistician Edgar Sydenstricker, the sociologist Bernhard J. Stern, the public health scientist C.-E. A. Winslow, and the medical historian Henry E. Sigerist. However, the term was not adopted by American medical schools because of the conservative views of the medical profession.

On the other hand, the term "social medicine" is now in the process of being replaced because it is too limiting—the field encompasses a variety of professional disciplines other than medicine, and

the term "public health" is becoming increasingly recognized as more accurate.

MILTON TERRIS

(SEE ALSO: *Future of Public Health; History of Public Health; Social Determinants; Social Health; Virchow, Rudolf*)

BIBLIOGRAPHY

Chadwick, E. (1965). *Report on the Sanitary Condition of the Labouring Population of Great Britain, 1842.* Edinburgh: Edinburgh University Press.

Coleman, W. (1982). *Death Is a Social Disease: Public Health and Political Economy in Early Industrial France.* Madison: University of Wisconsin Press.

Rosen, G. (1947). "What is Social Medicine? A Genetic Analysis of the Concept." *Bulletin of the History of Medicine* 21:674–733.

Terris, M. (1957). "Concepts of Social Medicine." *The Social Service Review* 31:164–178.

—— (1985). "The Distinction between Public Health and Community/Social/Preventive Medicine." *Journal of Public Health Policy* 6:435–439.

SOCIAL NETWORKS AND SOCIAL SUPPORT

It is widely recognized that social relationships and affiliations have powerful effects on physical and mental health. Although many social scientists from Emile Durkheim on have written about the critical role of social relationships in health outcomes, it was not until the 1970s that epidemiologists turned their attention to this issue.

In the first of these studies, in Alameda County, California (Berkman et al., 1979), men and women who lacked ties to others were 1.9 to 3.1 times more likely to die than those who had many contacts. A 1982 study in Tecumseh, Michigan (House et al., 1982), showed a similar association for men, but not for women, between social connectedness and participation and mortality risk. In the same year, D. Blazer reported similar results from a sample of elderly men and women in Durham County, North Carolina.

Schoenbach et al. (1986), in a study in Evans County, Georgia, used a measure of contacts modified from the Alameda County study and found risks to be significant in older white men and women even when controlling for risk factors, although some racial and gender differences were observed. In Sweden, the Goteborg study (Welin et al., 1985) showed that, in different cohorts of men, social isolation proved to be a risk factor for dying, independent of biomedical risk factors. A 1987 report by Orth-Gomér and Johnson reported significantly increased risks for men and women who have been socially isolated. Finally, in a study of men and women in eastern Finland, Kaplan and associates (1988) demonstrated that an index of social connections predicts mortality risk for men but not for women, independent of cardiovascular risk factors.

Several more recent studies, including the Established Populations for the Epidemiologic Study of the Elderly (EPESE) studies, confirm the continued importance of social relationships into late life. Furthermore, studies of large cohorts of men and women in a large health maintenance organization (Vogt et al., 1992) and male health professionals (Kawachi et al., 1996) suggest that social networks are, in general, more strongly related to mortality than to the incidence of disease. Studies in Danish men (Pennix et al., 1997) and Japanese men and women (Sugisawa et al., 1994) also indicate that social isolation and social support are related to mortality. Social networks and support have been found to predict a broad array of health outcomes, from survival after heart attacks to disease progression, functioning, and the onset and course of infectious diseases.

UPSTREAM AND DOWNSTREAM APPROACHES

Conceptually, social networks are embedded in a macrosocial environment in which large-scale social forces may influence network structure, which in turn influences a cascading causal process. Serious consideration of the larger macrosocial context in which networks form and are sustained is almost completely absent, and such consideration is needed in studies of social network influences on health.

Networks may operate through at least five primary pathways: (1) provision of social support, (2) social influence, (3) social engagement, (4) person-to-person contact, and (5) access to resources and material goods. These psychosocial and behavioral processes may influence even more proximate pathways to health status, including direct physiological stress responses, psychological states and traits, health-damaging or health-promoting behaviors such as tobacco consumption or physical activity, and exposure to infectious disease agents.

Most obviously, the structure of network ties influences health via the provision of social support. This framework immediately acknowledges that not all ties are supportive. Social support is typically divided into subtypes, including emotional, instrumental, appraisal, and informational support.

Perhaps even more important than social support are the ways in which social relationships provide a basis for intimacy and attachment. Intimacy and attachment have meaning not only for relationships that traditionally are thought of as intimate (e.g., between partners, between parents and children) but for more extended ties. For instance, when relationships are solid at a community level, individuals feel strong bonds and attachment to places (e.g., a neighborhood) and organizations (e.g., voluntary and religious organizations).

Social networks may also influence health via social influence. Shared norms about health behaviors (e.g., alcohol and cigarette consumption, treatment adherence) might be powerful sources of social influence with direct consequences for the behaviors of network members.

A third, and more difficult to define, pathway by which networks may influence health status is by promoting social participation and social engagement. Getting together with friends, attending social functions, group recreation, and church attendance are all instances of social engagement. Several studies suggest that social engagement is critical in maintaining cognitive ability (Bassuk et al., 1999) and reducing mortality (Glass et al., 2000).

Another pathway by which networks influence disease is by restricting or promoting exposure to infectious disease agents through person-to-person contact. What is perhaps most remarkable is that the same network characteristics that can be health-promoting can at the same time be health-damaging if they serve as vectors for the spread of infectious disease.

Little research has sought to examine differential access to material goods, resources, and services as a mechanism through which social networks might operate. This is unfortunate, given the existing work showing that social networks operate by regulating an individual's access to life opportunities by virtue of the extent to which networks overlap with other networks. In this way, networks operate to provide access, or to restrict opportunities, in much the same way that social status does.

LISA F. BERKMAN

(SEE ALSO: *Community Health; Cultural Identity; Inequalities in Health; Marginal People; Medical Sociology; Psychology, Health; Social Determinants; Sociology in Public Health*)

BIBLIOGRAPHY

Bassuk, S.; Glass, T.; and Berkman, L. (1999). "Social Disengagement and Incident Cognitive Decline in Community-Dwelling Elderly Persons." *Annals of Internal Medicine* 131:165–173.

Berkman, L., and Syme, S. (1979). "Social Networks, Host Resistance, and Mortality: A Nine-Year Follow-up of Alameda County Residents." *American Journal of Epidemiology* 109:186–204.

Berkman, L. F. (1995). "The Role of Social Relations in Health Promotion." *Psychosomatic Medicine* 57: 245–254.

Blazer, D. (1982). "Social Support and Mortality in an Elderly Community Population." *American Journal of Epidemiology* 115:684–694.

Cohen, S.; Underwood, S.; and Gottlieb, B. (2000). *Social Support Measures and Intervention.* New York: Oxford University Press.

Glass, T.; Dym, B.; Greenberg, S.; Rintel, D.; Roesch, C.; and Berkman, L. (2000). "Psychosocial Intervention in Stroke: The Families in Recovery from Stroke Trial (FIRST)." *American Journal of Orthopsychiatry* 70(2):169–181.

House, J.; Robbins, C.; and Metzner, H. (1982). "The Association of Social Relationships and Activities with Mortality: Prospective Evidence from the Tecumseh Community Health Study." *American Journal of Epidemiology* 116:123–140.

Kaplan, G.; Salonen, J.; Cohen, R.; Brand, R.; Syme, S.; and Puska, P. (1988). "Social Connections and Mortality from All Causes and Cardiovascular Disease: Prospective Evidence from Eastern Finland." *American Journal of Epidemiology* 128:370–380.

Kawachi, I.; Colditz, G. A.; Ascherio, A.; Rimm, E. B.; Giovannucci, E.; Stampfer, M. J. et al. (1996). "A Prospective Study of Social Networks in Relation to Total Mortality and Cardiovascular Disease in Men in the U.S.A." *Journal of Epidemiological Community Health* 50:245–251.

Orth-Gomer, K., and Unden, A. (1987). "The Measurement of Social Support in Population Surveys." *Social Science Medicine* 24:83–94.

Pennix, B. W.; van Tilburg, T.; Kriegsman, D. M.; Deeg, D. J.; Boeke, A. J.; and van Eijk, J. T. (1997). "Effects of Social Support and Personal Coping Resources on Mortality in Older Age: The Longitudinal Aging Study, Amsterdam." *American Journal of Epidemiology* 146:510–519.

Schoenbach, V.; Kaplan, B.; Freedman, L.; and Kleinbaum, D. (1986). "Social Ties and Mortality in Evans County, Georgia." *American Journal of Epidemiology* 123:577–591.

Seeman, T. (1996). "Social Ties and Health: the Benefits of Social Integration." *Annuals of Epidemiology* 6:442–451.

Seeman, T., and Berkman, L. (1988). "Structural Characteristics of Social Networks and Their Relationship with Social Support in the Elderly: Who Provides Support." *Social Science Medicine* 26(7):737–749.

Seeman, T.; Berkman, L.; Kohout, F.; LaCroix, A.; Glynn, R.; and Blazer, D. (1993). "Intercommunity Variation in the Association between Social Ties and Mortality in the Elderly: A Comparative Analysis of Three Communities." *Annals of Epidemiology* 3:325–335.

Sugisawa, H.; Liang, J.; and Liu, X. (1994). "Social Networks, Social Support and Mortality among Older People in Japan." *Journal of Gerontology* 49:S3–S13.

Vogt, T. M.; Mullooly, J. P.; Ernst, D.; Pope, C. R.; and Hollis, J. F. (1992). "Social Networks as Predictors of Ischemic Heart Disease, Cancer, Stroke, and Hypertension: Incidence, Survival and Mortality." *Journal of Clinical Epidemiology* 45:659–666.

Weiss, R. S. (1974). "The Provisions of Social Relationships." In *Doing unto Others,* ed. Z. Rubin. Englewood Cliffs, NJ: Prentice Hall.

Welin, L.; Tibblin, G.; Svardsudd, K.; Tibblin, B.; Ander-Peciva, S.; Larsson, B. et al. (1985). "Prospective Study of Social Influences on Mortality: The Study of Men Born in 1913 and 1923." *Lancet* 1:915–918.

SOCIAL WORK

In the public health arena, social workers are a valuable resource for the development of treatment plans for patients, for locating supportive resources, and in facilitating referrals. Under the auspices of government and non-government public health organizations and institutions, social workers often provide behavioral and social assessments along with mental health assessment, treatment, and short-term or ongoing case management. Social workers may also work in the community as planners or community organizers capable of engaging groups of people, neighborhoods, or entire communities to address social problems such as drug abuse or teen pregnancy. Social work is a distinct profession, requiring college training, and a masters degree is often a necessity. Many states license social workers, and in those states only those holding such licenses may legally provide social work services The possibilities of employment vary widely and include federal, state, and local government agencies; hospitals; and public health and not-for-profit organizations.

ROBERT P. LABBE

(SEE ALSO: *Assessment of Health Status; Community Health; Mental Health; Social Determinants; Social Health*)

SOCIETY FOR RISK ANALYSIS

The Society for Risk Analysis is an interdisciplinary scientific society focusing on the assessment, management, and communication of risks to human health, safety, and the environment. The society was founded in 1981, and its international membership includes social and behavioral scientists, engineers, biologists, chemists, ecologists, mathematicians, decision scientists, economists, policy analysts, and attorneys. The society is committed to research and education in risk-related fields and has helped develop the field of risk analysis and improve its credibility, viability, and utility.

The major aims of society are to foster and promote the knowledge and understanding of risk analysis and its applications; the exploration of policy, social, and economic implications of human health and environmental risk issues; the

advancement of new methods and technologies in the practice of risk analysis, and the provision of professional advice to policymakers regarding risk-related problems. Information about the society can be found at http://www.sra.org.

GAIL CHARNLEY

(SEE ALSO: *Benefits, Ethics, and Risks; Risk Assessment, Risk Management*)

SOCIETY OF TOXICOLOGY

Founders of the Society of Toxicology (SOT), incorporated in 1961, came from toxicology laboratories in academia, government, and the private sector. The driving force behind the founding of SOT was the lack of recognition being given to toxicologists by pharmacologists. The toxicologists were primarily involved in the safety assessment of chemicals and drugs, and they had a difficult time publishing their results. The toxicologists had a forum in the Gordon Research Conferences that initiated a series of conferences on toxicology and safety evaluation in 1954. The attendees of these conferences, and especially its early chairs, developed the concept of the SOT as a professional and learned scientific organization. In 1959 they held a small meeting to bring the society into being, and between 1959 and 1961 the founding members were selected. *Toxicology and Applied Pharmacology*, the first American journal dedicated to toxicology (and the original journal of the Society), and edited by Harry Hayes, Fredrick Coulston, and Arnold Lehman, was published.

Many of the founders of the SOT were colleagues, students, and collaborators of Professor E. M. K. Geiling, who is credited by many as the father of modern toxicology. Drs. Kenneth Du Bois (the first president of the SOT), Geiling, and Frances Kelsey published their *Textbook of Toxicology* in 1959. The National Institute of Environmental Health Sciences (NIEHS) has been a strong supporter of toxicology. It has funded toxicology training grants for several decades, and houses the National Toxicology Program. The SOT has grown because of the many toxicologists, both trainees and investigators, supported by the NIEHS.

The SOT is now an international professional and learned society. Several other countries have modeled their national toxicology societies after the SOT, and the SOT has developed regional chapters and specialty sections to accommodate its broad membership. The specialty sections have provided a venue to attract investigators from disciplines that were thought to be disparate from toxicology, and these investigators have spurred the toxicologists to address questions about the molecular mechanisms of toxicants. The SOT has also grown because of the support of many foundations and private donors. Each year at its annual meeting, now attended by over 4,000 scientists, the SOT presents several prestigious scientific awards and fellowships, sponsored by many donors, to students, postdoctoral fellows, and established investigators. The importance of the SOT is evidenced by its many members serving on critical local, national, and international committees, reviewing the impacts of chemicals, foods, and drugs on society.

MICHAEL GALLO

(SEE ALSO: *Toxicology*)

SOCIOLOGY IN PUBLIC HEALTH

Sociology as a discipline developed from theoretical writings of the nineteenth century and the first half of the twentieth century. The predominant theories stem from the work of Karl Marx, Emile Durkheim, Max Weber, Talcott Parsons, Robert Merton, and James Coleman. The influence of this rich theoretical foundation has manifested itself in major debates over the role of sociology as a science. European and American perspectives on sociology as a science differ, with the American perspective favoring sociology as a scientific discipline and emphasizing a more quantitative methodological approach than the European approach.

KEY CONCEPTS IN SOCIOLOGY

Several key concepts in sociology relate to its role in public health. Foremost is the emphasis on society rather than the individual. The individual is viewed as an actor within larger social processes. This distinguishes the field from psychology. The emphasis is on units of analysis at the collective level, such as the family, the group, the neighborhood, the city, the organization, the state, and the world. Of key importance is how the social fabric, or social structure, is maintained, and how social processes, such as conflict and resolution, relate to the maintenance and change of social structures. A sociologist studies processes that create, maintain, and sustain a social system, such as a health care system in a particular country. The scientific component of this study would be the concern with the processes regulating and shaping the health care system. Sociology assumes that social structure and social processes are very complex. Therefore its methodology is appropriately complex and often, particularly in American sociology, dominated by multivariate statistical methods of analysis. The advent of the computer in the second half of the twentieth century presented the field with the opportunity to work with very large bodies of data and complex variables.

MEDICAL SOCIOLOGY

Earlier social theorists, such as those noted above, did write on subjects of concern to medicine, health, and illness, but medical sociology, as a subdiscipline of sociology, developed in the post-World War II period. Early debates in medical sociology were concerned with the role of sociology as it relates to medicine: Should the field be critical and analytical, concerning itself with the sociology of medicine (i.e., examining how medicine works); or should it be largely applied, focusing on sociology as a handmaiden for medicine? Like many such formative debates, there could be no conclusive answer. However, the field has developed into two groups: those (largely within academic settings) which focus on the sociology of medicine; and those (primarily in schools of public health and governmental institutions) which focus on the application of sociology to medicine. Later debates related to whether the focus should be on health sociology or medical sociology. This debate has moved the field to a broader, more ecological, view of medicine and health.

SOCIOLOGY IN PUBLIC HEALTH

Public health has been and remains a very applied field. It is also characterized by a population-based approach to health, and statistical methods are deemed the appropriate underlying method for the field. It is viewed as a science that seeks to intervene, control, and prevent large-scale processes that negatively affect the public's health. By these criteria, there is a strong logical fit of sociological principles and practices within public health. Nonetheless, sociology has not been the key social science discipline in public health. That position has gone to psychology, where the emphasis on individual behavior resonates more with a biomedical model. Despite this, many of the primary concerns of present-day public health, with large-scale variables such as social capital, social inequality, social status, and health care organization and financing, remain topics best suited to the sociological perspective and methodology. The emphasis in public health is thus shifting toward a sociological perspective.

SOCIOLOGICAL CONCEPTS IN PUBLIC HEALTH

Sociology in public health is reflected in the myriad of sociological concepts that pervade the practice of public health. More than any other social science, sociology has the discussion of socioeconomic status at its very core. Social-class variation within society is the key explanatory variable in sociology—for everything from variation in social structure to differential life experiences of health and illness. Indeed, there appears to be overwhelming evidence that Western industrialized societies that have little variation in social class experience have far better health outcomes than societies characterized by wide social-class dispersion. In short, inequalities in health are directly related to social and economic inequalities. Much of later-twentieth-century public health is devoted to the reduction of these inequalities.

SOCIOLOGICAL METHODS IN PUBLIC HEALTH

Methodological concerns are critical to sociological research. The great debate in sociology has been on the relative merits and role of quantitative versus qualitative approaches. Both approaches are widely used and play a critical role for public health. Sociology has long recognized that the social world comprises both an objective and a subjective reality. For example, the objective reality of having cancer is accompanied by the subjective reality of the experience of cancer by the patient, and the patient's family and friends. Both realities are relevant to the sociological approach. The subjective, qualitative approach is generally discussed in the theory and methods concerned with illness behavior, but qualitative approaches are equally applicable to the understanding of social policy, world systems, and areas of sociology where statistical measurement is difficult or less relevant.

Within public health, surveillance is seen as a key approach to describing the distribution and dynamics of disease. In sociological approaches to public health, the role of social and behavioral factors in health and illness is central. Survey methodology has occupied a central place in sociological research since the middle of the twentieth century. The concern has been with the collection, management, analysis, interpretation, and use of large quantities of data obtained by direct interview with respondents. Social surveys are characterized by large random samples, complicated questionnaires, and the use of multivariate statistics for analysis. By their very nature, most sociological variables are complex to measure and to analyze. For example, the assessment of socioeconomic status of an individual requires the accurate measurement of several variables that sit within a larger social context. Socioeconomic status (SES) is regarded as a product of several components, including income, residence, education, and occupation. Determining the relative weight of each of these components is a major analytical problem. Thus, when considering the role of socioeconomic status on health care outcomes, there is no easy answer to what mechanism actually works to determine the observed relationship between SES and health.

SOCIOLOGY AND EVALUATION IN PUBLIC HEALTH

Because many sociological variables are at the so-called macro level, there is limited opportunity to intervene rapidly, directly, or simply. For example, the SES of a group is affected by complex components, such as education and occupation, that are part of the total life course of individuals within the group. Thus, to change the SES of a group would require significant redistribution of resources of the larger social structure. A significant period of time and concerted effort is needed to change such macro variables. This is, however, not dissimilar to many other challenges in public health, such as the long-term and time-consuming effort to change lifestyles and reduce behavioral risk factors related to chronic diseases.

The chief role of sociology in public health remains its evaluation of those macro components of society that affect public health at the population level. Such evaluations provide an understanding of why inequalities in health exist, and they help elaborate upon the mechanisms and processes that sustain these inequalities. This relates to the long-standing theoretical concern with social structure among sociologists. Further, sociology reveals the mechanisms for long-term changes that may lead to a reduction in health inequalities. The product of sociological thinking in public health is not immediate nor easily understood by those who seek quick and easy solutions to the suffering of humanity. Nonetheless, the long-term role of sociology in public health is to change and improve the public health.

DAVID V. MCQUEEN

(SEE ALSO: *Community Health; Medical Sociology; Psychology, Health; Social Determinants; Social Health*)

BIBLIOGRAPHY

Cockerham, W. C. (2000). *Medical Sociology*, 8th edition. Englewood Cliffs, NJ: Prentice Hall.

Coleman, J. S. (1994). *Foundations of Social Theory*. Cambridge, MA: Belknap Press.

Durkheim, E. (1982). *The Rules of Sociological Method*. New York: Free Press.

Marx, K. (1973). *Grundrisse: Foundations of the Critique of Political Economy*. New York: Vintage Books.

Merton, R. K. (1957). *Social Theory and Social Structure*. Glencoe, IL: Free Press.

Parsons, T. (1951). *The Social System*. Glencoe, IL: Free Press.

Weber, M. (1958). *From Max Weber: Essays in Sociology*. New York: Oxford University Press.

SPAN OF LIFE

See Life Expectancy and Life Tables

SPECIES EXTINCTION

Evolution is the interplay of the appearance of new life-forms and the disappearance of old ones. The appearance of new life-forms depends upon the availability of diverse habitats, relative stability of climatic regimes, and processes that allow genetic and behavioral modification to, in effect, isolate new life-forms from a common ancestor. When two populations can no longer interbreed, for whatever reason, they assume the status of separate species or subspecies. Historically, processes leading to the loss of life-forms have been related to changes in biophysical conditions, such as particularly rapid changes in climate. Of course it is seldom clear exactly what the causes of extinction are. Species extinction could arise from a combination of factors: changes in ecology; loss of critical habitat; pollution; overharvesting; or competition from an exotic (nonnative) species that is introduced into the ecosystem.

CAUSES AND CONSEQUENCES

The consequences of loss of species for ecosystem function depends upon the role played in the ecosystem by the species or group of species, and by the degree to which those roles are or could be assumed by other biotic components of the ecosystem. In general, the loss of a species in an ecosystem with naturally low species diversity is likely to have a larger consequence than the loss of a species in a more complex environment characterized by high species richness. There have been numerous theoretical and empirical investigations that have sought to validate this simple proposition. Unfortunately, owing to the natural complexity and diversity of ecosystems within the biosphere, no hard and fast rule on the consequences of the loss of species richness on ecosystem function has yet been accepted as above reproach.

What appears much clearer is the impact of human activity on species loss and accelerating species loss worldwide. There is a close parallel between early human migrations and the disappearance of large game species. Overexploitation of biological resources has continued to the present time, and numerous species have disappeared in regional environments as a consequence. For example the combination of overharvesting, pollution, and habitat loss (owing to shoreline restructuring) had much to do with the disappearance of the sturgeon, lake trout, and many other preferred species in the lower Great Lakes. (The introduction of exotic species, such as the sea lamprey, is also a factor.) Of greatest concern at the beginning of the twenty-first century is the potential for wholesale loss of species in some twenty-five hot spots around the world, as a consequence largely of habitat modifications (e.g., clearing tropical forests for agriculture, construction of large dams).

Biodiversity loss is one of the most consistent signs of ecosystem distress syndrome (EDS). Estimates range widely, but generally current estimates of species losses are ten-fold to one thousand-fold greater than historic levels, leading some to speculate that the earth is already entering a period of the sixth major extinction of life on the planet. This extinction, however, differs from the rest, in that the primary cause appears to be the effects of human activity. Humans appropriate more than 50 percent of global primary productivity. They have also altered the chemical composition of the atmosphere, triggering climate change, which in turn destabilizes ecological balance.

IMPLICATIONS FOR HUMAN HEALTH

Humans, as part of the web of life, are not immune to events that trigger the extinction of organisms on the profound scale that appears to be currently taking place; and the implications for human health are numerous and diverse.

Firstly, there are direct effects: for example, the loss of marine fisheries (over 70 percent of the major commercially fished marine stocks are overexploited and in decline), translates for many communities into a loss of reliable food supplies. This contributes to malnutrition—a rising problem, particularly in developing countries, where an estimated two billion people (approximately one-third of the global population) presently suffers from lack of adequate diet. Malnutrition reduces the longevity of a population both directly and indirectly by weakening the immune system, which renders the population more susceptible to diseases. Another direct impact is the loss of potential biological materials that are useful as medicines, both in traditional medicines and as ingredients in modern pharmacology. The loss of the inventory of biotic resources for medicinal purposes directly threatens human health. Finally, there is the loss of economic opportunity, and the loss of social cohesion that often accompanies a degrading environment. An impoverished socioeconomic condition generally is associated with a host of health threats, including substance abuse and violence.

Indirect effects are more difficult to pin down. Clearly, the loss of a significant portion of the species that inhabit a particular ecosystem has major implications for ecosystem functioning, including the provision of ecosystem services (such as production of food, regulation of hydrology, and pollination) that form part of the life-support system for humans and other species. Degradation of such environments through human activities, with a subsequent loss of species components, poses a host of threats to human health through the loss of critical ecosystem functions.

Loss of diversity of pathogens poses an entirely different set of issues. The history of European settlement in the Great Lakes is also a history of purposeful drainage of swamps and wetlands along the southwest shore of Lake Ontario in an effort (largely successful) to eliminate the mosquito vectors of malaria. In many parts of the world today, eradication of pathogens is part of a public health strategy which, in addition to the intended consequences, also degrades ecosystems. Worldwide, there has been a successful eradication of the smallpox virus. At the same time, the widespread use of antibiotics and pesticides is creating resistant strains (not new species) of pathogens and crop pests, thus contributing to an increase in genetic biodiversity. In this case, however, the increase in biodiversity is to the detriment of humans.

On balance, the impact of humans on biodiversity has resulted, through a variety of mechanisms and pathways, in increased human health burdens.

DAVID J. RAPPORT

(SEE ALSO: *Biodiversity; Ecosystems; Environmental Determinants of Health*)

BIBLIOGRAPHY

Grifo, F., and Rosenthal, J., eds. (1997). *Biodiversity and Human Health*. Washington, DC: Island Press.

May, R. M. (1985). "Evolution of Pesticide Resistance." *Nature* 315:12–13.

Myers, N. (1997). "Ecology: Mass Extinction and Evolution." *Science* 278:597–598.

Rapport, D. J.; Costanza, R.; Epstein, P. R.; Gaudet, C.; and Levins, R., eds. (1998). *Ecosystem Health*. Malden, MA: Blackwell Science.

Rapport, D. J.; Regier, H. A.; and Hutchinson, T. C. (1985). "Ecosystem Behavior under Stress." *American Naturalist* 125:617–640.

Rapport, D. J., and Whitford, W. G. (1999). "How Ecosystems Respond to Stress: Common Properties of Arid and Aquatic Systems." *BioScience* 49(3):193–203.

Vithousek, P. M.; Mooney, H. A.; Lubchenco, J.; and Melillo, J. M. (1997). "Human Domination of Earth's Ecosystems." *Science* 277:494–499.

SPORTS MEDICINE

Sports medicine is a multidisciplinary field involving physicians, physical therapists, athletic trainers, and other health care professionals trained in diagnosis, treatment, research, education, and prevention of athletic injuries. This team of professionals works together to enable an athlete to safely return to his or her sport as soon as possible after an injury or medical problem. These professionals also participate in research activities that further the understanding of different types of injuries and the human body's reaction to these injuries. Important facets of sports medicine are the pre-participation physical and the education of athletes, coaches, and parents in conditioning techniques in an attempt to prevent injuries and help athletes of all levels reach their full potential.

JOSEPH CONGENI

(SEE ALSO: *Physical Activity; Prevention; Primary Prevention*)

SPOUSAL VIOLENCE

See Domestic Violence

STAGES OF CHANGE

See Transtheoretical Model of Stages of Change

STANDARDIZATION (OF RATES)

Standardization (or adjustment) of rates is used to enable the valid comparison of groups (e.g., those studied in different places or times) that differ regarding an important health determinant (most commonly age). Although often presented in epidemiologic textbooks as a separate technique, it is in fact a specific application of the general methods to control for confounding factors. As such, many of the issues related to confounding and methods used to adjust for confounding can be applied to standardization. Historically, the need for age standardization was recognized well before the general concept of confounding was formalized. It has it roots in the earliest epidemiological studies—the first known reference to age standardization appeared in a publication by F. G. P. Neison in 1844. The most familiar application is in the presentation of age-standardized mortality or cancer incidence rates to explore temporal trends.

Two major approaches to standardization have been used, direct and indirect. Direct standardization is used when the study population is large enough that age-specific rates within the population are stable. When the population is small (or the outcome is rare), the number of events observed can be small. In that circumstance, indirect standardization methods can be used to produce a standardized mortality rate (SMR) or a standardized incidence rate (SIR).

Direct standardization is commonly used in reports of vital statistics (e.g., mortality) or disease incidence trends (e.g., cancer incidence). Indirect standardization has a played a major role in studies of occupational disease or studies of place- and time-limited environmental catastrophes. Indirect standardization was introduced as a tool before direct standardization (1844 vs. 1899).

The standard approach to explaining standardization involves the concepts of expected and "observed" counts. In direct standardization, one estimates the rate that would have been observed if

Table 1

Direct Age Standardization

Age Group	Number of cases	Number of deaths	Mortality rate	Reference Population	Expected number deaths
40-49	3,734	37	0.0099	1,000,000	9,900
50-59	1,887	94	0.0498	600,000	29,880
60-69	1,645	327	0.1988	200,000	39,760
Total	7,266	458	0.0630	1,800,000	79,540

SOURCE: Courtesy of author.

Table 2

Indirect Age Standardization

Age Group	Number of cases	Number of deaths	Mortality rate in Reference population	Expected number deaths
40-49	3,734	37	0.005	18.7
50-59	1,887	94	0.02	37.7
60-69	1,645	327	0.1	164.5
Total	7,266	458	0.0630	220.9

SOURCE: Courtesy of author.

the study population had had the same age structure as the reference group (e.g., the number of cases of disease that would be expected if the disease rates in the study population were applied to the reference population). In indirect standardization, one computes the number of cases of disease that would have been expected if the disease rates from the reference population had applied in the study population. Dividing the observed case count by the expected count yields the SMR. A more modern approach to standardization recognizes that these methods are computing weighted averages of the age-specific rates.

To perform a direct age standardization, one first has to select a reference population. This population is arbitrary, although conventionally one uses either the World Standard Population produced by the World Health Organization, or a census population count for the country in which the work is being conducted. Next, one computes the age-specific rates within the study group. Then, one multiplies these rates by the number of people in that age group in the reference population. These expected counts are summed and divided by the total population size of the reference population to yield the directly standardized rate. This is illustrated in the example shown in Table 1. The crude mortality rate is 63/1,000. Standardizing to the reference population gives an age-adjusted mortality rate of 79,540/1,800,000 = 44/1,000. The adjusted rate is lower than the crude rate is since the proportion of the reference population in the oldest age group (11%), which has the highest age-specific mortality rate, is only 50 percent of that found in the study population (22%). This adjusted rate can be directly compared to

adjusted rates from other years to detect trends in mortality.

Indirect standardization uses the reference population to provide age-specific rates. Within each age stratum, one multiplies the reference rate by the number of people in the study population to determine the number of cases that would have been expected if that were the rate in the study group. These expected numbers are added up across all age groups and divided into the observed number to yield the SMR. Values greater than 1 (or 100, as the SMR is commonly expressed multiplied by 100) indicate a higher mortality than expected. It is possible to compute an indirectly standardized rate, but this is much less common than SMR/SIRs. Unlike directly standardized rates, one can not compare SMRs across time or place. One can however, compare SMRs for different outcomes within the same study population. This is a significant limitation to the use of SMRs. In the example given in Table 2, the researcher observed 458 deaths. However, based on the age-specific rates in the reference population, only 221 deaths would have been expected, yielding an SMR of 2.07 (or 207) suggesting a higher mortality rate in the study population than in the reference population.

The use of standardized rates is controversial. Any summary measure can hide patterns that might have important public health implications. For example, with age standardization, one might fail to detect age-specific differences in risk across time or place. This might arise if a disease is displaying an increasing incidence due to a birth cohort effect (people at younger ages might have a higher risk in recent years compared to previous years, while older people could have the opposite pattern). An age-standardized rate could hide these trends. Despite this risk, standardized rates have been found to provide useful summary measures, especially when outcomes are rare and specific rates display wide random variability.

One of the biggest potential abuses of standardized rates is by health care planners who use the standardized rates to estimate demand for services. This is incorrect practice. The standardized rate reflects the number of new cases that would arise in a hypothetical population. The actual number of cases expected is given by the crude rate, which should always be employed in health care planning analyses.

GEORGE WELLS

(SEE ALSO: *Rates; Rates: Adjusted; Rates: Age-Adjusted; Rates: Age-Specific*)

STAPHYLOCOCCAL INFECTION

The ubiquitous *Staphylococcus aureus* causes several kinds of public health and clinical problems. It is the most common causative organism of boils, pimples, and other skin infections. When the staphylococcus grows in cream pies, potato salad, cooked meats, or other foodstuffs that have been prepared unhygienically, it produces a heat-stable, tasteless enterotoxin that causes severe and often explosive vomiting and diarrhea a few hours after ingestion—this is the most common cause of food poisoning outbreaks following communal feasts of many kinds.

Entirely different and more serious consequences can follow from a nidus (place of origin) of staphylococcal infection in hospitals, where the organism is often resistant to all common antibiotics. There have been many fatal outbreaks of "golden staph" infections, sometimes serious enough to lead to temporary closure of affected hospitals. Hospital-acquired (nosocomial) staphylococcal infection, due frequently to antibiotic-resistant organisms, causes septicemia, endocarditis, osteomyelitis, and pneumonia—any of which can be fatal, especially in debilitated patients.

Another manifestation of staphylococcal infection is toxic shock syndrome. This occurs because super-absorbent vaginal tampons provide an ideal culture medium for the organism, enabling it to produce large quantities of enterotoxin. (Toxic shock syndrome can also be caused by other organisms such as the streptococcus.) Other settings for institutionally acquired staphylococcal infection include nurseries and nursing homes, where vulnerable infants and elderly people can be exposed either to nosocomial or enterotoxic staphylococcal infection.

Prevention of institutionally acquired staphylococcal infection requires rigorous attention to personal hygiene on the part of all attending staff. The nasal mucosa is a common site for carriage of the staphylococcus, which can be detected by swabbing, and can be treated with topically applied antibiotic cream.

JOHN M. LAST

(SEE ALSO: *Antisepsis and Sterilization; Communicable Disease Control; Food-Borne Diseases; Nosocomial Infections; Streptococcal Infection*)

STARVATION

See Famine

STATE AND LOCAL HEALTH DEPARTMENTS

State and local health departments fulfill important governmental roles for protecting and assuring the health of the public. Health departments have a well-established, yet complex and slowly evolving, history in the United States. According to the Institute of Medicine's book *The Future of Public Health* (1988):

New ideas about causes of disease and about social responsibility stimulated the development of public health agencies and institutions. As environmental and social causes of diseases were identified, social action appeared to be an effective way to control diseases. When health was no longer simply an individual responsibility, it became necessary to form public boards, agencies, and institutions to protect the health of citizens. Sanitary and social reform provided the basis for the formation of public health organizations (p.62).

Baltimore, Maryland, established the first city health department in 1798. In general, city health departments were established before state health departments, and well before county health departments. State health agencies developed first in Massachusetts and then across the country during the latter half of the nineteenth century. As American ambivalence about government gave way to a desire for the benefits that local government intervention could provide to the public through sanitation and control of communicable disease, several more health departments were formed in the first half of the twentieth century. In 1953, Joseph Mountin reported that there were 1,239 local health departments in the United States. By 2000, there were state health agencies in every state, and approximately 2,832 local health departments nationwide. The state health departments, and many of the local health departments, were developed and have evolved independently. As a result, health departments vary considerably from state to state and from community to community in their organizational structure, responsibilities, funding mechanisms, performance of core services and competencies, and in the implications for agency accreditation and workforce certification.

DEFINITIONS

A state health department is a centralized unit of state government with overarching responsibility for protecting, assuring, and improving the health of the state's citizens. A unit of state government that matches this broad definition exists in each of the nation's fifty states. The National Association of County and City Health Officials (NACCHO), in collaboration with the Centers for Disease Control and Prevention (CDC), defines a local health department as "an administrative or service unit of local or state government, concerned with health, and carrying some responsibility for the health of a jurisdiction smaller than the state." This definition is very broad and is intended to be inclusive of units that vary in size, including local service units of a state health department. However, the definition does not take into consideration organizational capacity to perform basic or essential services. Units of local government that have health

departments include cities, towns, and counties (or equivalents), and there are combinations such as city-county and multiple county. Not all units of local government have health departments.

RESPONSIBILITIES AND ORGANIZATIONAL STRUCTURE

National standards or guidelines do not exist to delineate specific responsibilities for state and local health departments, and there is a wide degree of variation in their roles across the country. As suggested previously, some state health departments perform both state and local roles. In general, however, state health departments operate out of a central location, often the state capital, and represent the principal public sector locus of responsibility for health. The committee formulating the 1988 Institute of Medicine (IOM) report on public health recommended that states should be responsible for the following:

1. Assessment of health needs in the state based on statewide data collection.

2. Assurance of an adequate statutory base for health activities in the state.

3. Establishment of statewide health objectives, delegating power to localities as appropriate and holding them accountable.

4. Assurance of appropriate organized statewide effort to develop and maintain essential personal, educational, and environmental health services.

5. Provision of access to necessary services.

6. Solution of problems inimical to health.

7. Guarantee of a minimum set of essential health services.

8. Support of local service capacity, especially when disparities in local ability to raise revenue and/or administer programs requires subsidies.

9. Technical assistance, or direct action by the state to achieve adequate service levels.

Other responsibilities that are commonly fulfilled by state departments of health include the distribution of federal and state funds to local health departments and other service providers;

the assurance of contracts compliance and service quality; and maintenance of a variety of information and data sets, including records of births and deaths, infectious diseases, injuries, hospital admitting diagnoses, health care facilities, and health workforce information. Laboratory services—especially for more complex tests, and in support of smaller local health departments—and epidemiology services—including support of larger outbreaks of infectious diseases—are also provided by state health departments. In addition, states are responsible for agency and health workforce licensure, health planning and administration, and special research projects.

State departments of health are organized in a variety of ways. Some are cabinet-level departments, with the director reporting to the governor or governor's chief of staff. Some departments include responsibility for mental health, substance abuse, and other areas. Other state health departments are subunits of a larger organization such as a department of human services. These organizations are often responsible for the state's Medicaid agency, managed care, hospital and/or insurance regulation, welfare, and, in some cases, corrections.

The roles assumed by local health departments are dependent on the roles of the associated state health department, on the resources available to the local department, and on other local arrangements for services. While many provide environmental health services, local arrangements in some jurisdictions, for example, place such services in other departments of local government. In some states, larger local health departments may have responsibility for some hospital services. In general, larger local health departments serve larger communities, have more resources, and assume a broader array of responsibilities. Most local health departments, however, are small organizations. According to NACCHO, of the approximately 3,000 local health departments in the country in 1997, two-thirds served populations of 50,000 or less, with the median-sized health department having a staff of twenty.

Responsibilities of local health departments generally include the following:

- Monitoring for outbreaks of infectious diseases (e.g., measles, tuberculosis, meningococcal disease), and outbreak response when necessary.

- Health promotion.

- Nutrition programs (e.g., the Women, Infants, and Children [WIC] Program).

- Home visits for infectious disease follow-up, sudden infant death syndrome prevention, and child abuse prevention.

- Limited "personal health" services, including childhood and adult immunizations; sexually transmitted disease diagnosis, treatment, and follow-up; HIV/AIDS (human immunodeficiency virus/acquired immunodeficiency syndrome) testing, counseling, and support services; family planning; and well-baby services.

- Advocacy for and referral of people without health care resources.

- Inspection of eating establishments (e.g., restaurants, bars, fairs) and licensure of food handlers in such establishments to assure food safety.

- Inspection and approval prior to installation of private drinking water wells, septic tanks, and small scale sewage systems.

- Completion of community assessments to determine the strengths and needs of the communities in the jurisdiction.

- Collection and maintenance of vital statistics for the community.

Local health departments are structured in a variety of ways. County health departments are the most common. Such agencies are usually governed by a local board of health comprising the county commissioners (or equivalent) or a panel of citizens appointed by the commissioners. Other models include city health departments (usually governed by a city council), city-county health departments (with shared governance), and multijurisdictional health districts (often governed by stand-alone boards). In many instances, the local health department is governed by a board of political appointees, with few or no elected officials on the board.

In most states, particularly in the West, local public health agencies are usually units of local government. In about one-quarter of the states, nearly all of the local agencies are units of state government and are accountable to the state health department director. Even in these cases, however, the local health departments serving the larger cities is often locally governed. Finally, Native Americans living on reservations are usually served by tribal health departments governed by tribal governments.

In some states, significant portions of the population are not served by local public health services. Only one state, Rhode Island, has no local health departments. A number of counties in some states have no local health department presence. Other parts of the country, such as certain areas within Massachusetts and Connecticut, are served principally by very small local health departments with few employees and very little capacity. In at least one state, Pennsylvania, a few cities and/or counties are served by local health departments, while the majority of counties are served by small regional offices of the state health department. In New Jersey, the city, town, and an array of county and regional health departments provide services through the hundreds of separate boards of health representing each municipality in the state. To further complicate this configuration there exists autonomous municipal-level health departments functioning separately within the counties where county health departments operate.

This confusing and inconsistent organization of local public health services is strong evidence that the nation's local public health infrastructure is weak. The lack of uniform protection of the country's citizens from outbreaks of infectious diseases and other hazards represents potential harm to all residents. In the late 1990s this state of affairs led to the development of national performance standards, to congressional consideration of public health infrastructure needs, and to consideration of alternative methods of providing local public health services.

There are two major barriers to implementing significant improvements in the local public health system: disagreement about the relative importance of local control versus meaningful capacity, and availability of public resources. Some communities and states continue to operate under a tradition that places emphasis on local governance of operations rather than efficiency and service capacity. Other states have chosen to regionalize services or to share resources in order to achieve the capacity to provide essential services. Local offices of regional, multicounty health districts, for example, serve all counties in the state of Idaho. Multiple-county public health districts are employed to a significant degree in Michigan, Washington, and Utah as well. In some states, there is a significant level of resource sharing among smaller health departments (e.g., sharing health officers or administrators in Oklahoma and Washington).

FUNDING MECHANISMS

State and local health departments receive their funding primarily from governmental sources. In 1997, sources of the funds expended by state health departments included state funds (55 percent); federal funds (30 percent) and a variety of miscellaneous revenue sources (15 percent). Among local health departments in 1995, 46 percent of total funds came from state and federal sources, 34 percent from local sources, and 10 percent from Medicare and Medicaid, with fees and other sources accounting for the rest.

Public health accounts for very little of the nation's overall health budget. The overwhelming majority of health care dollars are directed to the treatment of illness and injuries, and particularly to those who are in their last year of life. Very little goes to prevention. Total health expenditures in the United States for 1991 were $752 billion. Expenditures by state health agencies and local health departments in that year represented only 1.9 percent of all health spending. (Discontinuation of a reporting system in the early 1990s eliminated collection of state and local public health expenditure data. Consequently, more recent data is not available.) For comparison purposes, 2.6 percent of all health spending was attributed to state and local health departments in 1978.

In terms of absolute expenditures, 1991 expenditures of state health agencies were $11.3 billion, more than double the level of expenditures in 1982. The 1991 total included $9.3 billion in direct expenditures and $1.9 billion in transfers to local health departments. Total combined state and local health department expenditures were $14 billion in 1991. Thus, although expenditures for state and local public health have increased over the past two decades, they account for the declining proportions of total national health expenditures.

Some of the categorical funding streams supporting state and local health departments have been capped, and others have decreased. Indeed, Congress and state legislatures provide resources for public health programming principally through categorical grants supporting relatively narrow, often disease–specific, uses of the appropriations. This shifting, disease-of-the-year approach to financing public health is difficult to administer, leaves large gaps, is not tied explicitly to the nation's objectives (e.g., Healthy People 2010), and limits the tailoring of programs to match local and state needs and priorities. In response to these limitations, state and local health departments in many parts of the country increasingly are looking to partnerships with foundations, businesses, and other community organizations to market public health and prevention programs, address infrastructure deficiencies, and initiate efforts to improve health status in their communities.

WORKFORCE REQUIREMENTS

The workforce employed by state departments of health varies from state to state. In some states, political appointees with little or no expertise in public health fill the executive positions. In others, there is a statutory requirement that physicians who are board certified in preventive medicine fill such positions. A typical state department of health employs a number of professionals to fulfill planning, data analysis, contract compliance, epidemiology and laboratory functions, technical assistance, and other state functions. Typical employees include physicians, nurses, nurse practitioners, dentists, veterinarians, nutritionists, health educators, planners, social workers, epidemiologists, laboratory technicians, biostatiticians, computer technicians, and communications specialists.

As with state health departments, the workforce requirements of local health departments vary widely. The executives of about 35 percent of local agencies have medical degrees (a few states still require that local health directors be licensed physicians). Other professional positions most commonly found in local health departments include nurses, environmental health specialists (sanitarians), health educators, and nutritionists. In addition, larger health departments often employ physicians, nurse practitioners, epidemiologists, dentists, dental hygienists, social workers, outreach workers, planners, and computer specialists.

It has been estimated that between 50 percent and 80 percent of public health workers in state and local agencies have no formal training in the field. A number of resources for workforce development have evolved to address this concern. The Health Resources and Services Administration (HRSA) provides grants for postgraduate studies and public health residencies. The CDC provides a broad range of training, accessible by mail, Internet, satellite downlinks, and on-site classes. The number of accredited schools of public health rose by 20 percent between 1990 and 2000, increasing from twenty-four to twenty-nine schools located around the country. Many have begun providing continuing education offerings for public health professionals. Several offer graduate degrees in public health through courses of study designed for midcareer workers.

In addition, in 1999, both CDC and HRSA received funds for training the existing public health workforce. In July 2000, HRSA announced grants to eight Public Health Training Centers (PHTC's), which provide assistance to workers in 28 states. In September 2000, CDC's four Centers for Public Health Preparedness (CPHPs) awards were announced. Although the PHTCs and CPHPs are funded separately by the two agencies, both require a partnership with an accredited school of public health.

Many essential practice skills, however, are not typically addressed in traditional public health training. Work completed in the late 1990s, for example, showed that, of public health workers across the range of professions, most needed training in leadership, communication, and management. A number of resources to address these needs developed during the 1990s. For example, the Public Health Leadership Institute was established in 1991 through a partnership of California universities with funding from the CDC. Public health workers in nearly every state now have access to smaller state or regionally based leadership institutes. In the late 1990s, the CDC, the

HRSA, the W. K. Kellogg Foundation, and the Robert Wood Johnson Foundation funded basic management skills training for teams of middle and upper management workers from local health departments. This pilot program is provided through the University of North Carolina School of Public Health.

CORE FUNCTIONS AND ESSENTIAL SERVICES

In 1988 the Institute of Medicine published its landmark report, *The Future of Public Health*. This report identified a number of problems with the public health system, including an appalling lack of resources, a confused mission, poor leadership, and a prevailing view among policymakers that public health challenges like infectious diseases, unsafe food, and contaminated drinking water were all resolved. The report concluded with its most frequently quoted phrase, "public health is in disarray."

The IOM report has contributed significantly to the practice of public health. It proposed a simple but powerful mission statement: "to fulfill society's interest in assuring conditions in which people can be healthy" (p. 17). The report also proposed a more comprehensive operational framework for governmental public health with the elucidation of three core functions: assessment, policy development, and assurance (see Figure 1).

The assessment function requires public health agencies "to regularly and systematically collect, assemble, analyze, and make available information on the health of the community, including statistics on health status, community health needs, and epidemiologic and other studies of health problems" (p. 7). The report emphasized that "this basic function of public health cannot be delegated." Within a decade of the report's release, about 70 percent of local health departments had completed assessments of the communities they serve. Many have developed fairly sophisticated subunits of their organization to conduct assessment activities on an ongoing basis.

A number of assessment tools evolved in the early 1990s. Those most commonly used through the decade included Assessment Protocol for Excellence in Public Health (APEXPH) (developed by the National Association of County and City Health

Figure 1

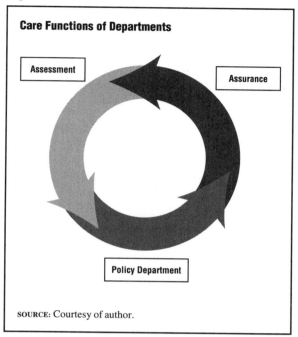

SOURCE: Courtesy of author.

Officials, in cooperation with the CDC), Planned Approach To Community Health (PATCH) (developed by the CDC), and Model Standards (developed by the American Public Health Association and others).

The second core function, policy development, was portrayed as what policymakers, particularly in government, do with the results of assessments. If an assessment defined the problems of a community, the policy development process would yield priorities and produce plans to address the problems. In the words of the report, public health agencies should "serve the public interest in the development of comprehensive public health policies by promoting the use of the scientific knowledge base in decision-making about public health and by leading in developing public health policy. Agencies must take a strategic approach, developed on the basis of a positive appreciation for the democratic political process" (p. 8).

The assurance function called for public health agencies "to assure their constituents that services necessary to achieve agreed upon goals are provided, either by encouraging actions by other entities (private or public), by requiring such action through regulation, or by providing services directly" (p. 8). This function might be seen as the implementation step, following policy development. Thus, the three core functions are tightly linked with one another, with assessment leading to policy development, resulting in assurance, leading again to assessment to evaluate the results and continue the process.

While the core functions represented a new framework for considering the practice of public health, the framework was rather sparse in detail and did little to explain the practice to those outside public health. In 1994, the Public Health Functions Steering Committee, chaired by the Surgeon General, adopted the Ten Essential Public Health Services. While based on the core functions, the more expansive list is more precise in describing specific capacities that all levels of governmental public health should have.

Development of the core functions and the essential services had a profound impact on the practice of public health through the 1990s. State and local health departments have dramatically increased the number and the level of involvement of partners in conducting assessments, developing policy, and in assuring the delivery of services. In some locales, the partnerships have led to innovation in how services are delivered, loosening two long-held perspectives: that only public health agencies can serve the poor, and that "public health is what public health departments do."

Many local and state agencies began placing increased emphasis on population-level services in the mid-1990s. In many instances, this resulted in contracts or other arrangements with private-sector providers to provide personal health services for disenfranchised populations. In place of direct service delivery, local and state health departments increasingly conducted community assessments, developed local and state priorities and plans, participated in the development of healthy communities, and addressed such issues as community violence prevention, injury prevention, and safer sex practices. In some locales, "public health" has been redefined to mean "that which the community does collectively to protect and improve the health of its residents." In such communities, the role of the state and local health departments is principally to provide financial and technical resources, and to convene and guide local process.

PERFORMANCE MEASUREMENT AND ACCREDITATION

The 1990s heralded a call for increased accountability of governmental agencies, and for greater emphasis on outcomes. Florida developed performance standards, and several other states developed standards as a component of statewide accreditation. Illinois, in conjunction with its IPLAN program, also developed a certification system for local health departments.

In the late 1990s, the CDC, in partnership with NACCHO, the Association of State and Territorial Health Officials, the National Association of Local Boards of Health, the Public Health Foundation, and the American Public Health Association, conducted an effort to develop national performance standards for local and state public health systems and for standards related to governance. The National Public Health Performance Standards Program (NPHPSP), is based on three principles: (1) public health must be accountable to its constituencies; (2) public health professionals need a system for ensuring that the provision of essential public health services meets a defined level of quality; and (3) the public health decision-making process must be based on strong scientific evidence. The standards use the essential services as categories of services. By early 2000 this program was still in its infancy, and the standards were being tested in several states. The objective was to implement the program nationally on a voluntary basis early in the first decade of the twenty-first century.

By the end of the twentieth century, public health leaders were having serious discussions about the need for accreditation of state and local health departments. Some pointed out that public health is the last health arena with no accreditation available, and that some form of accreditation is needed to assure quality and accountability. Others expressed concerns about the feasibility of accreditation, given the huge diversity in organizational capacity and jurisdictional structures. It is clear that the discussions will continue, and that the NPHPSP will likely serve as the basis for an accreditation system, should one evolve.

Many people have decried the lack of a certification program for public health workers, particularly in light of the small percentage of the workforce that has had formal training in public health.

While some of the specific professions comprising the public health workforce have their own licensure or certification (e.g., MDs, RNs, registered sanitarians), none necessarily assure or contribute to overarching public health competency. Efforts to explore the potential for this type of certification were beginning in January 2000.

THOMAS L. MILNE
CAROL K. BROWN

(SEE ALSO: *Accreditation of Local and State Health Departments; Community Health; Director of Health; Essential Public Health Services; Mobilizing for Action through Planning and Partnerships; National Association of County and City Health Officials; National Association of Local Boards of Health; Official U.S. Health Agencies*)

BIBLIOGRAPHY

Core Public Health Functions Steering Committee (1994). *Public Health in America*. Washington, DC: Office of Disease Prevention and Health Promotion, USDHHS.

Gebbie, K., and Hwang, I. (1998). *Preparing Currently Employed Public Health Professionals for Changes in the Health System*. New York: Columbia University School of Nursing.

Institute of Medicine, Committee on the Future of Public Health (1998) *The Future of Public Health*. Washington, DC: National Academy Press.

Mountin, J., and Flook, E. (1953). *Guide to Health Organizations in the United States*. Washington, DC: U.S. Public Health Service.

National Association of County Health Officials (1990). *National Profile of Local Health Departments, 1989*. Washington, DC: NACHO.

National Association of County and City Health Officials (1995). *National Profile of Local Health Departments, 1992–93*. Washington, DC: NACHO.

Siegel, M., and Doner, L. (1998). *Marketing Public Health*. Gaithersburg, MD: Aspen Publishers.

Turnock, B. J. (1997). *Public Health: What It Is and How It Works*. Gaithersburg, MD: Aspen Publishers.

STATE PROGRAMS IN TOBACCO CONTROL

The goal of state or provincial tobacco-control programs is to reduce the death and disease caused by tobacco use, the single most preventable cause of death and disease in developed societies. Annually, tobacco use causes more than 400,000 deaths in the United States, at a cost of approximately $50 billion to $73 billion in medical expenses alone. Comprehensive tobacco-control programs combine a variety of strategies and tactics to prevent the initiation of tobacco use, to promote smoking cessation, to protect the nonsmoker from environmental tobacco smoke (ETS), and to identify and eliminate disparities in tobacco use and disease among different population groups. The Centers for Disease Control and Prevention (CDC) recommends that state tobacco-control programs be comprehensive, sustainable, and accountable. The term "tobacco control" has come to mean both the control and the prevention of tobacco use, and includes all forms of tobacco.

State tobacco-control programs underwent an evolution during the 1990s. Prior to 1990, state programs focused on individual cessation programs offered in group settings, dissemination of self-help materials for quitting, and the distribution of information via public-service campaigns. During the 1990s, state tobacco-control programs shifted away from the provision of education and services as a means to achieve individual behavioral change. The next generation of programs was designed to impact whole populations by addressing political, social, and environmental factors that support the use or nonuse of tobacco. This also marked a shift away from a focus on individual responsibility for tobacco use to documenting and exposing tobacco industry tactics to market their product. The tobacco industry spends an estimated $5 billion annually in advertising and promotion aimed at sustaining or increasing tobacco use in the United States.

California led this evolution when, in 1988, voters passed Proposition 99, which raised the tobacco excise tax by twenty-five cents and dedicated approximately $90 million annually for tobacco control. The California program initiated a statewide social change to indirectly influence current and potential future tobacco users by creating a social milieu and legal climate in which tobacco was less desirable, less acceptable, and less accessible. The state tobacco-control program did this in part by implementing an unprecedented, hard-hitting media campaign that placed responsibility for the problem of tobacco use on the shoulders of the tobacco industry. While the program was intended to prevent individuals from suffering the health consequences of smoking, the program made it clear that this could not be achieved without holding the tobacco industry accountable for its actions and the products it sold. In the 1990s, Massachusetts, Arizona, and Oregon passed voter referendums earmarking increases in the tax on tobacco products for comprehensive tobacco-control programs.

In addition to implementing hard-hitting media campaigns, these states focused on changing norms regarding tobacco use at the community level through the support of local coalitions. In 1991, the National Cancer Institute partnered with the American Cancer Society to launch the American Stop Smoking Intervention Study (ASSIST). ASSIST's goal was to build a capacity within seventeen health departments to prevent and reduce tobacco use, primarily through the application of policy-based approaches that would alter the sociopolitical environment. Interventions included media advocacy to increase pro-tobacco-control media coverage, strengthening support for clean indoor air laws, reducing youth access to tobacco products, limiting tobacco advertising and promotion, increasing tobacco taxes, and increasing the demand for smoking-cessation services.

In 1993, the CDC Office on Smoking and Health (OSH) established funding for state-based programs for the District of Columbia and the thirty-two states that were not part of the ASSIST project. CDC funding provided state health departments with a core capacity to create a nucleus of trained staff, to conduct assessments and collect data, to develop program plans, and to establish coalitions and partnerships that later would be instrumental in implementing tobacco-control programs. At the conclusion of the ASSIST project, in 1999, the CDC established the National Tobacco Control Program, which provides approximately $57 million annually in funding to the fifty states. The National Tobacco Control Program supports the implementation of several program elements, including community interventions, counter-marketing, program policy, and evaluation and surveillance. These program elements combine to achieve changes in the four goal areas.

In 1999, the CDC issued *Best Practices for Comprehensive Tobacco Control Programs*, which drew upon evidence from the analyses of the past decade's comprehensive state tobacco-control programs to support nine specific elements of a comprehensive program. CDC recommends that states establish tobacco control programs that contain the following elements:

- Community programs to reduce tobacco use

- Chronic disease programs to reduce the burden of tobacco-related disease

- School programs

- Enforcement

- Statewide programs

- Counter-marketing

- Cessation programs

- Surveillance and evaluation

- Administration and management

Approximate annual costs to implement all of the recommended program components have been estimated to range from $7 to $20 per capita in small states (population under 3 million), $6 to $17 per capita in medium-sized states (population 3 million to 7 million), and $5 to $16 per capita in larger states (population over 7 million).

Three other publications have summarized the results from comprehensive state tobacco-control programs. The Institute of Medicine, National Research Council report *State Programs Can Reduce Tobacco Use* (2000) concluded that state programs can make a difference. In 2000, Surgeon General David Satcher released the first-ever Surgeon General's Report on the effectiveness of various methods to reduce tobacco use—educational, clinical, regulatory, economic, and social. The report offers a science-based blueprint for achieving the *Healthy People 2010* objectives to reduce tobacco use and its health impact. Also in 2000, the Task Force on Community Preventive Services released a report and recommendations on strategies to reduce exposure to ETS and to increase smoking cessation.

The evidence that state comprehensive tobacco control programs work is demonstrated by:

- Major reductions in the consumption of tobacco

- Reduction in the prevalence of tobacco use

- Increases in medical coverage for cessation efforts

- Declines in the initiation of tobacco use

- A growing number of places that are 100 percent smoke-free

- Declines in the illegal sale of tobacco

- Greater restrictions on the promotion and marketing of tobacco

- Additional regulation of tobacco products

- Increase in the price of tobacco products

The states that have implemented tobacco control programs have achieved varying degrees of these outcomes, as well as others, depending on amount of funding and length of time necessary to implement programs. After a decade of implementing California's programs there is evidence that long-term health outcomes can also be achieved. Two studies released in December 2000 indicate that California's declines in lung cancer rates and in heart disease deaths can be associated with the impact of the comprehensive tobacco-control programs.

Another major evolution occurred within state tobacco-control programs during the 1990s. The accumulation of a half century of work by researchers, policymakers, states, economists, advocates and many others resulted in the states suing the tobacco industry to reclaim Medicaid costs incurred by the states for treating patients with tobacco-related illnesses. Mississippi was the first to file such a lawsuit, and the first to settle. Florida, Texas, and Minnesota also settled individually with the tobacco industry. The other forty-six states reached a collective agreement with the tobacco industry, known as the Master Settlement Agreement (MSA), which would provide an estimated $206 billion over twenty-five years to the states. In 1998, Florida and Mississippi committed $100 million and $64 million, respectively, in settlement funds to prevent tobacco use. This presents a historic opportunity to secure state funding for tobacco control.

Jeffrey P. Koplan, director of the Centers for Disease Control and Prevention, has characterized tobacco control as one of the greatest public health achievements of the twentieth century, and as one of the greatest challenges of the twenty-first. The *Healthy People 2010* goal of achieving a 12 percent prevalence rate has been reached by only one population segment—those individuals with sixteen years or more of education.

The states have demonstrated that tobacco use can be reduced. The next steps are to assure that the states have the resources to plan, conduct, and evaluate comprehensive tobacco-control programs. A state's ability to carry out such programs will be dependent on the social, economic, and political context that supports the use or nonuse of tobacco products. But it also includes such factors as past experiences with tobacco-control programs, the level of knowledge and skill of the practitioners, the commitment and resolve of state leadership, collaboration with others, adequate funding to support all the components of a program, and the commitment to long-term funding.

DEARELL NIEMEYER
MELISSA ALBUQUERQUE

(SEE ALSO: *Addiction and Habituation; Cancer; Cardiovascular Diseases; Chewing and Smokeless Tobacco, Snuff; Clean Indoor Air Ordinances; Environmental Tobacco Smoke; Office on Smoking and Health; Smoking Behavior; Smoking Cessation; Smuggling Tobacco; Tobacco Control; Tobacco Sales to Youth, Regulation of*)

BIBLIOGRAPHY

Advocacy Institute (2000). *Making The Case: State Tobacco Control Policy Briefing Papers.* Washington, DC: Advocacy Institute Tobacco Control Project.

American Cancer Society (2000). *Communities of Excellence in Tobacco Control: A Community Planning Guide.* Atlanta, GA: ACS National Office.

California Department of Health Services, Tobacco Control Section (1998). *A Model for Change: The California Experience in Tobacco Control.* Sacramento, CA: Department of Health Services.

—— (2000). *Communities of Excellence in Tobacco Control: Community Planning Guide.* Sacramento, CA: Department of Health Services.

—— (2000). *Toward a Tobacco-Free California: Strategies for the 21st Century, 2000–2003.* Sacramento, CA: Department of Health Services.

Campaign for Tobacco-Free Kids (2000). *Show Us the Money: An Update on States's Allocation of the Tobacco*

Settlement Funds. Available at http://www.tobaccofreekids.org.

Centers for Disease Control and Prevention (1999). *Best Practices for Comprehensive Tobacco Control Programs.* Atlanta, GA: CDC. National Center for Chronic Disease Prevention and Health Promotion, Office on Smoking and Health.

—— (1999). *Chronic Disease and Health Promotion, Adapted from the MMWR, Tobacco Topics 1990–1999.* Atlanta, GA: CDC. National Center for Chronic Disease Prevention and Health Promotion.

—— (1999). *State Tobacco Control Highlights.* Atlanta, GA: CDC National Center for Chronic Disease Prevention and Health Promotion, Office on Smoking and Health.

—— (2000). "Decline in Lung Cancer Rates—California, 1988–1997." *Morbidity and Mortality Weekly Report* 40(47):1066–1069.

—— (2000). "Strategies for Reducing Exposure to Environmental Tobacco Smoke, Increasing Tobacco-Use Cessation, and Reducing Initiation in Communities and Health-Care Systems. A Report on Recommendations of the Task Force on Community Preventive Services." *Morbidity and Mortality Weekly Report* 49(RR-12):1–11.

Firchtenberg, C. M., and Glantz, S. A. (2000). "Association of the California Tobacco Control Program with Declines in Cigarette Consumption and Mortality from Heart Disease." *New England Journal of Medicine* 343(24):1772–1777.

Institute of Medicine, National Research Council (2000) *State Programs Can Reduce Tobacco Use.* Washington, DC: National Academy Press. Available at http://www.nop.edu/html/state_tobacco.

Partnership for Prevention (2000). *Priorities in Prevention, Real Reform vs. Rhetoric in Tobacco Prevention.* Washington, DC: Author.

Stillman, F.; Hartman, A.; and Graubard, B. (1999). "The American Stop Smoking Intervention Study: Conceptual Framework and Evaluation Design." *Evaluation Review* 23(3):259–280.

U.S. Department of Health and Human Services (1991). *Strategies to Control Tobacco Use in the United States: A Blueprint for Public Health Action in the 1990s.* Washington, DC: National Institutes of Health, National Cancer Institute.

—— (1995). *Community-Based Interventions for Smokers: The COMMIT Field Experience.* Washington, DC: National Institutes of Health, National Cancer Institute.

—— (1998). *Tobacco Use among U.S. Racial/Ethnic Minority Groups–African Americans, American Indians and Alaska Natives, Asian American and Pacific Islanders, and Hispanics: A Report of the Surgeon General.* Atlanta, GA: CDC, National Center for Chronic Disease Prevention and Health Promotion, Office on Smoking and Health.

—— (2000). *Healthy People 2010: Understanding and Improving Health,* 2nd edition. Washington, DC: U.S. Government Printing Office.

—— (2000). *Reducing Tobacco Use: A Report of the Surgeon General.* Atlanta GA: CDC, National Center for Chronic Disease Prevention and Health Promotion, Office on Smoking and Health.

Wakefield, M., and Chaloupka, F. J. (1999). *Effectiveness of Comprehensive Tobacco Control Programs in Reducing Teenage Smoking: A Review.* Chicago, IL: University of Illinois at Chicago.

STATISTICS FOR PUBLIC HEALTH

Nearly every day statistics are used to support assertions about health and what people can do to improve their health. The press frequently quotes scientific articles assessing the roles of diet, exercise, the environment, and access to medical care in maintaining and improving health. Because the effects are often small, and vary greatly from person to person, an understanding of statistics and how it allows researchers to draw conclusions from data is essential for every person interested in public health. Statistics is also of paramount importance in determining which claims regarding factors affecting our health are not valid, not supported by the data, or are based on faulty experimental design and observation.

When an assertion is made such as "electromagnetic fields are dangerous," or "smoking causes lung cancer," statistics plays a central role in determining the validity of such statements. Methods developed by statisticians are used to plan population surveys and to optimally design experiments aimed at collecting data that allows valid conclusions to be drawn, and thus either confirm or refute the assertions. Biostatisticians also develop the analytical tools necessary to derive the most appropriate conclusions based on the collected data.

ROLE OF BIOSTATISTICS IN PUBLIC HEALTH

In the Institute of Medicine's report *The Future of Public Health*, the mission of public health is defined as assuring conditions in which people can be healthy. To achieve this mission three functions must be undertaken: (1) assessment, to identify problems related to the health of populations and determine their extent; (2) policy development, to prioritize the identified problems, determine possible interventions and/or preventive measures, set regulations in an effort to achieve change, and predict the effect of those changes on the population; and (3) assurance, to make certain that necessary services are provided to reach the desired goal—as determined by policy measures—and to monitor how well the regulators and other sectors of the society are complying with policy.

An additional theme that cuts across all of the above functions is evaluation, that is, how well are the functions described above being performed.

Biostatistics plays a key role in each of these functions. In assessment, the value of biostatistics lies in deciding what information to gather to identify health problems, in finding patterns in collected data, and in summarizing and presenting these in an effort to best describe the target population. In so doing, it may be necessary to design general surveys of the population and its needs, to plan experiments to supplement these surveys, and to assist scientists in estimating the extent of health problems and associated risk factors. Biostatisticians are adept at developing the necessary mathematical tools to measure the problems, to ascertain associations of risk factors with disease, and creating models to predict the effects of policy changes. They create the mathematical tools necessary to prioritize problems and to estimate costs, including undesirable side effects of preventive and curative measures.

In assurance and policy development, biostatisticians use sampling and estimation methods to study the factors related to compliance and outcome. Questions that can be addressed include whether an improvement is due to compliance or to something else, how best to measure compliance, and how to increase the compliance level in the target population. In analyzing survey data, biostatisticians take into account possible inaccuracies in responses and measurements, both intentional and unintentional. This effort includes how to design survey instruments in a way that checks for inaccuracies, and the development of techniques that correct for nonresponse or for missing observations. Finally, biostatisticians are directly involved in the evaluation of the effects of interventions and whether to attribute beneficial changes to policy.

UNDERSTANDING VARIATION IN DATA

Nearly all observations in the health field show considerable variation from person to person, making it difficult to identify the effects of a given factor or intervention on a person's health. Most people have heard of someone who smoked every day of his or her life and lived to be ninety, or of the death at age thirty of someone who never smoked. The key to sorting out seeming contradictions such as these is to study properly chosen groups of people (samples), and to look for the aggregate effect of something on one group as compared to another. Identifying a relationship, for example, between lung cancer and smoking, does not mean that everyone who smokes will get lung cancer, nor that if one refrains from smoking one will not die from lung cancer. It does mean, however, that the group of people who smoke are more likely than those who do not smoke to die from lung cancer.

How can we make statements about groups of people, but be unable to claim with any certainty that these statements apply to any given individual in the group? Statisticians do this through the use of models for the measurements, based on ideas of probability. For example, it can be said that the probability that an adult American male will die from lung cancer during one year is 9 in 100,000 for a nonsmoker, but is 190 in 100,000 for a smoker. Dying from lung cancer during a year is called an "event," and "probability" is the science that describes the occurrence of such events. For a large group of people, quite accurate statements can be made about the occurrence of events, even though for specific individuals the occurrence is uncertain and unpredictable. A simple but useful model for the occurrence of an event can be made based on two important assumptions: (1) for a group of individuals, the probability that an event occurs is the same for all members of the group; and (2) whether or not a given person experiences the event does not affect whether others do. These assumptions are known as (1) common distribution for events, and (2) independence of events. This simple model can apply to all sorts of public health issues. Its wide applicability lies in the freedom it affords researchers in defining events and population groups to suit the situation being studied.

Consider the example of brain injury and helmet use among bicycle riders. Here groups can be defined by helmet use (yes/no), and the "event" is severe head injury resulting from a bicycle accident. Of course, more comprehensive models can be used, but the simple ones described here are the basis for much public health research. Table 1 presents hypothetical data about bicycle accidents and helmet use in thirty cases.

It can be seen that 20 percent (2 out of 10) of those not wearing a helmet sustained severe head injury, compared to only 5 percent (1 out of 20) among those wearing a helmet, for a relative risk of four to one. Is this convincing evidence? An application of probability tells us that it is not, and the reason is that with such a small number of cases, this difference in rates is just not that unusual. To better understand this concept, the meaning of probability and what conclusions can drawn after setting up a model for the data must be described.

Probability is the branch of mathematics that uses models to describe uncertainty in the occurrence of events. Suppose that the chance of severe head injury following a bicycle accident is one in ten. This risk can be simulated using a spinning disk with the numbers "1" through "10" equally spaced around its edge, with a pointer in the center to be spun. Since a spinner has no memory, spins will be independent. A spin will indicate severe head injury if a "1" shows up, and no severe head injury for "2" through "10." The pointer could be spun ten times to see what could happen among ten people not wearing a helmet. The theory of probability uses the binomial distribution to tell you exactly what could happen with ten spins, and how likely each outcome is. For example, the probability that we would not see a "1" in ten spins is .349, the probability that we will see

Table 1

	Wearing helmet	Not wearing helmet
Severe head injury	1	2
Not severe head injury	19	8

SOURCE: Courtesy of author.

exactly one "1" in ten spins is .387, exactly two is .194, exactly three is .057, exactly four is .011, exactly five is .001, with negligible probability for six or more. So if this is a good model for head injury, the probability of two or more people experiencing severe head injury in ten accidents is .264.

A common procedure in statistical analysis is to hypothesize that no difference exists between two groups (called the "null" hypothesis) and then to use the theory of probability to determine how tenable such an hypothesis is. In the bicycle accident example, the null hypothesis states that the risk of injury is the same for both groups. Probability calculations then tell how likely it is under null hypothesis to observe a risk ratio of four or more in samples of twenty people wearing helmets and ten people not wearing helmets. With a common risk of injury equal to one in ten for both groups, and with these sample sizes, the surprising answer is that one will observe a risk ratio greater than four quite often, about 16 percent of the time, which is far too large to give us confidence in asserting that wearing helmets prevents head injury.

This is the essence of statistical hypothesis testing. One assumes that there is no difference in the occurrences of events in our comparison groups, and then calculates the probabilities of various outcomes. If one then observes something that has a low probability of happening given the assumption of no differences between groups, then one rejects the hypothesis and concludes that there is a difference. To thoroughly test whether helmet use does reduce the risk of head injury, it is necessary to observe a larger sample—large enough so that any observed differences between groups cannot be simply attributed to chance.

SOURCES OF DATA

Data used for public health studies come from observational studies (as in the helmet, use example above), from planned experiments, and from carefully designed surveys of population groups. An example of a planned experiment is the use of a clinical trial to evaluate a new treatment for cancer. In these experiments, patients are randomly assigned to one of two groups—treatment or placebo (a mock treatment)—and then followed to ascertain whether the treatment affects clinical outcome. An example of a survey is the National Health and Nutrition Examination Survey (NHANES) conducted by the National Center for Health Statistics. NHANES consists of interviews of a carefully chosen subset of the population to determine their health status, but chosen so that the conclusions apply to the entire U.S. population.

Both planned experiments and surveys of populations can give very good data and conclusions, partly because the assumptions necessary for the underlying probability calculations are more likely to be true than for observational studies. Nonetheless, much of our knowledge about public health issues comes from observational studies, and as long as care is taken in the choice of subjects and in the analysis of the data, the conclusions can be valid.

The biggest problem arising from observational studies is inferring a cause-and-effect relationship between the variables studied. The original studies relating lung cancer to smoking showed a striking difference in smoking rates between lung cancer patients and other patients in the hospitals studied, but they did not prove that smoking was the cause of lung cancer. Indeed, some of the original arguments put forth by the tobacco companies followed this logic, stating that a significant association between factors does not by itself prove a causal relationship. Although statistical inference can point out interesting associations that could have a significant influence on public health policy and decision making, these statistical conclusions require further study to substantiate a cause-and-effect relationship, as has been done convincingly in the case of smoking.

A tremendous amount of recent data is readily available through the Internet. These include already tabulated observations and reports, as well as access to the raw data. Some of this data cannot be accessed through the Internet because of confidentiality requirements, but even in this case it is sometimes possible to get permission to analyze the data at a secure site under the supervision of employees of the agency. Described here are some of the key places to go for data on health. Full Internet addresses for the sites below can be found in the bibliography.

A comprehensive source can be found at Fedstats, which provides a gateway to over one hundred federal government agencies that compile publicly available data. The links here are rather comprehensive and include many not directly related to health. The key government agency providing statistics and data on the extent of the health, illness, and disability of the U.S. population is the National Center for Health Statistics (NCHS), which is one of the centers of the Centers for Disease Control and Prevention (CDC). The CDC provides data on morbidity, infectious and chronic diseases, occupational diseases and injuries, vaccine efficacy, and safety studies. All the centers of the CDC maintain online lists of their thousands of publications related to health, many of which are now available in electronic form. Other major governmental sources for health data are the National Cancer Institute (which is part of the National Institutes of Health), the U.S. Bureau of the Census, and the Bureau of Labor Statistics. The Agency for Healthcare Research and Quality is an excellent source for data relating to the quality, access, and medical effectiveness of health care in the United States. The National Highway and Traffic Safety Administration, in addition to publishing research reports on highway safety, provides data on traffic fatalities in the Fatality Analysis Reporting System, which can be queried to provide data on traffic fatalities in the United States.

A number of nongovernmental agencies share data or provide links to online data related to health. The American Public Health Association provides links to dozens of databases and research summaries. The American Cancer Society provides many links to data sources related to cancer. The Research Forum on Children, Families, and the New Federalism lists links to numerous studies and data on children's health, including the National Survey of America's Families.

Table 2

	Wearing helmet	Not wearing helmet
Severe head injury	5	10
Not severe head injury	95	41

SOURCE: Courtesy of author.

Table 3

	Wearing helmet	Not wearing helmet	Row totals
Severe head injury	9.934	5.066	15
Not severe head injury	90.066	45.933	136
Column totals	100	51	151

SOURCE: Courtesy of author.

Much of public health is concerned with international health, and the World Health Organization (WHO) makes available a large volume of data on international health issues, as well as provides links to its publications. The Center for International Earth Science Information Network provides data on world population, and its goals are to support scientists engaged in international research.

The Internet provides an opportunity for health research unequaled in the history of public health. The accessibility, quality, and quantity of data are increasing so rapidly that anyone with an understanding of statistical methodology will soon be able to access the data necessary to answer questions relating to health.

ANALYSIS OF TABULATED DATA

One of the most commonly used statistical techniques in public health is the analysis of tabled data, which is generally referred to as "contingency table analysis." In these tables, observed proportions of adverse events are compared in the columns of the table by a method known as a "chi-square test." Such data can naturally arise from any of the three data collection schemes mentioned. In our helmet, for example, observational data from bicycle accidents were used to create a table with helmet use defining the columns, and head injury, the rows. In a clinical trial, the columns are defined by the treatment/placebo groups, and the rows by outcome (e.g., disease remission or not). In a population survey, columns can be different populations surveyed, and rows indicators of health status (e.g., availability of health insurance). The chi-square test assumes that there is no difference between groups, and calculates a statistic based on what would be expected if no

difference truly existed, and on what is actually observed. The calculation of the test statistic and the conclusions proceed as follows:

1. The expected frequency (E) is calculated (assuming no difference) for each cell in the table by first adding to get the totals for each row, the totals for each column, and the grand total (equal to the total sample size); then for each cell we find the expected count: E = (rowtotal)(columntotal)/(grandtotal).

2. For each cell in the table, let O be the observed count, and calculate: $(O-E)^2/E$.

3. The values from step 2 are summed over all cells in the table. This is the test statistic, X.

4. If X exceeds 3.96 for a table with four cells, then the contingency table is said to be statistically "significant." If the sample and the resulting analysis is repeated a large number of times, this significant result will happen only 5 percent of the time when there truly is no difference between groups, and hence this is called a "5 percent significance test."

5. For tables with more than two rows and/or columns different comparisons values are needed. For a table with six cells, we check to see if X is larger than 5.99, with eight cells, we compare X to 7.81, and for nine or ten cells we compare X to 9.49.

6. This method has problems if there are too many rows and columns and not enough observations. In such cases, the table should be reconfigured to have a smaller

Table 4

	Wearing helmet	Not wearing helmet
Severe head injury	2.450	4.805
Not severe head injury	0.270	0.530

SOURCE: Courtesy of author.

Table 5

	Low blood-lead level	High blood-lead level
Low soil-lead level	63	37
High soil-lead level	37	63

SOURCE: Courtesy of author.

number of cells. If any of the E values in a table fall below five, some of the rows and/or columns should be combined to make all values of E five or more.

Suppose a larger data set is used for our helmet use/head injury example (see Table 2).

It is worthwhile noting that the proportions showing head injury for these data are almost the same as before, but that the sample size is now considerably larger, 151. Following the steps outlined above, the chi-square statistic can be calculated and conclusions can be drawn:

1. The total for the first column is 100, for the second column 51, for the first row 15, and for the second row 136. The grand total is 151, the total sample size. The expected frequencies, that is the "Es," assuming no difference in injury rates between the helmet group and the no helmet group, are given in Table 3. It is quite possible for the Es to be non-integer, and if so, we keep the decimal part in all our calculations.

2. The values for $(O-E)^2/E$ are presented in Table 4.

3. X=8.055

4. Because this exceeds 3.84, we have a significant association between the helmet use and head injury, at the 5 percent level.

The chi-square procedure presented here is one of the most important analytic techniques used in public health research. Its simplicity allows it to be widely used and understood by nearly all professionals in the field, as well as by interested third parties. Much of what we know about what

makes us healthy or what endangers our lives has been shown through the use of contingency tables.

STUDYING RELATIONSHIPS AMONG VARIABLES

A major contribution to our knowledge of public health comes from understanding trends in disease rates and examining relationships among different predictors of health. Biostatisticians accomplish these analyses through the fitting of mathematical models to data. The models can vary from a simple straight-line fit to a scatter plot of X-Y observations, all the way to models with a variety of nonlinear multiple predictors whose effects change over time. Before beginning the task of model fitting, the biostatistician must first be thoroughly familiar with the science behind the measurements, be this biology, medicine, economics, or psychology. This is because the process must begin with an appropriate choice of a model. Major tools used in this process include graphics programs for personal computers, which allow the biostatistician to visually examine complex relationships among multiple measurements on subjects.

The simplest graph is a two-variable scatter plot, using the y-axis to represent a response variable of interest (the outcome measurement), and the x-axis for the predictor, or explanatory, variable. Typically, both the x and y measurements take on a whole range of values—commonly referred to as continuous measurements, or sometimes as quantitative variables. Consider, for example, the serious health problem of high blood-lead levels in children, known to cause serious brain and neurologic damage at levels as low as 10 micrograms per deciliter. Since lead was removed from gasoline, blood-levels of lead in children in

Figure 1

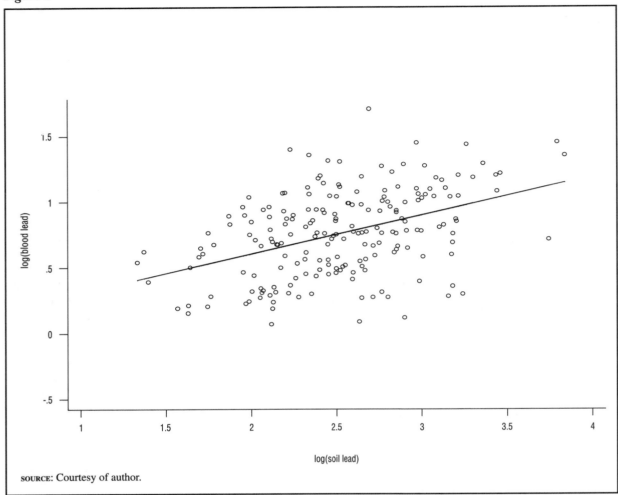

SOURCE: Courtesy of author.

the United States have been steadily declining, but there is still a residual risk from environmental pollution. One way to assess this problem is to relate soil-lead levels to blood levels in a survey of children—taking a measurement of the blood-lead concentration on each child, and measuring the soil-lead concentration (in milligrams per kilogram) from a sample of soil near their residences. As is often the case, a plot of the blood levels and soil concentrations shows some curvature, so transformations of the measurements are taken to make the relationship more nearly linear. Choices commonly used for transforming data include taking square roots, logarithms, and sometimes reciprocals of the measurements. For the case of lead, logarithms of both the blood levels and of the soil concentrations produce an approximately linear

relationship. Of course, this is not a perfect relationship, so, when plotted, the data will appear as a cloud of points as shown in Figure 1.

This plot, representing two hundred children, was produced by a statistical software program called Stata, using, as input, values from a number of different studies on this subject. On the graph, the software program plotted the fitted straight line to the data, called the regression equation of y on x. The software also prints out the fitted regression equation: $y = .29x + .01$. How does one interpret this regression? First, it is not appropriate to interpret it for an individuals; it applies to the population from which the sample was taken. It says that a increase of 1 in log (soil-lead) concentration will correspond, on average, to an increase in log (blood-lead) of .29. To predict the average blood-lead level given a value for soil lead, the entire equation is used. For example, a soil-lead level of 1,000 milligrams per kilogram, whose log is three, predicts an average log blood-lead level of .29×3 + .01 = .57, corresponding to a measured blood level of 7.6 micrograms per deciliter. The main point is that, from the public health viewpoint, there is a positive relationship between the level of lead in the soil and blood-lead levels in the population. An alternative interpretation is to state that soil-lead and blood-lead levels are positively correlated.

We note that many calculators, and all statistical software for personal computers, can calculate the best line for a given data set. Commercially available statistical software packages such as Stata, SAS, and SPSS can be purchased in versions for both IBM and Macintosh PCs. One comprehensive package, EpiInfo 2000, may be acquired free from CDC and can be downloaded on the Internet.

As in the case of contingency tables, the significance of the regression can be tested. In this case, as in all of statistics, statistical significance does not refer to the scientific importance of the relationship, but rather to a test of whether or not the observed relationship is the result of random association. Every statistical software package for personal computers includes a test of significance as part of its standard output. These packages, and some hand calculators, along with the line itself, will produce an estimate of the correlation between the two variables, called the correlation coefficient, or "r." If t is larger than 2, or smaller than -2, the regression is declared significant at the 5 percent level. For the data in Figure 1, r is 0.42. This number can very easily be used to test for the statistical significance of the regression through the following formula:

$$t = r\sqrt{\frac{n-2}{1-r^2}} = 0.42\sqrt{\frac{198}{.8236}} = 6.51$$

The number "r" calculated this way must lie between -1 and +1, and is often interpreted as a measure of how close to a straight line the data lie. Values near ±1 indicate a nearly perfect linear relationship, while values near 0 indicate no linear relationship. It is important not to make the mistake of interpreting r near 0 as meaning there is no relationship whatever—a curved relation can lead to low values of r.

The relationship between soil-lead and blood-lead could be studied using the contingency table analysis discussed earlier. For each child, both the soil-lead levels and the blood-lead levels could be classified as high or low, choosing appropriate criteria for the definitions of high and low. This too would have shown a relationship, but it would not be as powerful, nor would it have quantified the relationship between the two measurements as the regression did. Choosing a cutoff value for low and high on each measurement that divides each group into two equal-size subgroups as shown in Table 5.

The chi-square statistic calculated from this table is 13.5, which also indicates an association between blood-lead level and soil-lead levels in children. The conclusion is not as compelling as in the linear regression analysis, and a lot of information in the data has been lost by simplifying them in this way. One benefit, however, of this simpler analysis is that we do not have to take logarithms of the data and worry about the appropriate choice of a model.

Regression is a very powerful tool, and it is used for many different data analyses. It can be used to compare quantitative measurements on two groups by setting x = 1 for each subject in group one, and setting x = 2 for each subject in group two. The resulting analysis is equivalent to the two-sample t-test discussed in every elementary statistics text.

The most common application of regression analysis occurs when an investigator wishes to relate an outcome measurement y to several x variables—multiple linear regression. For example, regression can be used to relate blood lead to soil lead, environmental dust, income, education, and sex. Note that, as in this example, the x variables can be either quantitative, such as soil lead, or qualitative, such as sex, and they can be used together in the same equation. The statistical software will easily fit the regression equation and print out significance tests for each explanatory variable and for the model as a whole. When we have more than one x variable, there is no simple way to perform the calculations (or to represent them) and one must rely on a statistical package to do the work.

Regression methods are easily extended to compare a continuous response measurement across several groups—this is known as analysis of variance, also discussed in every elementary statistics text. It is done by choosing for the x variables indicators for the different groups—so-called dummy variables.

An important special case of multiple linear regression occurs when the outcome measurement y is dichotomous—indicating presence or absence of an attribute. In fact, this technique, called logistic regression, is one of the most commonly used statistical techniques in public health research today, and every statistical software package includes one or more programs to perform the analysis. The predictor x-variables used for logistic regression are almost always a mixture of quantitative and qualitative variables. When only qualitative variables are used, the result is essentially equivalent to a complicated contingency table analysis.

Methods of regression and correlation are essential tools for biostatisticians and public health researchers when studying complex relationships among different quantitative and qualitative measurements related to health. Many of the studies widely quoted in the public health literature have relied on this powerful technique to reach their conclusions.

WILLIAM G. CUMBERLAND
ABDELMONEM A. AFIFI

(SEE ALSO: *Bayes' Theorem; Biostatistics; Chi-Square Test; Epidemiology; Probability Model; Rates; Rates: Adjusted; Sampling; Survey Research Methods; T-Test*)

BIBLIOGRAPHY

Afifi, A. A., and Clark, V. A. (1996). *Computer-Aided Multivariate Analysis*, 3rd edition. London: Chapman and Hall.

Armitage, P., and Berry, G. (1994). *Statistical Methods in Medical Research*. Oxford: Blackwell Science.

Doll, R., and Hill, A. B. (1950). "Smoking and Carcinoma of the Lung. Preliminary Report." *British Medical Journal* 13:739–748.

Dunn, O. J., and Clark, V. A. (2001). *Basic Statistics*, 3rd edition. New York: John Wiley and Sons.

Glantz, S. A., and Slinker, B. K. (2001). *Primer of Applied Regression and Analysis of Variance*. New York: McGraw-Hill.

Hosmer, D. W., and Lemeshow, S. (2000). *Applied Logistic Regression*. New York: John Wiley and Sons.

Institute of Medicine. Committee for the Study of the Future of Public Health (1988). *The Future of Public Health*. Washington, DC: National Academy Press.

Kheifets, L.; Afifa, A. A.; Buffler, P. A.; and Zhang, Z. W. (1995). "Occupational Electric and Magnetic Field Exposure and Brain Cancer: A Meta-Analysis." *Journal of Occupational and Environmental Medicine* 37:1327–1341.

Lewin, M. D.; Sarasua, S.; and Jones, P. A. (1999). "A Multivariate Linear Regression Model for Predicting Children's Blood Lead Levels Based on Soil Lead Levels: A Study at Four Superfund Sites." *Environmental Research* 81(A):52–61.

National Center for Health Statistics (1996). *NHANES: National Health and Nutrition Examination Survey*. Hyattsville, MD: Author.

Thompson, D. C.; Rivara, F. P.; and Thompson, R. S. (1996). "Effectiveness of Bicycle Safety Helmets in Preventing Head Injuries—A Case-Control Study." *Journal of the American Medical Association* 276:1968–1973.

STATISTICAL SOFTWARE

Dean, A. G.; Arner, T. G.; Sangam, S.; Sunki, G. G.; Friedman, R.; Lantinga, M.; Zubieta, J. C.; Sullivan, K. M.; and Smith, D. C. (2000). *EpiInfo 2000, A Database and Statistics Program for Public Health Professionals, for Use on Windows 95, 98, NY, and 2000 Computers*. Atlanta, GA: Centers for Disease Control and Prevention.

The SAS System for Windows, Version 8.1. Cary, NC: SAS Institute.

SPSS Version 10.1 for Windows. Chicago, IL: SPSS.

Stata Statistical Software: Release 6.0. College Station, TX: StataCorp.

LINKS FOR DATA SOURCES

Agency for Healthcare Research and Quality: http://www.ahcpr.gov/data/.

American Cancer Society: http://www.cancer.org/.

American Public Health Association: http://www.apha.org/public_health/.

Bureau of Labor Statistics: http://stats.bls.gov/datahome.htm.

Center for International Earth Science Information Network: http://www.ciesin.org/.

Centers for Disease Control and Prevention: http://www.cdc.gov/scientific.htm.

Fedstats: http://www.fedstats.gov.

National Cancer Institute: http://cancernet.nci.nih.gov/statistics.shtml.

National Center for Health Statistics: http://www.cdc.gov/nchs/.

National Highway and Traffic Safety Administration: http://www-fars.nhtsa.dot.gov/.

National Institutes of Health: http://www.nih.gov.

National Survey of America's Families: http://newfederalism.urban.org/nsaf/cpuf/index,htm.

Research Forum on Children Families and the New Federalism: http://www.researchforum.org/.

U.S. Bureau of the Census: http://www.census.gov.

World Health Organization: http://www.who.int/whosis.

STOCHASTIC MODEL

See Probability Model

STRATIFICATION OF DATA

In public health, "stratification" is defined as the process of partitioning data into distinct or nonoverlapping groups. These distinct groups can represent, among other things, treatment regimens, geographical regions, or study centers. Although this definition is seemingly straightforward, stratification is a term that can be used to characterize either the design of a study (e.g., stratified sampling), or alternatively, an analytic approach (stratified analysis) that can be applied to data that has already been collected. In both cases, stratification is used because the study population consists of subpopulations or subdomains that are of particular interest to the researcher.

Stratified sampling is an approach used to ensure that an adequate number of individuals or entities are sampled so that comparisons of a parameter of interest can be made between two or more groups (strata) within a population. For example, a social worker may be interested in comparing the prevalence of drug use between those who live on the streets and the general population. This could be evaluated by sampling a sufficient number of individuals in each of the two groups and performing the relevant statistical test to determine whether the prevalence of drug use was equal in these two groups. In such a study, sampling is best approached using a stratified design because different recruitment strategies are needed to collect data from these two groups. That is, it is unlikely that homeless individuals could be contacted using telephone or voting lists. In some cases, data can only be divided into strata after it has been collected—this technique is referred to as poststratificition. For example, a health professional might be interested in determining differences in cigarette smoking between male and female smokers in order to devise a program to reduce smoking in teenagers. Such information could readily be extracted from an existing health survey that collected information on the smoking habits of both sexes.

As described at the outset, stratification is an important analytic tool in studies of public health. As an illustration, investigators conducting a study of smoking and lung cancer may elect to stratify study participants by gender in order to determine whether the females are more susceptible to the effects of smoking than males. Notable differences in the risk of lung cancer due to smoking between men and women would indicate that gender modifies the effect of cigarette smoking on the risk of developing lung cancer. In this instance, the terms "effect-modifier" or "interaction variable" could be applied to describe the role of gender on the relation between smoking and lung cancer.

Stratified analysis can also be used to assess whether the variable upon which the strata are based confounds the relationship between the outcome and the factor of primary interest. A confounding variable is a factor that is associated with both the factor of primary interest and the outcome under study. The inability to control for a confounding variable will bias inferences drawn between the factor of the primary interest and the outcome variable. With stratified analysis, if the overall effect using missing data pooled from the different strata is approximately equal to the stratum-specific estimates of effect, this indicates that the stratification variable does not confound the result. Alternatively, if the stratum-specific estimates of risk are similar to each other, yet different from the risk estimate based using the entirety of the data, then this indicates that the stratification variable is a confounder.

Stratification can also be used within the context of a randomized control trial. For example, in some clinical studies, patients may be divided into subgroups (strata) based on factors that are thought to be related to outcome. Within each strata, patients could randomly be assigned to different treatment groups (e.g., placebo or treatment). This analytic approach would permit the effectiveness of the different treatments to be compared within each stratum, while also ensuring the treatment and control groups are similar with respect to the postulated risk factors upon which the stratification was based.

PAUL J. VILLENEUVE

(SEE ALSO: *Sampling; Statistics for Public Health; Survey Research Methods*)

BIBLIOGRAPHY

Malec, D. (1998). "Stratified Sampling." In *Encyclopedia of Biostatistics*, eds. P. Armitage and T. Colton. New York: John Wiley.

Rothman, K. J., and Greenland, S. (1998). *Modern Epidemiology*, 2nd edition. New York: Lippincott Williams & Wilkins.

STREET VIOLENCE

Violence is the "intentional use of physical force against another person or against oneself, which either results in, or has a high likelihood of resulting in, injury or death" (Rosenberg, O'Carroll and Powell 1992, p. 3071). Violence is typically categorized according to the relationship between the victim and the perpetrator, as well as the location in which it takes place.

In general, street violence refers to the use of physical force by individuals or groups within public spaces, the result of which may involve injury or death. This definition is quite broad and includes the forms of violence that are most often addressed by public health practitioners and researchers, particularly gang and youth violence, which often take place in the street or other open areas.

Although statistics for violent crimes do not always specify the location of the incident, approximately one third of violent crimes occur in a street or open area. School-related violence has gained widespread media attention and concern; however, many violent acts committed by adolescents take place off of school property. In 1999, over one-third (35%) of U.S. high school students had been in a physical fight, while only one in seven students had a physical fight on school property. Homicides of school-age individuals are even less likely to take place on school property. Between 1992 and 1994, less than 1 percent of homicides of school-age persons occurred on school property, with the majority occurring on streets.

Street violence takes a variety of different forms, including actual or threatened homicide, rape and sexual assault, robbery (with or without injury), and assault. Although not all street violence is gang related, the relationship of gangs to homicide makes street violence a public health issue. Over 94 percent of U.S. cities with populations over 100,000 have street gangs, and many smaller and more rural cities report street gang activity. Membership in a street gang increases the risk of violent death by 60 percent.

Recognition of violence, including street violence, as a public health priority is relatively recent. In 1979, the Surgeon General's report *Healthy People* included interpersonal violence as one of fifteen priority areas for improving the health of the U.S. population. More objectives for improving the public's health through reducing violence have been included in the updated versions, *Healthy People 2000* (Public Health Service, 1991) and *Healthy People 2010* (Public Health Service, 2000). These objectives target health status (e.g., reduce homicide rates), risk reduction (e.g., reduce weapons carrying and physical fighting among adolescents), and services (increase the proportion of schools that offer conflict-resolution programs).

Violence, particularly among youth, is a public health priority because it causes premature death, injury, and disability. Homicide is the second leading cause of death for people aged 15 to 24 years, and is the leading cause of death for African-American males aged 15 to 24 years.

Street violence may also result in serious nonfatal injury and temporary or permanent disability. Among youth, violence is a leading cause of nonfatal injuries, second only to motor vehicle accidents. In 1994, an estimated 1.4 million people were treated in hospital emergency departments for violence-related injuries. Nearly one-half of all the injuries treated occurred in public buildings or on the street. Of all of the injuries treated, one-third were cuts or stab wounds and 5 percent were gunshot wounds. Severe injuries to children due to intentional shootings also typically occur in streets or other open areas.

Street violence also results in financial burdens. Injuries may result in days missed from work or school, causing victims to lose wages and/or academic progress. Injuries resulting in permanent disability may further affect the social, emotional, and economic consequences for victims. Society too, bears the financial burden of violence-related injuries. Acute care and rehabilitation for injuries can cost thousands of dollars, and not all patients have adequate money or insurance to cover the costs. Unpaid medical costs are passed on to hospitals and taxpayers.

STREET VIOLENCE PREVENTION

Public health utilizes three levels of prevention: primary, secondary, and tertiary. Primary prevention strategies aim to prevent a problem (i.e., violent acts) before it occurs. The goal of secondary prevention is to prevent further injury. Tertiary prevention aims to limit the extent of disability after an injury has taken place. Criminal justice strategies for violence prevention are often in the secondary category. By removing individuals who have already become violent, criminal justice attempts to reduce the likelihood of further injuries or deaths caused by the already violent person. Public health strategies, specifically primary prevention strategies, make an essential contribution to criminal justice efforts because they may keep individuals from committing violent acts in the first place.

The public health approach utilizes health-event surveillance and epidemiology to determine who are the victims and perpetrators of violence-related injuries and where and when violence-related injuries occur. The answers to these questions tell public health researchers and practitioners where to direct prevention efforts.

Adolescents currently have the highest and most rapidly increasing rates of lethal and nonlethal violence. As youth are at much greater risk of being victims or perpetrators of street violence, they are an important audience for violence prevention programs. Further, because males, African–American and Hispanic youth, and residents in poor urban neighborhoods are more likely to engage in and be victims of street violence, prevention programs are also developed specifically for these populations.

In order to develop effective prevention programs and policies, public health must first determine what factors cause individuals to commit violent acts. Public health surveillance and epidemiology identify risk characteristics. However, not all individuals with these characteristics engage in violence. Public health researchers use a variety of theories from different disciplines (e.g., psychology, sociology, criminology) and scientific research to determine what factors either increase or decrease the risk that individuals will commit violent acts and what factors are possible to change through prevention programs. Psychosocial (proviolence attitudes, low self-control) and behavioral (drug selling, weapons carrying) characteristics may also increase youths' risk for engaging in violent behaviors such as street violence.

Characteristics of social and physical environments are also a factor in street violence. Social environments include exposure to violence or violence-promoting attitudes through families, peers, schools, neighborhoods, and even media (e.g., television). Adolescents who have been victims or witnesses of violence are more likely to engage in violent behaviors. In addition, children raised by individuals with poor parenting skills, those living in high-crime and dangerous urban neighborhoods, and those exposed to or involved in gangs are more likely to engage in violent behaviors. Young people living in urban areas may be more likely to engage in gang- and nongang-related violence because in areas with poor economic and educational opportunities, violence may become a way to gain respect and status.

Some violence-prevention programs target children and adolescents identified as having aggressive behaviors and attitudes and try to change these behaviors and attitudes before they develop into more violent behaviors. These programs attempt to promote self-esteem, problem solving, and development of nonviolent attitudes and interpersonal skills in high-risk children and adolescents.

While prevention strategies targeting individuals are important, they may fail to reach some individuals. It is not always easy to identify which individuals will later engage in violent behaviors. Other public health strategies for reducing violence focus on community or even societal level changes as well as individuals. These changes affect everyone, not just those successfully identified as being at high-risk. As availability of firearms has been associated with the risk of violence, policies that reduce the overall availability of weapons on the street may help reduce firearm injuries and deaths. Changes in the physical structures (e.g., improved lighting, limitations in through-traffic) can also reduce rates of violent street crimes within neighborhoods. Policies that promote economic and educational opportunities may help young people resist the pressures to join gangs in order to achieve self-esteem and respect in dangerous high-crime neighborhoods.

Some of the most promising prevention programs attempt to change a variety of factors; that is, they attempt to intervene not only with individuals, but also with families, schools, and neighborhoods. For instance, the Seattle Social Development Project promotes positive development of children and youth by training teachers and parents in classroom and family management strategies that promote problem solving, effective communication, conflict resolution skills, self-esteem, and autonomy. The program is designed to promote children's bonding to schools and parents (or other positive adult role models), so they will be better able to resist pressures to engage in a variety of health-compromising behaviors, including violence. Children who participated in this program throughout elementary and middle school were found to be less likely than those who did not participate to have engaged in violent behaviors by the time they were eighteen years old.

Prevention of street violence requires the collaboration and cooperation of public health professionals with those in other academic disciplines, law enforcement, and social policy positions. Prevention programs need to be rigorously evaluated to determine the most effective strategies to prevent individuals from engaging in street violence. In addition, legal and policy strategies could reinforce public health efforts to help alleviate the human, social, and economic costs of street violence.

RALPH DICLEMENTE
CATLAINN SIONEAN

(SEE ALSO: *Adolescent Violence; Crime; Gun Control; Healthy Communities; Healthy People 2010; Homicide; School Health; Social Determinants; Urban Health; Violence; Youth Risk Behavior Surveillance System*)

BIBLIOGRAPHY

Anderson, E. (1999). *Code of the Street: Decency, Violence, and the Moral Life of the Inner City.* New York: W. W. Norton.

Centers for Disease Control and Prevention (2000). *Morbidity and Mortality Weekly Report.* CDC Surveillance Summaries. June 9, 2000.

Hawkins, J. D.; Catalano, R. F.; Kosterman, R.; Abbott, R.; and Hill, K. G. (1999). "Preventing Adolescent Health-Risk Behaviors by Strengthening Protection During Childhood." *Archives of Pediatrics and Adolescent Medicine* 153:226–234.

Herrenkohl, T. I.; Maguin E.; Hill, K. G.; Hawkins, J. D., Abbott, R. D.; and Catalano, R. F. (2000). "Developmental Risk Factors for Youth Violence." *Journal of Adolescent Health* 6(3):176–186.

Hutson, H. R.; Anglin, D.; Kyriacou, D. N.; Hart, J.; and Spears, K. (1995). "The Epidemic of Gang-Related Homicides in Los Angeles County from 1979 through 1994." *Journal of the American Medical Association* (13):1031–1036.

Kachur, S. P.; Steenes, G. M.; Powell, K. E.; Modzeleski, W.; Stephens, R.; Murphy, R. et al. (1996). "School-Associated Violent Deaths in the United States, 1992 to 1994." *Journal of the American Medical Association* (22):1729–1733.

Li, G.; Baker, S. P.; DiScala, C.; Fowler, C.; Ling, J.; and Kelen, G. D. (1996). "Factors Associated with the Intent of Firearm-Related Injuries in Pediatric Trauma Patients." *Archives of Pediatrics & Adolescent Medicine* 150(11):1160–1165.

Public Health Service (U.S.) (1991). *Healthy People 2000: National Health Promotion and Disease Prevention Objectives.* Washington, DC: Government Printing Office.

Public Health Service (U.S.). Department of Health and Human Services (2000). *Healthy People 2010* (Conference Edition in Two Volumes). Washington, DC: Government Printing Office.

Rachuba, L.; Stanton, B.; and Howard, D. (1995). "Violent Crime in the United States. An Epidemiologic Profile." *Archives of Pediatrics & Adolescent Medicine* 149(9):953–960.

Rand, M. R. (1997). *Violence-Related Injuries Treated in Hospital Emergency Departments.* Bureau of Justice Statistics Special Report, NCJ-156921. Washington, DC: U.S. Department of Justice.

Resnick, M. D.; Bearman, P. S.; Blum, R. W.; Bauman, K. E.; Harris, K. M.; Jones, J. et al. (1997). "Protecting Adolescents from Harm: Findings from the National Longitudinal Study on Adolescent Health." *Journal of the American Medical Association* 278(10):823–832.

Rosenberg, M. L.; and Fenley, M. A., eds. (1991). *Violence in America: A Public Health Approach.* London: Oxford University Press.

Rosenberg, M. L.; O'Carroll, P. W.; and Powell, K. E. (1992). "Let's Be Clear: Violence Is a Public Health Problem." *Journal of the American Medical Association* 267(22):3071–3072.

Zavoski, R. W.; Lapidus, G. D.; Lerer, T. J.; Burke, G.; and Banco, L. I. (1999). "Evaluating the Impact of a Street Barrier on Urban Crime." *Injury Prevention* 5(1):65–68.

STREPTOCOCCAL INFECTION

Among the large family of streptococci, the most dangerous is group A hemolytic streptococcus, formerly known as *Streptococcus pyogenes*, the pus-producing streptococcus. This is responsible for several diseases that in the past have had great public health importance, and still do in developing countries. *Streptococcus pyogenes* was the principal cause of puerperal sepsis, or childbed fever, once a leading cause of death in the immediate postpartum period when delivery of the baby introduced virulent pathogenic organisms into the birth canal and uterus. Streptococcal tonsillitis is a precursor of rheumatic fever and acute nephritis when the toxin produced by the invading pathogens provokes an autoimmune response. Streptococcal infection also causes scarlet fever, formerly a common and sometimes deadly infection of early childhood.

All these diseases have become rare since the discovery and development of chemotherapy and antibiotics to which the streptococcus is sensitive. However, streptococcal infection has not become extinct. Erysipelas, a skin infection, remains common; streptococcal septicemia occurs occasionally; and the rare but dramatic streptococcal cellulitis, known as flesh-eating disease, captures headlines when it attacks, disfigures, and sometimes kills a previously healthy young adult. Humans are the main reservoir of infection, which is transmitted person-to-person by direct contact or droplet spread, with a brief incubation period of one to three days.

Outbreaks of all these forms of streptococcal infection occur when social and economic conditions deteriorate, as in post–Soviet Russia and its satellites, and in many of the world's combat zones where hygiene and public health facilities are rudimentary or have deteriorated to the stage of being ineffectual. Treatment of streptococcal infection relies on antibiotics, and prevention requires good hygiene, cleanliness, and education about ways to minimize the risks of transmission of this and other pathogens.

JOHN M. LAST

(SEE ALSO: *Antibiotics; Communicable Disease Control; Contagion; Drug Resistance; Maternal and Child Health; Staphylococcal Infection*)

STRESS

Over the course of evolution, the human mind and body have developed means of handling stressful situations. Over the short term, such stress response pathways are highly adaptive, allowing a person to manage his or her resources in order to navigate the crisis; in some cases, however, these processes go awry and result in pathology. Chronic stress is becoming increasingly problematic in the United States as workers work longer and harder hours. Approximately one-third of all workers report that they are in high-stress jobs, and that not only is stress implicated in 15 percent of all disability claims, the number of stress-related absences is increasing. Such prolonged exposure to stress can also result in consequences in the form of physical illness. Alternatively, a severe acute stressor may result in a stress-response syndrome such as an acute stress disorder or a post-traumatic stress disorder.

In acute stress, the mind and body respond with a fight or flight response that involves activation of the sympathetic nervous system and release of stress hormones such as cortisol. Psychologically, this increases the organism's alertness and response time. Physiologically, these changes provide the organism with the energy needed to meet the emergency. Such intense activation helps the organism in the short term, but prolonged activation of this system creates problems in that it may increase the risk of certain disease states, and, once set into motion, chronic stress responses may be difficult to extinguish. This has led some researchers to investigate potential mediating factors such as personality. For example, a correlation has been established between a personality characterized by hostile competitiveness (type A) and increased risk of myocardial infarction (heart attack).

An acute stressor or psychological trauma, such as a life-threatening circumstance, presents a person with new information that may be difficult to assimilate. In an attempt to adapt, the person will typically alternate between contemplation of the stressor and avoidance of reminders of the event. Such a cycle allows for dose-by-dose psychological processing of the event. Difficulties in adaptation may present as an acute stress disorder that manifests itself as an extreme version of this cycle. People with such a disorder may have intrusive remembrances, nightmares, or even flashbacks of the stress event. These can alternate with emotional numbing, interpersonal alienation, and extreme avoidance of traumatic reminders. A diagnosis of postraumatic stress disorder (PTSD) is made if these symptoms persist longer than one month. Studies suggest that approximately 0.5 percent of men and 1.3 percent of women meet criteria for PTSD over their lifetime. A larger percentage (approximately 15%) of subjects were found to have some symptoms but did not meet criteria for the full disorder.

At present, psychotherapy is the mainstay of treatment for stress response syndromes. A variety of approaches exist, but they share a common goal of assisting the patient with conscious contemplation of the event in such a way that it may be assimilated and anxiety responses extinguished. Care must be taken to create an environment of safety and to avoid retraumatization, which may occur with overly rapid exposure to traumatic memories. Patients experience decreased feelings of guilt and shame as they learn that they responded to the trauma as adequately as possible. Contemplation of the event in therapy may lead to further benefits, including an enhanced understanding of the meaning of the event in the larger context of the individual's life.

Psychopharmacologic treatment may be a useful adjunct for specific symptom clusters such as associated anxiety, depression, and insomnia. The prognosis for treatment is good and is improved if the patient was without preexisting psychiatric comorbidity and if the treatment occurs in close proximity to the event. Brief treatment is frequently helpful in restoring a patient to a baseline level of functioning, but longer-term treatment may be necessary if exposure to the stressor was chronic or occurred in childhood.

Stress response systems have developed in humans as an adaptive mechanism to assist individuals in times of crisis. These systems, however, may also result in physical or psychological pathology. Chronic overactivation of the stress response may predispose an individual to greater risk for physical illnesses such as heart disease. Overly intense exposure to an acute stressor may result in a stress response syndrome with potentially disabling consequences. Treatment is, however, available and may return individuals to their previous level of functioning. A subset of patients even report a sense of enhanced insight into their lives as a result of the trauma.

JAMES POWERS
STUART J. EISENDRATH

(SEE ALSO: *Mental Health*)

BIBLIOGRAPHY

Eisendrath, S. J., and Feder, A. (1995). "The Mind and Somatic Illness: Psychological Factors Affecting Physical Illness." In *Review of General Psychiatry*. ed. H. H. Goldman. Norwalk CT: Appleton & Lang.

Horowitz, M. J. (1997). *Stress Response Syndromes: PTSD, Grief and Adjustment Disorders,* 3rd edition. Northvale, NJ: Aranson.

Van der Kolk, B. A.; McFarlane, A. C.; and Weisaeth, L. (1996). *Traumatic Stress: The Effects of Overwhelming Experience on Mind, Body and Society.* New York: Guilford Press.

STROKE

Stroke, or cerebrovascular accident (CVA), is the third leading cause of death (after heart disease and cancer) in the United States and the industrialized countries of the world. The term "stroke," which comes from subjects being suddenly "struck down" with neurological deficits, is commonly used by both professional and lay groups. Efforts are being made to replace the term with "brain attack" to dramatize its analogous effects to a "heart attack," the term used for myocardial infarction. The term "cerebrovascular accident" is used interchangeably with stroke ("accident" indicates the catastrophic nature of strokes, not a traumatic origin as the term implies). More than 600,000 strokes occur annually in the United States, according to the American Heart Association, and stroke prevalence (number of living stroke victims) is approximately 4.5 million with an annual cost in 1997, both direct and indirect, of over $40 billion.

Stroke refers to the usually sudden onset of a neurological deficit, such as hemiparesis (weakness on one side of the body), or aphasia (impairment of language comprehension and production), which can be attributed to either the occlusion or rupture of a cerebral vessel. Resulting specific neurological symptoms and signs are determined by the area of the brain that is affected, and since the complex functions of the brain are either localized in specialized areas or diffusely distributed, stroke symptoms may similarly be localized or generalized in nature. For example, the long pathway of motor fibers can be interrupted, with resulting hemiparesis involving various cerebral arteries or their branches, such as the anterior, middle, or vertebrobasilar arteries. Occlusion of smaller arterioles which feed smaller areas of brain may result in more isolated effects, such as pure sensory or motor hemiparesis. On the other hand,

occlusion or rupture of vessels in "silent" areas of the brain, as in the frontal or parietal cortex, can lead to subtle nonfocal symptoms reflected in impaired cognition, executive function, or memory. Other symptoms of impaired specialized brain functions from strokes include apraxia (impairment in the execution of motor actions), and agnosia (loss of ability to recognize familiar objects). Leukoaraiosis, or increased T2-signal intensity, on magnetic resonance imaging (MRI) of brain white matter results predominantly from small-vessel disease, and this syndrome is associated with increased risks for strokes and dementia.

ISCHEMIC STROKES

The causes of arterial occlusion, or ischemic strokes, are multiple. The most frequent is atherosclerotic disease of extracranial and/or intracranial arteries; the former is more common in Caucasians, while the latter is more frequent among African Americans and Asians. A thrombus (stationary blood clot) formed on atherosclerotic plaques in these locations, as well as on the aorta, can dislodge and embolize to occlude a distal artery. Strokes due to atherosclerosis account for approximately two-thirds of all strokes. If seen within three hours of stroke onset, treatment with tissue plasminogen activator (tPA), a thrombolytic agent, may substantially improve a patient's neurological outcome. Otherwise, therapeutic efforts are aimed at optimizing cerebral blood flow to ischemically impaired brain tissue, providing neural protection to avert brain damage, and maximizing neurorehabilitation. Research on stem cell and neural progenitor cell implantation into an ischemically damaged brain to promote recovery is a recently promising area of stroke research.

Transient Ischemic Attacks (TIAs). Strokes may be heralded by transient neurological deficits, called transient ischemic attacks (TIAs), such as temporary blindness of one eye (amaurosis fugax), hemiparesis, or aphasia. Most frequently, TIAs occur with significant atherosclerotic disease of the extracranial carotid arteries. Control of risk factors for atherosclerosis, such as hypertension, smoking, diabetes mellitus, elevated cholesterol, stress, and, perhaps, sedentary lifestyle, will hopefully minimize strokes from this cause to an irreducible minimum. For significant extracranial disease (>70% diameter stenosis [constriction] at the carotid bifurcation), carotid endarterectomy in competent surgical hands has been shown to reduce stroke recurrence significantly. Aspirin and other antiplatelet drugs in nonsurgical candidates can prevent subsequent strokes.

Cardiogenic strokes. Ischemic strokes can be caused by emboli from the heart as a result of more than a dozen cardiac disorders, the most common being arrhythmias, particularly atrial fibrillation (AF). Suspected cardiogenic strokes require workup, including transthoracic and transesophageal echocardiography (TTE and TEE), which can detect valvular pathologies, wall-motion abnormalities, thrombi, and patent foramen ovale (PFO). This group, in aggregate, may account for up to a quarter or more of all ischemic strokes. For AF, the treatment of choice to prevent embolic strokes is long-term anticoagulation. Patients who are not anticoagulation candidates should be treated with antiplatelet drugs. Conditions such as PFO can be treated medically with anticoagulation; surgical and percutaneous options are also available for PFO closure.

Lacunar Strokes. These strokes refer to small branch occlusions (noted previously), and include discrete syndromes such as pure sensory and motor hemiparesis. Lacunar strokes result primarily from chronic sustained hypertension, and the pathological change is "lipohyalinosis" of arterioles. This syndrome may account for 10 to 15 percent of all strokes. Adequate control of hypertension should prevent this condition.

Two final categories of diseases-causing ischemic strokes are more frequently considered in younger persons, especially those under fifty-five years of age, and involve arteries and blood elements. For the former, vessel diseases other than atherosclerosis include inflammatory processes, such as the arteritides; migraine; dissection—either spontaneous or traumatic; moyamoya syndrome; fibromuscular disorders; MELAS syndrome (mitochondrial encephalopathy, lactic acidosis, and stroke-like symptoms) and a few others. For the latter, blood-element disorders include clotting, and platelets and erythrocyte abnormalities. The most common clotting disorders are resistance to protein C activation—most frequently due to Factor V Leiden mutation (506Q); antiphospholipid syndrome, which includes the lupus anticoagulant

and anticardiolipin antibodies; reduced antithrombin III; protein C & S deficiencies; plus a few others. Treatment of vascular disorders is tailored to the individual condition; for example, migraine is treated with prophylactic agents, which prevent vasospasm; arteritides with steroids and immunosuppressive agents; and moyamoya syndrome with a variety of bypass surgical procedures. Many of the hypercoagulable or prothrombotic conditions are treated with long-term anticoagulation.

INTRACEREBRAL AND SUBARACHNOID HEMORRHAGES

Rupture of vessels include two large categories. The more common is intracerebral hemorrhage (ICH), which results from chronic sustained hypertension and accounts for approximately 10 percent of all strokes. An infrequent cause of ICH is amyloid angiopathy; its cause (and cure) is unknown. A second category of vessel rupture is subarachnoid hemorrhage (SAH), most frequently due to aneurysmal rupture, but occasionally from arteriovenous malformations. SAH accounts for about 5 percent of all strokes. Gene and molecular pathological markers to identify persons at risk will hopefully provide interventional tools to both prevent and treat subjects at risk before aneurysmal rupture.

ICH occurs in five brain sites, most commonly in the putamen. With substantial cerebellar ICH in a noncomatose patient, surgical evacuation can be life-saving. The only other site that may benefit from surgery is polar or white matter ICH. In neurologically viable patients, SAH can be treated successfully with surgical extirpation of the aneurysm, or with a variety of endovascular procedures, such as aneurysmal obliteration.

PUBLIC HEALTH IMPORTANCE OF STROKES

As the third leading cause of death and disability, there are important public health implications for strokes, especially since many of the stroke syndromes are preventable. This is particularly true for those due to atherosclerosis, which is the most common cause of strokes. Except for increasing age, all of the risk factors for atherosclerosis can be either controlled or eliminated. To accomplish this goal, better strategies to educate and motivate the general public are vital.

In addition to controlling risk factors, a better understanding of the nature of stroke symptoms by the public is required for expeditious corrective and therapeutic measures, much as has happened with the public's general awareness of chest pain as a symptom of a potential heart attack. Investigations on proteomic and gene expression profiles for strokes to identify individuals at increased risk for strokes will hopefully provide public health planners with an even more powerful tool to intervene effectively for stroke prevention, the ultimate best treatment of strokes.

FRANK YATSU

(SEE ALSO: *American Heart Association; Atherosclerosis; Cardiovascular Diseases; Transient Ischemic Attacks*)

BIBLIOGRAPHY

Barnett, H. J. M.; Mohr, J. P.; Stein, B.; and Yatsu, F. M., eds. (1998). *Stroke: Pathophysiology, Diagnosis & Management.* Philadelphia, PA: Churchill-Livingstone.

STRUCTURE ACTIVITY RELATIONSHIPS

A structure-activity relationship (SAR) is used to determine the primary, secondary, and tertiary structure of chemicals as a means of ascertaining the relationship between the effects of different compounds on biological systems. The history of SARs is over 150 years old and goes back to the laboratory of Louis Lewin, who, in the nineteenth century, developed the early chlorinated methane derivatives chloroform, carbon tetrachloride, and dichloromethane. The many derivatives of benzene (toluene, xylene, and others) also fall into this category. Once the organic chemists and medicinal chemists began to understand the impact of chemical structure on biological systems, the rudimentary basis of SARs commenced. By the 1920s, the chemistry of disinfectants, pesticides, and some drugs was based on SAR.

A classic example of an early SAR was the discovery of the benefits of acetylsalicylic acid (aspirin) and its near congeners, acetaminophen and salicylate. Another early classic example of a SAR was the development of DDT and its analogs and congeners. Several organochlorine pesticides are members of this broad family. The organophosphate insecticides are derivatives of the nerve gases. They were structurally engineered to be less toxic than nerve gases but to work by the same basic mechanism.

Modern SAR analysis is used to develop almost all drugs. Once the prototype drug is discovered and its three-dimensional characteristics determined, the chemists and structural biologists can then use the SAR to better understand the interaction between the drug and the affected protein or membrane.

The role of the SAR in public health has evolved in a manner similar to drugs. Based on seminal work carried out by many investigative teams, the key structural determinants of a large class of toxicants have been identified. For example, many of the determinants of carcinogenic activity have been characterized and published. Investigators can then use the SAR to examine a novel chemical structure to see if it contains one or more of the determinants of carcinogenicity. The ability to use SARs allows for a tier approach to carcinogenicity testing. The mutagenic potential of several classes of chemicals has also been cataloged to the extent that SARs can be used to examine novel molecules. There is a developing database to use SARs for the determination of skin and eye irritants. In each of these cases the effective use of SARs saves time, resources, and animals. As new and better methods of determining the three-dimensional structure of genes and proteins become available, the importance of SARs for toxicology will be critical. Coupling SARs with gene and protein structure should allow the investigator to determine the exact site of action of a toxicant. Understanding the function of any given gene (functional genomics) or protein (functional proteomics) can then be used to determine toxicity and risk.

MICHAEL GALLO

(SEE ALSO: *Carcinogen Assessment Groups; Carcinogenesis; Toxicology*)

SUBSTANCE ABUSE, DEFINITION OF

Public health has an opportunity to address the issues of substance use, abuse, and dependency across all age groups in the community since it occurs in all age groups. Substance abuse prevention and treatment professionals are acutely aware that alcohol and other drugs have a destructive impact on a person's physical, mental, and social development. Research and experience in the field of public health correlates the etiology of most criminal justice, family, and employment problems with alcohol and drug use. The role of the substance abuse professional in a public health setting is to promote the understanding and treatment of addiction as disease with sensitivity and in collaboration with other relevant community resources.

RONALD J. ZUMPANO

SUDDEN INFANT DEATH SYNDROME (SIDS)

Sudden infant death syndrome (SIDS) was defined in the United States in 1989 by a conference of the National Institute of Health as the sudden death of an infant under one year of age that remains unexplained after a thorough case investigation, including performance of a complete autopsy, examination of the death scene, and a review of the clinical history. Most cases occur between three weeks and six months of age. The cause of SIDS is, by definition, unknown. One current theory is that ineffective respiration may cause the infant to stop breathing. Placing infants on their back when they sleep reduces the incidence of SIDS by approximately 30 to 40 percent. A number of factors increase the incidence of SIDS. These include (1) the use of waterbeds and soft bedding; (2) sleeping on the stomach; (3) infants born of mothers who smoke or use drugs; (4) young, unmarried mothers of low socioeconomic status; (5) male infants; and (6) prematurity and low birth weight. There is no genetic cause of SIDS, and immunizations do not cause SIDS. An autopsy must be performed to exclude abuse,

injury, infection, or metabolic disease. These diagnoses remove the cases from the SIDS category.

MARVIN S. PLATT

(SEE ALSO: *Child Mortality; Perinatology*)

BIBLIOGRAPHY

DiMaio, D. J., and DiMaio, V. J. (1993). *Forensic Pathology*. Boca Raton, FL: CRC Press.

Hauck, F. R., and Hunt, C. E. (2000). "Sudden Infant Death Syndrome in 2000." *Current Problems in Pediatrics* 30:237–268.

Spitz, W. U. (1993). *Medicolegal Investigation of Death*, 3rd edition. Springfield, MA: Charles C. Thomas.

SUICIDE

Suicide is defined as the act of deliberately taking one's own life. It occurs most often in response to a crisis such as a death or the loss of a relationship or job. During a crisis people experience a wide range of feelings, and each person's response to crisis is different. It is normal to feel frightened or anxious or depressed. If a person feels overwhelmed or unable to cope, he or she may try to commit suicide.

Almost all people who kill themselves either suffered from depression or had substance abuse problems. People who are lonely and isolated or who have histories of previous suicide attempts are also at greater risk for attempting suicide.

In 1996, approximately 31,000 people died of suicide in the United States. Suicide is the eighth leading cause of death overall, and the third leading cause of death among American teenagers. In Canada, suicide is second only to motor-vehicle accidents as a cause of death among adolescents.

The suicide rate is twice the murder rate among those aged 15 to 24, and it has increased dramatically in recent years. Each year, two thousand adolescents commit suicide in the United States. The highest suicide rates in the United States are found in white men over age 85. Men are more than four times as likely as women to die by suicide, yet women are more likely to make a nonlethal suicide attempt.

Suicide is a major public health problem. The need for a public health approach to suicide can be found in the African-American community, where the suicide rate among youths more than doubled between 1980 and 1995. Further, the number of suicides in the United States outnumbered homicides in 1995. Each year, firearms are used as many times for suicide as they are for murder. In some other countries, 71 percent of all firearm deaths are suicide.

Attempted and completed suicides result in enormous social, economic, and medical costs. Suicide is very disruptive to the quality of life of survivors and their families and friends. In 1995 it was estimated that in the United States each suicide attempt costs approximately $33,000. The cost of a completed suicide has been estimated at almost $400,000. These estimates were derived from factors including the expense of hospitalization, medication, and more general social costs.

Public health professionals have a major role to play in addressing the problem of suicide. Public health programs and policies can play a part before, during, and after completed or attempted suicides. First, public health programs are an important aspect of the prevention of suicide. Education campaigns can be used to increase knowledge and to change people's attitudes, beliefs, and values about suicide, and about people who may have attempted suicide. People may have distorted ideas about suicidal persons. For example, it is a myth that people who commit suicide never talk about it first. Most people provide important warning signs that can help to reduce the risk of suicide.

Health education can be combined with counseling or support programs. These programs can be provided by trained public health professionals or by peer counselors. For example, teenagers can be trained to provide counseling and support for other teens. Suicide awareness or prevention programs can be delivered in a variety of settings such as schools, churches, or in the community as a whole. They can also be delivered in psychiatric settings.

A second aspect of the prevention of suicide lies in judging or assessing a person's risk for suicide. Public health professionals such as nurses or doctors can help to prevent completed suicides by identifying people who may be thinking about or planning to try to commit suicide. They can also provide support through crisis or suicide-prevention counseling.

Public health can also play a valuable role during a suicide attempt. A suicide attempt is often a person's response to a crisis, or to a time when they feel overwhelmed or hopeless. Public health professionals can help during a suicide attempt through suicide-prevention counseling. This type of short-term counseling involves providing support and guidance to an individual who is suicidal. Its purpose is to decrease the person's emotional pain, to make sure that the person is safe, and to help develop a plan for coping. Sometimes suicide-prevention counseling includes connecting a person to community or health services. These services can then provide longer-term support.

Suicide prevention counseling is a valuable tool for public health. It is relatively low-cost, flexible, and simple to provide. A wide variety of health professionals, including doctors, nurses, psychologists, and social workers, can be taught to help people with suicide-prevention counseling techniques. These services can be provided in a wide variety of places or settings, including hospitals, community clinics, and telephone-based crisis centers or helplines. Suicide-prevention services provide an important link between the community and the formal health care system.

Public health professionals who work in suicide prevention and counseling are faced with a growing variety of issues and clients. Most communities are home to an increased number of people from a wide variety of cultural and ethnic backgrounds. There are also more older people in society. New issues that might trigger a suicide attempt include elder abuse, racism or discrimination, bullying, or gay bashing. Police officers, firemen, paramedics, and others are being trained to deliver on-the-spot suicide prevention counseling.

There is also a role for public health following a completed or attempted suicide. A suicide attempt or death can have a traumatic effect on the quality of life of survivors and their families and friends. Public health programs can provide important support services to survivors of a suicide attempt and their families.

Public health is only one important part of society's response to suicide as a health and social problem. There is also a role for law enforcement, the education system, the government, and the formal health care system in prevention, treatment, and follow-up to a suicide attempt.

Law enforcement (police officers) and public health professionals can cooperate to help suicidal persons. Police officers are often the first ones on the scene of a suicide attempt. They may act to prevent a suicidal person from hurting themselves (or someone else) through suicide prevention counseling. The may detain someone who is at high risk for suicide and refer him or her to appropriate public health resources.

Legislators can also help to address the challenges of suicide by creating policies or laws to support the development of public health programs and the training of public health professionals. They can also work to change society's attitude toward suicide and suicidal people. One example of this type of work is the fact that in many countries suicide is no longer illegal. Attempting suicide is seen as a mental health issue, not a crime. In 1999 the United States Public Health Service issued the first-ever Surgeon General's Report on Mental Health, as well as a Call to Action on Suicide Prevention, charting out this new approach to suicide.

The educational and health care systems also have a role to play in the prevention, treatment, and follow-up to a suicide attempt. Schools provide access to most young people and provide a place for delivering suicide prevention or awareness programs. They can also teach young people to recognize the warning signs of a potential suicide attempt in their friends, to provide peer counseling, and how to get immediate help and support. This is important because young people are at higher risk of attempting suicide than most adults.

The formal health care system (hospitals, clinics, doctor's offices) can play an important role in two main ways. First, people who are suicidal may come to an emergency room or a physician's office. In these cases, the health system serves as a "first-response" and crisis service. Second, once a person has been identified by a public health or law enforcement professional as suicidal, they may need to be hospitalized for a period of time. Health professionals can provide medications and further counseling or support to a suicidal person and their family.

Once a suicidal person is released from a hospital, public health professionals may make home visits or provide follow-up support through a community-based clinic. The prevention of suicide and the provision of support to people who are suicidal play an important and increasing role in the health of individuals, families, and communities. The most comprehensive national strategies on suicide have been developed by Finland, Norway, Australia, New Zealand, and Sweden.

C. JAMES FRANKISH
ROBBIN JEFFEREYS

(SEE ALSO: *Crisis Counseling; Gun Control; Hotlines, Helplines, Telephone Counseling; Mental Health; School Health; Social Work; Violence*)

BIBLIOGRAPHY

Carter, C., and Baume, P. (1999). "Suicide Prevention: A Public Health Approach." *Australian and New Zealand Journal of Mental Health Nursing* 8:45–50.

Harwitz, D., and Ravizza, L. (2000). "Suicide and Depression." *Emergency Medical Clinics of North America* 18:263–271.

Lester, D. "Estimating the True Economic Cost of Suicide." *Perceptual and Master Skills* 80:746.

Office of the Surgeon General (1999). *Mental Health: A Report of the Surgeon General.* Washington, DC: U.S. Public Health Service.

Potter, L. B.; Powell, K. P.; and Kachur, S. P. (1995). "Suicide Prevention from a Public Health Respective." *Suicide and Life Threatening Behavior* 25:82–91.

U.S. Public Health Service (1999). *The Surgeon General's Call to Action to Prevent Suicide.* Washington, DC: U.S. Public Health Service.

SULFUR-CONTAINING AIR POLLUTANTS (PARTICULATES)

Sulfur oxides are an important class of air pollutants. They include sulfur dioxide, sulfuric acid, and various forms of sulfate. The major determinant of total sulfur oxide production is the sulfur content of fossil fuels, which tends to be highest in coal and lowest in natural gas. Sulfur dioxide, a gas, was found to be associated with mortality and morbidity in London during periods of heavy smog and during other air pollution episodes. While in retrospect the problem had been present for decades and perhaps centuries, it was not demonstrated epidemiologically until the 1950s. This led in the 1960s to effective control measures, including a switch to fuels with lower sulfur content and the banning of many local point sources, such as coal used for heating homes. However, toxicological studies, including controlled human exposures, could not substantiate the epidemiological association of low levels of sulfur dioxide with adverse health effects. It soon became apparent that the causal relation was primarily with sulfuric acid and sulfates, and that atmospheric sulfur dioxide was both a precursor of these particulate forms of sulfur oxides, and a surrogate measure for their air concentrations.

Sulfur dioxide can be oxidized in the atmosphere to particulate sulfates, the oxidation being abetted by oxidant smog conditions, which also lead to ozone formation and to particulate forms of nitric oxides. This oxidation can occur many kilometers downwind from the emission source, which accounts for the occurrence of acid rain in relatively pristine rural areas. The toxicity of particulate sulfates depends upon the physical and chemical attributes of the inhaled particles. Size is particularly important, with only smaller particles being inhaled deeply into the lung, a recognition that has led to a change in the U.S. particulate standard, which originally was based solely on the total weight of all airborne particles. This was changed to a standard that only measured particles with a median diameter of less than 10 microns; a new proposed standard will only measure particles with a median diameter less than 2.5 microns.

Also important to toxicity is the chemical form of the sulfur oxide; that is, particles that are more acidic or more soluble in the lung tend to be more toxic. Recent epidemiological studies have shown an association of morbidity and mortality with atmospheric levels of particles much lower than previously reported. The adverse health effects include increases in mortality of the elderly and those with preexisting heart and lung conditions, as well as increases in the incidence of respiratory disease (including asthma attacks), in children. These new findings are the basis for the more stringent particulate standard recently proposed by the U.S. Environmental Protection Agency,

which will require additional, costly control measures. This controversial proposed standard is complicated by the lack of sufficient clarity in the epidemiological and toxicological data. It has been difficult to separate out which chemical type or source of particles is most important, a situation that greatly complicates devising control strategies. Evidence suggests that adverse health effects are due to a gas-aerosol complex consisting of many air pollutant components, among which sulfur oxides play a significant role.

BERNARD D. GOLDSTEIN

(SEE ALSO: *Acid Rain; Airborne Particles; Air Quality Index; Ambient Air Quality [Air Pollution]; Atmosphere; Inhalable Particles [Sulfates]; Pollution; Smog [Air Pollution]; Total Suspended Particles [TSP]*)

BIBLIOGRAPHY

Bates, D. V., and Sizto, R. (1987). "Air Pollution and Hospital Admissions in Southern Ontario: The Summer Haze Effects." *Environmental Research* 43:317–331.

Dockery, D. W.; Pope, C. A.; Xu, X. et al. (1993). "An Association between Air Pollution and Mortality in Six U.S. Cities." *The New England Journal of Medicine* 329(24):1753–1759.

SUN EXPOSURE

See Sunscreens *and* Ultraviolet Radiation

SUNSCREENS

Sunscreens can be categorized as chemical sunscreens, physical blockers, or a combination of both. Chemical sunscreens contain UV-absorbing molecules that filter and limit the amount of ultraviolet (UV) radiation exposure at the skin. The most widely used chemical sunscreens in the United States contain para-aminobenzoic acid (PABA) or its derivatives, cinnamates, benzophenones, anthranilates, or salicylates. Some individuals develop allergic contact dermatitis to these compounds in sunscreens. These compounds predominantly absorb short-wave UV light (UVB) although chemicals that contain benzophenones and dibenzoylmethane (Parsol 1789) have also been developed recently to filter long-wave UV light (UVA).

Physical blockers utilize particles that reflect and scatter UV light. The more common physical blockers include titanium dioxide, zinc oxide, magnesium oxide, magnesium silicate (talc), kaolin, iron derivatives, barium sulfate, and red petrolatum. The older, opaque formulations had limited cosmetic appeal; newer blockers, however, have been combined with chemical sunscreens to give a more elegant appearance. In 1978, the Food and Drug Administration classified sunscreens as drugs and thus established standards for toxicity and quality control. The efficacy of sunscreens is measured in terms of the Sun Protection Factor (SPF). The SPF is defined as the ratio of the doses of artificial sunlight required to cause minimal skin redness with and without sunscreen. Individuals who burn easily, who are on photosensitizing medications, or who have light-sensitive diseases should diligently use sunscreens with SPFs between 15 and 30. Reapplication after prolonged sweating or swimming is recommended. Although sunscreens can provide protection against sunburns, its role in skin cancer protection remains a controversial issue. Some, but not all, studies have found an increased risk of cutaneous melanoma with sunscreen use. The most likely explanation is the individuals who use sunscreen tend to stay out longer in the sun, thereby increasing photocarcinogenesis.

HENSIN TSAO

(SEE ALSO: *Food and Drug Administration: Skin Cancer; Ultraviolet Radiation*)

SURGEON GENERAL

Since 1871, the Surgeon General of the United States has been the nation's leading spokesman on matters of public health. In that year, Dr. John Woodworth was appointed as the first supervising surgeon (later renamed surgeon general). Woodsworth established a cadre of medical personnel, called the Commissioned Corps, to administer the Marine Hospital System. This corps was established along military lines to be a mobile force of professionals subject to reassignment to meet the needs of the U.S. Public Health Service (PHS).

Prior to 1968, the surgeon general was the head of the PHS, and all program, administrative, and financial management authorities were supervised by the surgeon general, who reported directly to the secretary of health, education, and welfare. In 1968, pursuant to a reorganization plan issued by President Lyndon B. Johnson, the secretary delegated responsibility for the PHS to the assistant secretary for health. The position of surgeon general became that of a principal deputy to the assistant secretary for health, with responsibility for advising and assisting on professional medical matters. In addition, a primary role developed in which the surgeon general became the PHS spokesperson on certain health issues.

In 1987, the Office of the Surgeon General (OSG) was established as a staff office within the Office of the Assistant Secretary for Health at the department of United States Health and Human Services (USDHHS). Concomitant with this action, the surgeon general again became responsible for management of the personnel system for the Commissioned Corps, which is now a nearly 6,000-person cadre of public health professionals who are on call twenty-four hours a day, seven days a week for deployment in case of national health emergencies. (The surgeon general does not directly supervise all commissioned officers; most of whom work in the PHS or other federal agencies and report to agency line managers who may or may not be in the corps.) In carrying out these responsibilities, the surgeon general reports to the assistant secretary for health, who is the principal advisor to the secretary on public health and scientific issues.

Today, the surgeon general's duties also include the following:

- Providing leadership and management oversight for PHS Commissioned Corps involvement in departmental emergency preparedness and response activities.

- Protecting and advancing the health of the nation through educating the public; advocating for effective disease-prevention and health-promotion programs and activities; and providing a highly recognized symbol of national commitment to protecting and improving the public's health.

- Articulating scientifically based health-policy analysis and advice to the president and the secretary of health and human services on the full range of critical public health and health-system issues facing the nation.

- Providing leadership in promoting special departmental health initiatives, including tobacco and HIV (human immunodeficiency virus) prevention efforts, both domestically and internationally.

- Elevating the quality of public health practice in the professional disciplines through the advancement of appropriate standards and research priorities.

- Fulfilling statutory and customary departmental representational functions on a wide variety of federal boards and governing bodies of nonfederal health organizations, including the Board of Regents of the Uniformed Services University of the Health Sciences, the National Library of Medicine, the Armed Forces Institute of Pathology, the Association of Military Surgeons of the United States, and the American Medical Association.

DAVID SATCHER

(SEE ALSO: *United States Department of Health and Human Services [USDHHS]; United States Public Health Service [USPHS]*)

SURVEILLANCE

Health surveillance is the ongoing, systematic use of routinely collected health data to guide public health action in a timely fashion. Surveillance systems count health events (e.g., deaths from a disease or new cases of a disease) and health services (e.g., visits to a doctor, hospital admissions, vaccination, surgery, provision of prescription drugs) as they occur. Some systems collect information on risk factors related to various diseases, including foods, water supply, drug use, and travel, while other systems measure health behaviors (e.g., smoking, alcohol and drug use, nutrition) and environmental factors (e.g., air, food, or

water quality) independently of any health events associated with them

At the local level, health authorities receive detailed health information, often including names and addresses, because they have a mandate to provide services such as water testing, immunization, education, or referral to health agencies and services. As local authorities pass data to regional and national health departments, the data become less detailed. National data are usually anonymous. After collation, local, provincial, and national health departments tabulate, graph, and map cases in an effort to identify patterns of disease or risk factors, and to guide their actions. Routine reports normally include total case counts for specific time periods and populations, grouped by characteristics such as age, sex, or residence. Where population denominators are known, incidence rates of diseases are reported. With the wider availability of the Internet, many developed countries have implemented automated systems for the exchange, mapping, and analysis of surveillance data.

The first health surveillance activity is attributed to John Graunt, who first summarized causes of death in London in 1662. Today, surveillance exists for many infectious and chronic diseases, injuries, adverse reactions to drugs and vaccines, behavioral risk factors, and animal diseases. Most countries publish national data on a weekly or monthly basis for communicable diseases, and annually for causes of death. The World Health Organization (WHO) publishes causes of death and data on a few diseases on a global basis, using internationally accepted case definitions. In these ways, health surveillance provides health departments and related agencies with ongoing measurements of health of populations. Surveillance data have the same value to health departments and other interested groups (such as drug companies) as financial data do to commercial enterprises.

In the twentieth century, there were significant gains in global health as a result of immunization, made possible because routine surveillance of infectious diseases identified the important causes of childhood infections. Furthermore, continued surveillance after the introduction of vaccines has monitored the effectiveness of immunization programs. Perhaps the most impressive example of this was the WHO program for the elimination of smallpox. This program used intensive worldwide surveillance to identify all suspected cases of smallpox. Specialized teams then confirmed the diagnosis and instituted immunization programs in the population surrounding each case. Surveillance data were also used by many countries to justify elimination of routine smallpox vaccination programs as the number of new cases diminished. This program of public health action directed by surveillance led to the eventual elimination of this devastating disease in 1977.

JAMES HOCKIN

(SEE ALSO: *Assessment of Health Status; Epidemiology; Graunt, John; Information Technology; Internet; Notifiable Diseases; Registries; Surveys*)

BIBLIOGRAPHY

Teutsch, S. M., and Churchill, R. E., eds. (1999). *Principles and Practices of Public Health Surveillance.* New York: Oxford University Press.

World Health Organization (1992). *International Statistical Classification of Diseases and Related Health Problems* (ICD-10), 10th revision. Geneva: Author.

SURVEY RESEARCH METHODS

A survey is a method of collecting information about a human population. In a survey, direct (or indirect) contact is made with the units of the study (e.g., individuals, organizations, communities) by using systematic methods of measurement such as questionnaires and interviews.

Many surveys are conducted around the world each year. While the purpose, topics, and size of these surveys varies, similar steps are followed in the planning, development, and implementation of each. These steps are described below, with an example from an existing survey, the Youth Risk Behavior Survey, which is taken every two years by the Centers for Disease Control and Prevention (CDC).

Identify the Purpose. To determine the purpose of a survey, two questions must be asked: (1) what information is wanted or needed, and (2) where can this information be found. A researcher may want to describe a population or program,

plan a new program, or evaluate an existing one. Survey questions might address scientific issues (e.g., "What is the prevalence of cigarette smoking in the United States?"), social marketing issues (e.g., "How do adolescents respond to a new public service announcement?"), or broad public opinion (e.g., "Should schools teach sex education?").

Information may be obtained from a specific group (e.g., high school students in a city or women of childbearing age in a state) or a broader group (e.g., adults in the United States). The population of interest (unit of study) can be identified in a country, state, city, or local area. For example, the purpose of the Youth Risk Behavior Survey (YRBS) is to provide information on priority health-risk behaviors among students in grades nine through twelve throughout the United States.

Develop the Questionnaire. Once the purpose of the survey and population of interest are determined, a questionnaire must be developed. The questionnaire should be designed to provide the information being sought. It is important to determine which topics are essential, and previous questionnaires can be reviewed to identify questions that can be used for each topic. Reviewing previous questionnaires will also help determine the best format (e.g., multiple choice, open-ended) and question order. Questionnaires should start with easy questions rather than sensitive or hard to remember questions. If it is necessary to translate the questionnaire into multiple languages, the quality of the translation can be checked by having it "back-translated" into the original language.

Pilot testing the questionnaire using focus groups or small samples of respondents in the population of interest will determine the acceptability of the questionnaire to typical respondents and how long it takes them to complete it. A cognitive lab test of the questionnaire is also useful for determining problems with question comprehension, flow, and understanding of response options. Internal review board or other approvals should be obtained prior to survey administration.

The questionnaire for the YRBS contains eighty-six multiple-choice questions measuring six categories of behaviors: tobacco use, dietary behaviors, physical activity, alcohol and other drug use, sexual behaviors, and behaviors that may result in unintentional injuries or violence.

Identify the Setting. Surveys are usually conducted in households, schools, health care facilities, or worksites. It is important to pick the location where the population of interest can be accessed most easily and where it can be most fully represented. Because of the need to obtain information from students in grades nine through twelve, the YRBS is conducted in schools.

Identify the Mode. Within each setting, data can be obtained in three ways: through personal interviews, through self-administered questionnaires, or by reviewing records. Personal interviews are conducted by an interviewer who records the respondent's answers on a questionnaire or directly into a computer. Personal interviews are done in person or by telephone.

Self-administered questionnaires can be "paper and pencil" or electronic in nature. Paper and pencil questionnaires are brought to the respondent by a data collector or mailed to the respondent. Electronic questionnaires use computer-assisted self-interviewing technology. The questions are answered either on a lap top computer that is brought to the respondent or on a web site which the respondent can access. Record review is typically done on-site, but also can be done electronically if the records are stored on a web site or local area network.

Selecting the appropriate combination of setting and mode is important and should be based on the survey topic and population of interest, as well as answers to the following questions:

- Which approach will produce the most valid and reliable data? For youth, sensitive topics are often best measured in a school setting using a paper and pencil self-administered questionnaire.

- Which approach will yield the highest response rate? Household surveys often produce the highest response rate for general population surveys.

- How much will the survey cost to conduct? Household surveys are generally the most expensive.

- How long will the survey take to complete? Telephone surveys, such as public opinion polls, often are the fastest.

The YRBS uses a paper and pencil self-administered questionnaire, which is provided to students by a data collector.

Select the Sample. The quality of the sample often determines the quality of the data. Samples of convenience or volunteer samples produce data representative only of persons who participate in the survey. Scientifically selected samples can be representative of a larger population and are used to generalize findings to persons beyond those who participate in the survey.

To identify the appropriate sample for a survey, the survey topic, population of interest, setting, and mode must all be considered. Once this is done, the next step is to select an appropriate sampling frame from which to draw the sample. The sampling frame is a list of all the members of the population of interest. It should be as current and inclusive as possible. Existing databases may be available, or it may be necessary to construct a sampling frame. For the sample design, many possibilities exist (e.g., simple random sample, stratified sample, cluster sample). The YRBS uses a sampling frame of all public and private high schools in the United States and a three-stage cluster sample design to produce a nationally representative sample of students in grades nine through twelve.

Conduct the Fieldwork. Fieldwork begins with obtaining clearance or approval to conduct the survey. It may be necessary to seek clearance or approval not only from respondents (e.g., students), but also gatekeepers to the respondent (e.g., school administrators and parents). Data collection protocols must also be developed. The goal is to standardize data collection as much as possible to assure quality control throughout the fieldwork, to obtain a high response rate, and, often, to protect the privacy of respondents.

Selection of data collectors or field staff is also important. It is best to select persons appropriate for the content of the survey and the demographic characteristics of the population of interest (e.g., female interviewers for surveys on reproductive health issues among women). Formal training of data collectors or field staff will help them become familiar with the questionnaire format, content, mode of data collection, data collection protocol, and quality control procedures.

Before the YRBS is conducted, clearance is obtained from school administrators and parents. Then, trained data collectors are sent to each school to collect data according to the survey protocol. Because of the sensitive nature of the questionnaire, special procedures are used to protect student privacy.

Enter, Edit, and Prepare Data for Analysis. Since the 1980s, data entry has become easier due to advances in electronic data input. Previously, most survey data were entered manually by key punching and then reentered to assure accuracy. Today, most survey data collected using questionnaires are scanned electronically into a data set. Data collected via computer-assisted interviewing are automatically entered into a data set. Once entered, the data are edited for out-of-range responses, simple consistency, and logic errors. Then the sample is weighted to adjust for nonresponse, varying probabilities of selection, and sample characteristics. Weighting is necessary to ensure that the data are representative of the entire population of interest.

YRBS questionnaire booklets are scanned to produce the data file. Basic out-of-range and consistency edits are run and a weighting factor is applied to each student record to adjust for nonresponse and for varying probabilities of selection.

Conduct Analyses. Analyses are done using a software package that incorporates the sample design. Several software packages have been developed to analyze complex survey data (e.g., STATA, SUDAAN, and Westvar). Without these packages, accurate standard errors cannot be produced. Analyses are used to answer the questions that were originally developed to identify the purpose and population of interest for the survey. They should be kept as simple as possible to enhance the usefulness of the data for multiple audiences. To analyze YRBS data, SAS and SUDAAN are used to compute prevalence estimates and 95 percent confidence intervals for priority health risk behaviors among high school students.

Write and Disseminate Reports. Survey data are often used to improve policies and programs. Consequently, key decision makers need to be able to access and understand the data. In addition to formal research papers, other methods can be used to share survey results, such as press releases, fact sheets or pamphlets, or Internet materials. If the needs and interests of the target audience are considered, it will enhance the likelihood they will act on the results. YRBS data are disseminated in MMWR Surveillance Summaries, fact sheets, a CD-Rom (YOUTH '99), on the CDC web site (at http://www.cdc.gov/nccdphp/dash/yrbs), and in numerous professional journals.

CHARLES W. WARREN
LAURA KANN

(SEE ALSO: *Behavioral Risk Factor Surveillance System; Census; Cohort Study; Data Sources and Collection Methods; National Health Surveys; Sampling; Statistics for Public Health; Surveillance; Surveys*)

BIBLIOGRAPHY

Centers for Disease Control and Prevention (2000). *Youth Risk Behavior Surveillance System–At-A-Glance.* Atlanta, GA: Author.

—— (2000). "CDC Surveillance Summaries, June 9, 2000." *Morbidity and Mortality Weekly Report* 49(SS-5)-1–96.

SURVEYS

The word "survey" comes from the Latin *sur* (over) and *videre* (to see), and it eventually came to mean a general or comprehensive view of anything. Studies that involve the systematic collection of data about populations are usually called surveys. This is especially true when they are concerned with large or widely dispersed groups of people. When they deal with only a fraction of a total population—a fraction representative of the total—they are called sample surveys. The term "sample survey" should ideally be used only if the part of the population studied is selected by accepted statistical methods.

Surveys can be classified broadly into two types—descriptive and analytical. In a descriptive survey the objective is simply to obtain certain information about large groups. In an analytical survey, comparisons are made between different subgroups of the population in order to discover whether differences exist among them that may enable researchers to form or verify hypotheses about the forces at work in the population.

Surveys differ in terms of purpose, subject matter, coverage, and source of information. In the field of epidemiology, surveys have been used to study the history of the health of populations, diagnose community health, study the working of health services, complete the clinical history of chronic diseases, search for the cause of health and disease, contribute to the formation of health care policy, and to evaluate the effects of different approaches to the organization of health services. More recently, health-survey data have been identified as a key resource for the development of health indicators, such as alcohol consumption and the prevalence of smoking, in the twenty-first century. The Health for All initiative of the World Health Organization is a policy that can be translated into three operational goals: increase in life expectancy and sustainable life; improved equity in health between and within countries; and access for all to sustainable health systems. Efforts have been made to promote standards for international comparability of such health indicators.

WAYNE MILLAR

(SEE ALSO: *National Health Surveys; Sampling; Survey Research Methods*)

BIBLIOGRAPHY

Bradburn, N. M., and Sudman, S. (1988). *Polls and Surveys–Understanding What They Tell Us.* San Francisco: Jossey-Bass Publishers.

Festinger, L., and Katz, D., eds. (1966). *Research Methods in the Behavioral Sciences.* New York: Holt, Rinehart and Winston.

Morris, J. N. (1975). *Uses of Epidemiology,* 3rd edition. London: Churchill Livingston.

Moser, C. A., and Kalton, G. (1989). *Survey Methods in Social Investigation,* 2nd edition. Aldershot, UK: Gower Publishing Company.

SUSTAINABLE DEVELOPMENT

The term "sustainable development" was popularized in 1987 by the World Commission on Environment and Development. It refers to a systematic approach to achieving human development in a way that sustains planetary resources, based on the recognition that human consumption is occurring at a rate that is beyond Earth's capacity to support it. Population growth and the developmental pressures spawned by an unequal distribution of wealth are two major driving forces that are altering the planet in ways that threaten the long-term health of humans and other species on the planet.

Human health is dependent on the healthy functioning of the earth's ecosystem. These systems would be overwhelmed if all of the earth's inhabitants were to match the consumption patterns of wealthier nations. Sustainable development requires alterations in the lifestyle of the wealthy to live within the carrying capacity of the environment. To achieve sustainability there is a need for holistic responses to global issues such as urbanization and energy overconsumption, and there is a need for better measures of ecological and social sustainability. While sustainable development is a prerequisite for the long-term health of humans, it will not be possible to achieve sustainability in much of the world unless the toll of major health scourges, such as malaria and HIV (human immunodeficiency virus) infection, is significantly reduced.

BERNARD D. GOLDSTEIN

(SEE ALSO: *Atmosphere; Brownfields; Carson, Rachel; Climate Change and Human Health; Ecosystems; Environmental Justice; Environmental Movement; Equity and Resource Allocation; International Health; Pollution; Urban Health; Urban Sprawl*)

BIBLIOGRAPHY

McMichael, A. J.; Smith, K. R.; and Corvalan, C. F. (2000). "The Sustainability Transition: A New Challenge." *Bulletin of the World Health Organization* 78(9):1067.

McMichael, A. J., and Powles, J. W. P. (1999). "Human Numbers, Environment, Sustainability, and Health." *British Medical Journal* 319:977–980.

United Nations Conference on Environment and Development (1992). *Rio Declaration on Environment and Development.* Nairobi: United Nations Environment Programme.

SUSTAINABLE HEALTH

The concept of health as a sustainable state became part of the health lexicon in the last two decades of the twentieth century. It is related to the idea of environmental sustainability and makes explicit the notion that humans and other living creatures on earth are interdependent. If human affairs are conducted in such a way as to sustain life-supporting ecosystems in a stable state of equilibrium, then humans will survive and flourish. If, however, a local, regional, or global ecosystem is degraded beyond the point where it is sustainable, then the health and survival of humans in that ecosystem cannot be sustained. As Maurice King, a research fellow at the University of Leeds, explained, the population is then caught in a demographic trap. Without external food aid or out-migration, people in such an ecosystem will starve. Sometimes a nation, tribe, or ethnic group that is demographically trapped will attempt to fight its way out. The evidence supporting a direct causal relationship between environmental stress and violent armed conflict has been documented by Thomas Homer-Dixon. The ultimate cause of such conflict is an imbalance between the number of people and the resources that are available to sustain them.

Sometimes it is difficult to say which comes first, environmental (i.e., ecosystem) pressure or population pressure. A previously stable and sustainable ecosystem may be irretrievably changed by natural forces such as a volcanic eruption, but human activity and population pressure are the most common causes. Human activities may be unwise agricultural practices—like over-grazing a savannah with sparse rainfall, excessive irrigation that alters the soil chemistry, or destruction of food-producing land for strip mining or hydroelectric dam development—or warfare that destroys what had previously been a stable agricultural ecosystem or depletes arable land of the workforce needed to maintain it. The end result is a vicious cycle; unsustainable pressure on life-supporting ecosystems and a progressively deteriorating state of population health.

Sustainable health is often linked to sustainable population growth (or a steady-state population). In the second half of the twentieth century, some countries in Africa and South Asia experienced a rate of population growth that exceeded the capacity of regional and local ecosystems to sustain them. In the Sahel, an arid zone in northwestern Africa, a sequence of droughts and occasional flash floods led to overgrazing on a fragile savannah that was unsuitable for any form of agricultural development to begin with. As a result, the region became a desert and the people began to starve. Their predicament was eased by extensive out-migration, but even so, in the intermittent crises of severe food shortages and regional famines in which many died, they were dependent upon food aid from other parts of the world.

Human communities require several kinds of resources to survive in a healthy state. The absolute essentials are secure and safe water, food, and shelter. Other factors that help create sustainable health include peace, freedom from oppression, protection from infection, secure work, and economic stability. To achieve these states, people (especially girls and women) require the ability to control their own destiny, including their reproductive capacity and the ability to care adequately for themselves and for their dependent infants and others unable to take care of themselves. This ability in turn requires insight and understanding that are acquired through education. Literacy, therefore, is another essential prerequisite for sustainable health. Early in the twenty-first century, all these prerequisites are lacking in some parts of the world, especially in several countries in sub-Saharan Africa, where health is emphatically not sustainable. In these countries, the environment is severely stressed and is being further degraded by ill-judged agricultural practices and destructive extraction of mineral resources such as diamonds, as well as a lack of concern for indigenous fauna and flora, leading to catastrophic loss of biodiversity. Increasing numbers of children and young adults are illiterate, many having spent their entire lives engaged in armed conflict. The HIV/AIDS (human immunodeficiency virus/acquired immunodeficiency syndrome) epidemic is cutting a terrible swath through the population, creating a generation of orphans who are being raised by aging and infirm grandparents. Malaria kills more than a million people every year in Africa, mostly children. Manifestly, health is not sustainable in much of the African continent, south of the Sahara, and the situation is getting worse.

In this setting, several kinds of action are urgently required to achieve sustainable health. Violent armed conflicts must be ended, which requires peace enforcement—a stage beyond peacekeeping, which has in the past been the main focus of United Nations peacekeeping forces. Populations must be educated so they gain an understanding of their situation and what must be done to improve it. Massive public health endeavors are required to control the HIV/AIDS pandemic, to control malaria and other tropical infectious diseases, and, with almost equal urgency, to control infectious and nutritional deficiency diseases, especially among children. Agricultural and animal husbandry practices must be made compatible with the environment, the climate, the topography, and the culture. Political stability must be achieved, and the infrastructure of organized urban and rural societies (communications, banking, a legal framework, etc.) must be established. The above catalogue is incomplete, but enough has been outlined to emphasize the holistic nature of sustainable health.

In the industrial nations of Western Europe, North America, Japan, and Oceania—and those nations that are in the process of industrializing (India, Thailand, Brazil)—sustainable health is closer to being achieved, but it is threatened by forces as diverse as religious fundamentalism, which is often associated with obscurantism (opposition to the spread of knowledge), and the subversion of democratic institutions by special interest groups. The gap between rich and poor grows ever wider; and while good health may be sustainable among those who are well off enough to afford good housing and medical care, the increasing proportion of people who are not economically secure face enormous obstacles to good health. In Eastern Europe and the former Soviet Union, some industrial environments are, as C. Hertzman has shown, a grave danger to health, especially women's reproductive health and child health. If the dire predictions of the Intergovernmental Panel on Climate Change are correct, the entire earth is in a precarious state that puts in doubt the long-term sustainability of all life.

JOHN M. LAST

(SEE ALSO: *Carrying Capacity; Climate Change and Human Health; Economics of Health; Ecosystems; Environmental Determinants of Health; Famine; Health; Health Maintenance; Inequalities in Health; War*)

BIBLIOGRAPHY

Hertzman, C. (1995). *Environment and Health in Central and Eastern Europe; A Report for the Environmental Action Programme for Central and Eastern Europe.* Washington, DC: World Bank.

Homer-Dixon, T. F.; Boutwell, J. H.; and Rathjens, G. W. (1993). "Environmental Stress and Violent Conflict." *Scientific American* 268:38–45.

King, M. (1990). "Health as a Sustainable State." *Lancet* 336:664–667.

McMichael, A. J.; Haines, A.; and Kovats, S. (1996). *Climate Change and Human Health.* Geneva: World Health Organization.

SYDENHAM, THOMAS

Thomas Sydenham (1624–1689) is often referred to as the English Hippocrates because of the emphasis, in his medical practice and teachings, of the importance of bedside observation. His writings, controversial in his day, condemned theorizing in medicine and taught that the understanding of disease and its treatment should be based on observation of the evolution of signs and symptoms in groups of patients over time, and on the observed responses of patients to medicines and treatments. His importance in public health stems principally from his interest in classifying febrile diseases and his study of epidemic patterns of fevers in London over many years. He concluded that febrile diseases were not merely idiosyncratic humoral responses to environmental stimuli, but distinct species of disease whose expression was greatly dependent on atmospheric and seasonal influences.

In treatment, Sydenham avoided the heavy use of drugs characteristic of his time, challenged prevailing approaches to the treatment of smallpox, and was a strong advocate of physical exercise and diet as therapy. He was perhaps the first influential physician to embrace Peruvian bark (quinine) in the treatment of ague (malaria), and one of the first to treat anemia with iron. In spite of his opposition to academic theorizing and experimental approaches in medicine, he was close to many of English scientists of the time, including Robert Boyle, Christopher Wren, Robert Hooke, and philosopher John Locke (also a physician), who was a devoted student of his medical teachings.

Sydenham's unconventional, even revolutionary, approach to medicine cannot easily be divorced from his involvement in the seventeenth-century Puritan rebellion against the British crown. The Sydenham family, Dorsetshire landowners, were strong supporters of Parliament and Cromwell in the English civil war of the 1640s. All five Sydenham brothers (Thomas was the youngest) and their father served as officers in Cromwell's rebel army. Thomas was wounded, two of his brothers were killed, their mother was murdered by Royalist troops, and the eldest brother, William, became a leading figure in Cromwell's protectorate. Sydenham's unpopularity with leading physicians during the period of Restoration in which he practiced may in part have been the consequence of his political history, as well as his lack of a full classical education, attributable to the interruption of his Oxford education by military service. His two major works, *Methodis Curandis Febres* (1666) and *Observationes Medicae* (1676), are thought to have been written in English and translated by a Latin scholar for publication.

NIGEL PANETH

BIBLIOGRAPHY

Dewhurst, K. (1966). *Dr. Thomas Sydenham (1624–1689): His Life and Original Writings.* London: Wellcome Historical Medical Library.

SYDENSTRICKER, EDGAR

Edgar Sydenstricker (1881–1936) was a pioneer public health statistician, an eloquent advocate of measures aimed at enhancing the health of the American people, and an inspiring teacher who impressed on his students the importance of recognizing their social responsibility to attack and solve intractable public health problems. He was born in Shanghai, China, the son of American Presbyterian missionary parents, and educated at Fredericksburg College in Virginia. After working as a journalist for two years, he then studied political economy at the University of Chicago before commencing a lifetime of public health service, concentrating on the problems of the poor and the underprivileged.

Sydenstricker worked in the United States Public Health Service (PHS), for the League of Nations, and for the Milbank Memorial Fund. In

the PHS he worked initially with Joseph Goldberger on studies of pellagra, then in 1920 he was appointed chief of the Office of Statistical Investigations. In this office, he initiated many investigations, the best known of which was the Hagerstown Morbidity Survey, which began in 1921. This could be regarded as a precursor of the U.S. National Health Survey. Related surveys followed, using the same methods of intermittent or continuous observation, including surveys on the costs of medical care. In collaboration with the Metropolitan Life Insurance Company, he produced detailed statistical analysis of the information contained in the medical examination records of policy holders. In 1923, Sydenstricker developed some of these studies at an international level for the League of Nations while on leave from the PHS. During the Great Depression, he conducted studies of the effects of poverty and deprivation on health. He died suddenly at age fifty-four of a cerebral hemorrhage.

JOHN M. LAST

(SEE ALSO: *Goldberger, Joseph; United States Public Health Service [USPHS]*)

BIBLIOGRAPHY

Kasius, R. V., ed. (1974). *The Challenge of Facts: Selected Public Health Papers of Edgar Sydenstricker.* New York: Milbank Memorial Fund.

SYPHILIS

Syphilis is a sexually transmitted disease (STD) caused by *Treponema pallidum*, a spirochete that can be transmitted during vaginal, anal, or oral sex. An estimated 70,000 syphilis cases occur in the United States annually.

Without treatment, syphilis in adults progresses through four stages: primary, secondary, latent, and tertiary. Persons with syphilis are most infectious during the primary and secondary stages. Primary syphilis is marked by an infectious sore (chancre) that resolves on its own. Without treatment, syphilis bacteria spread through the bloodstream and lead to the secondary stage, which is characterized by a skin rash and systemic symptoms. These symptoms can come and go over one to two years, during which an infected person can infect others. If untreated, the infection progresses to a latent stage. Symptoms disappear, and the disease is no longer infectious, but the bacteria remain in the body and can damage vital organs. In about a third of untreated persons, the results of the internal damage show up years later in the tertiary stage. Symptoms include paralysis, blindness, dementia, impotence, joint damage, heart problems, tumors, and deep sores. The damage can be serious enough to cause death. An untreated pregnant woman in an infectious stage of syphilis can pass the infection to her developing fetus.

Syphilis bacteria can be detected by laboratory examination of material from infectious sores. A safe, accurate, and inexpensive blood screening test is also available. Syphilis is treatable with penicillin. Persons who engage in sexual behaviors that place them at risk of STDs should use latex or polyurethane condoms every time they have sex and limit the number of sex partners. Pregnant women should be screened for syphilis. Infected persons should notify all sex partners so they can receive treatment.

ALLISON L. GREENSPAN
JOEL R. GREENSPAN

(SEE ALSO: *Sexually Transmitted Diseases*)

BIBLIOGRAPHY

Centers for Disease Control and Prevention (1998). "1998 Guidelines for Treatment of Sexually Transmitted Diseases." *Morbidity and Mortality Weekly Report* 47(RR-1):28–41.

Sparling, P. F. (1999). "Natural History of Syphilis." In *Sexually Transmitted Diseases,* 3rd edition. eds. K. Holmes, P. Mardh, P. Sparling et al. New York: McGraw-Hill.

SYSTEMS THINKING

Systems thinking is a way of looking at organizations that emphasizes the interconnections between parts of an organization and external environments. It is also a method for solving organizational problems and helping organizations change. Systems thinking is especially appropriate in the field of public health because public health managers and leaders work in large, complex organizations whose success depends upon the cooperation of other organizations and institutions. As applied to organizations, systems thinking was made popular by Peter Senge's 1994 book, *The Fifth Discipline*; but a systems approach is also the basis of theories in many fields, from biology to psychology.

The central concepts in systems thinking are interconnections, feedback, and time delays. Systems thinking encourages managers to identify the larger pattern of interconnections, or causal links, of which problems are a part. Thus, a problem to solve is seen as a symptom of an underlying pattern. Feedback refers to the kind of cause-and-effect relationship found among system elements. Systems thinking proponents identify two types of cause-and-effect relationships, reinforcing and balancing relations. An example of a reinforcing relationship is when, as staff workload increases, so also does job dissatisfaction, which leads to absenteeism, which in turn leads to even higher workloads. An example of a balancing relation is the short–term solution of rewarding individual high performers on the staff. The effect seems to be that morale improves and absenteeism goes down. The concept of time delays must be factored in, however, for in the long run, individual rewards pit staff members against each other, lowering morale and aggravating the underlying problem, which in this case might be excessive workloads and lack of team development.

Interorganizational relations also exhibit system properties. For example, public health managers often rely on coalitions of citizens and local organizations to achieve community health goals. Systems thinking directs the public health manager's attention to the pattern of interconnections between organizations and citizen groups that lead to the success, or failure, of initiatives.

JOHN C. LAMMERS

(SEE ALSO: *Community Organization; Leadership; Planning for Public Health*)

BIBLIOGRAPHY

Kauffman, D. L. (1980). *Systems One: An Introduction to Systems Thinking.* Minneapolis, MN: S. A. Carlton.

Senge, P. M. et al. (1994). *The Fifth Discipline Fieldbook: Strategies and Tools for Building a Learning Organization.* New York: Doubleday.

T

TAMOXIFEN

Tamoxifen, a selective estrogen-receptor modulator, is an oral medication exhibiting both estrogen agonist and antagonist effects. Tamoxifen can be used to treat advanced breast cancer, to decrease the risk of recurrence of early-stage breast cancer, and for breast cancer prevention. Patients with an early-stage breast cancer with expression of the estrogen or progesterone receptors, or for whom no receptor result is known, benefit from five years of tamoxifen treatment. This treatment has been shown to decrease the annual risk of recurrence of breast cancer, and to decrease the risk of contralateral breast cancer by 47 percent. Tamoxifen has been studied as breast cancer prevention in patients at elevated risk of developing breast cancer (five-year risk of 1.66% or higher), decreasing the chance of developing an invasive or noninvasive breast cancer by approximately 50 percent. Newer antiestrogens, such as raloxifene, may have fewer side effects and similar effectiveness. Studies are underway to determine their effectiveness.

CLIFFORD HUDIS
ARTI HURRIA

(SEE ALSO: *Breast Cancer; Breast Cancer Screening; Preventive Medicine*)

BIBLIOGRAPHY

Osborne, C. K. (1998). "Tamoxifen in the Treatment of Breast Cancer." *New England Journal of Medicine* 339:1609–1618.

TAXATION ON TOBACCO

During the final third of the twentieth century, taxes imposed on tobacco products, especially cigarettes, became a principal weapon in the war against tobacco-produced disease. A series of studies by economists demonstrated convincingly that increases in cigarette prices, driven by increases in cigarette taxes, reduced cigarette smoking. In particular, several studies indicated that tax-induced price increases were particularly effective in discouraging smoking by young people. Students of tobacco-control policy became convinced that taxation was one of the most effective tools available to policy makers to reduce smoking and hence its enormous toll on human health.

EXCISE TAXES

Each of the fifty U.S. states, the ten provinces of Canada, and their federal governments, as well as most countries throughout the world, impose product-specific taxes on cigarettes and, less frequently, on other tobacco products. Often called excise taxes, product-specific taxes are used sparingly by most governments. Rather, when they tax products at all, they typically do so with a general tax applied to all products, called sales taxes in the United States. Excise taxes are applied most frequently to three specific types of products: tobacco products, alcoholic beverages (wine, beer, and spirits), and gasoline.

Excise taxes are often motivated by the expectation that they will yield sizable revenues to governmental units, primarily because consumer demand for such products is relatively insensitive to their price. Alternatively (or sometimes concurrently), excise taxes are motivated by legislators' desire to reduce consumption of products deemed by society to be undesirable. Thus, in the case of cigarettes and alcoholic beverages, excise taxes are sometimes referred to as "sin taxes."

EFFECTS OF CIGARETTE TAXES

Historically, cigarette excise taxation has been motivated by both concerns. The demand for cigarettes is only modestly responsive to price changes. The consensus estimate is that, in developed countries, for every 10 percent increase in price, the quantity of cigarettes demanded by consumers will fall by about 4 percent. When one considers, however, that cigarette taxes constitute only a fraction of total cigarette price, one realizes that large increases in cigarette tax rates can simultaneously generate significant increases in governmental revenues and a substantial decrease in smoking. Thus, tobacco taxation gives governments the opportunity to do well in terms of enriching their treasuries while improving public health.

Studies suggest that smoking by young people is especially sensitive to cigarette price increases. In general, the older the age group considered, the less price responsive it appears to be. This makes considerable intuitive sense because, compared to younger smokers, older smokers tend to be more addicted and to have more disposable income to spend on cigarettes. The general consensus is that youth are approximately twice as price responsive as adults. Thus, a 10 percent increase in cigarette price should decrease smoking by youth by about 8 percent. As a consequence, many legislators and public health policy makers have called for increased cigarette taxation as a means of discouraging youth smoking.

By the end of the twentieth century, virtually all comprehensive tobacco control plans have included substantial increases in tobacco taxes as a fundamental component. Such plans call for increases in cigarette taxes as a means of both discouraging children from smoking and raising funds to pay for other tobacco control measures, such an antismoking education. In addition to being an effective deterrent to youth smoking, cigarette taxation offers an attractive political feature: Proposed cigarette tax increases are often popular with voters, including many smokers, especially when the revenues generated by the tax increases are directed toward prevention of youth smoking.

LIMITATIONS

Tobacco taxation is not devoid of controversy, however. Whenever a tobacco tax increase is proposed, opponents argue that the tax increase will be regressive, imposing a larger financial burden on the poor than on the rich. This is especially true because larger proportions of the poor population smoke than of the rich. The more highly educated population, which tends to be more affluent as well, has quit smoking in dramatic numbers in response to health education messages concerning the dangers of smoking.

Although the regressivity argument merits serious consideration, its importance should not be exaggerated. The impact is blunted by the fact that low-income smokers are more price responsive than high-income smokers, thus giving up smoking—and its concomitant impact on disease— in greater proportions than is the case among the rich. In public health circles, this progressively distributed health benefit is viewed as ample justification to promote increased tobacco taxation wherever and whenever possible. As a tool for tobacco control, substantial taxation may have no peer.

KENNETH E. WARNER

(SEE ALSO: *Enabling Factors; Smuggling Tobacco; Tobacco Control*)

BIBLIOGRAPHY

Chaloupka, F. J., and Warner, K. E. (2000). "The Economics of Smoking." In *Handbook of Health Economics,* eds. A. J. Culyer and J. P. Newhouse. Amsterdam: Elsevier Science.

Grossman, M., and Chaloupka, F. J. (1997). "Cigarette Taxes: The Straw to Break the Camel's Back." *Public Health Reports* 112(4):290–297.

Warner, K. E.; Chaloupka, F. J.; Cook, P. J.; Manning, W. G.; Newhouse, J. P.; Novotny, T. E.; Schelling, T. C.; and Townsend, J. (1995). "Criteria for Determining an Optimal Cigarette Tax: The Economist's Perspective." *Tobacco Control* 4(4):380–386.

TEENAGE PREGNANCY

In the United States, 900,000 adolescents (fifteen- to nineteen-year-olds) became pregnant in 1996. While this was 15 percent lower than in 1994, it is still higher than any other developed country. There are twice as many teenage pregnancies in the United States each year as there are in England, Wales, or Canada, and eight times as many as in Japan. These figures include live births (accounting for approximately half of the total of 900,000), induced abortions, and fetal losses due to miscarriages and still births.

In 1996, the pregnancy rate was twice as high among non-Hispanic black and Hispanic teens as among non-Hispanic white teens. By 2003, the under-18 Hispanic and non-Hispanic black population will be greater than 50 percent of the adolescent population. These figures are important in planning pregnancy-prevention programs.

Teen pregnancy is one serious consequence of early initiation of sexual activity. Other serious consequences include an increased likelihood of late or no prenatal care, unattended births, reduced educational attainment, and decreased employment opportunities. Infants of teenage mothers are at greater risk of low birth weight and increased infant mortality. Thirteen percent of infants born to 15 year olds have a low birth weight, compared to 7 percent of infants born to mothers in their twenties. Infants of mothers 13 to 14 years old have an infant mortality rate of 17 per 1000 live births, compared to the rate of 10 per 1000 live births for those 15 to 19 years old, and a rate of only 4.5 per 1000 live births for all mothers in the United States. Children of teenage mothers are more likely to perform poorly in school, more likely to drop out of school, and less likely to attend college. Overall problems related to teen pregnancies cost taxpayers an estimated $7 billion per year.

After three decades of steady increases, the proportion of teenagers 15 to 19 years old who were sexually active decreased by 50 percent during the mid 1990s. In addition, condom use at first intercourse increased from 18 percent in 1975 to 54 percent in 1995.

Socioeconomic factors and limited life options, rather than ethnic or cultural background, place many youth at higher risk for unintended pregnancy. Early attempts at preventing teen pregnancies often ignored the complex relationship between development, environment, and behavior. Neither those programs that focus on increasing knowledge, nor abstinence-only programs have been effective in reducing the rate of unintended pregnancies. Adolescent behaviors are shaped by the desire to broaden horizons, interact with peers, or try out adult roles and behaviors. If early sexual behavior is the only perceived option to achieve these objectives, teens may well choose it.

As our society moves forward, a more comprehensive approach to reducing adolescent pregnancy is needed. Many risk behaviors, including early and unprotected intercourse, are linked and share common motivations. Programs designed to prevent pregnancy need to address these other behaviors as well. A variety of life choices need to be available for teens, and programs need to address real economic barriers if the unintended teen pregnancy rate in the United States is to be reduced.

JAMES J. FITZGIBBON

(SEE ALSO: *Abortion; Condoms; Ethnicity and Health; Family Planning Behavior; Infant Health; Infant Mortality Rate; Maternal and Child Health; Perinatology; Pregnancy; Prenatal Care*)

BIBLIOGRAPHY

Brindis, C. (1999). "Building for the Future: Adolescent Pregnancy Prevention." *Journal of JAMWA* 54(3):129–132.

Hoffman, S. (1998). "Teenage Childbearing Is Not So Bad After All, or Is It? A Review of the New Literature." *Family Planning Perspectives* 30(5):236–239.

MacKay, A. P.; Fingerhut, L. A.; and Duran, C. R. (2000). Adolescent Health Chartbook. Hyattsville, MD: National Center for Health Statistics.

Mainard, R. A. (1996). *Kids Having Kids: Robinwood Foundation Special Report on the Cost of Adolescent Childbearing.* New York: Robinwood Foundation.

TEENAGE SMOKING

See Adolescent Smoking *and* Smoking Behavior

TEENAGE VIOLENCE

See Adolescent Violence

TEETH

See Oral Health

TERATOGENS

Teratogens are those chemicals that lead to structural and/or functional birth defects. The effects of teratogenic compounds are time dependent as well as dose dependent. Time dependency is a function of the differences in development of particular organs and systems during pregnancy. The original definition of teratogens was narrow and referred to those chemicals, drugs, and diseases that led to structural and functional abnormalities observed in early life. The classic therapeutic human teratogen is thalidomide. This drug, a sedative developed in the late 1950s and early 1960s, induced serious birth defects in babies whose mothers had taken the drug during the critical period of organogenesis of the limbs (second trimester of pregnancy). The babies were born with several defects, including missing or stumped limbs (phocomelia), cleft palate and lip, and other defects. This abnormality affected over 10,000 babies worldwide and led to the testing of all new drugs (and eventually some pesticides and commodity chemicals) for teratogenic potential. Several maternal diseases, such as German measles, hypothyroidism, and syphilis, to name a few, are teratogenic.

The definition of a teratogen has been expanded as knowledge increases about the mechanism of action of additional chemicals. A broader definition of a teratogen now encompasses defects other than simply structural changes and includes the transplacental carcinogen, diethylstilbestrol.

Of great import are the retinoic acid derivatives, such as 13-cis-retinoic acid, that remain teratogenic years after a woman has taken the drug. This type of teratogen is very difficult to predict from animal studies and the scientific community must rely on mechanistic studies to assess risk.

Since the central nervous system, including the brain, completes development after birth, late pregnancy exposure to many toxicants can have serious adverse effects on the developing nervous system. Many of the heavy metals affect these systems and have been shown to be very teratogenic. The classic example is methylmercury, which induces a multitude of defects, the most devastating of which are those of the central nervous system.

Hence, teratogens are any class of xenobiotics that induce structural or functional changes in offspring when consumed by the mother during or before pregnancy.

MICHAEL GALLO

(SEE ALSO: *Congenital Anomalies; Mercury; Pregnancy*)

TERRORISM

Terrorism refers here to the public health consequences and the methods for prevention of the purposeful use of violence or threats of violence by groups or individuals in order to serve political or personal agendas. This article does not include what has been termed "state terrorism," the use of violence by a nation-state without clear necessity for self-defense and without the authorization of the United Nations.

EXAMPLES OF TERRORISM

Use or threat of use of violence has long caused concern among those responsible for public health. Examples include indiscriminate violence, such as the 1993 bombing of the World Trade Center in New York City and the 1995 bombing of the Federal Building in Oklahoma City, and targeted violence, such as attacks on facilities for the termination of pregnancy or on those who work in such facilities. The primary responsibility for response to the health consequences of such violence has resided largely in emergency medical services and the primary responsibility for prevention in agencies concerned with public order and safety, such as the police and the Federal Bureau of Investigation.

Recent instances of use or threatened use of biological or chemical agents in terrorism have raised interest in the role of public health agencies and public health personnel in primary or secondary prevention. Documented episodes, although extremely rare, have been dramatic. In Japan, the chemical warfare agent Sarin was released by the Aum Shinrikyo cult in Matsumoto in 1994 and in the Tokyo subway in 1995. In 1984, an Oregon cult allegedly contaminated salad bars with a biological agent, salmonella. These episodes, and recent hoaxes concerning anthrax release, have led to well publicized, costly responses by public health and public safety officials. Chemical terrorism could include the purposeful contamination of water and food supplies or the aerosolization of toxicants within enclosed public spaces. Biological terrorist actions could include purposeful contamination with infectious materials, as well as the purposeful release of insects or other vectors infected with a transmissible disease.

AVAILABILITY OF CHEMICAL AND BIOLOGICAL WEAPONS

Underlying concern about bioterrorism is the long history of use of chemical and biological weapons (CBW) in war. Since World War II, worldwide military forces have built up major stockpiles of such weapons and tested them at a number of sites around the world. Although the Biological Weapons Convention (BWC) and the Chemical Weapons Convention (CWC) outlawed the development, production, stockpiling, and transfer of these weapons, large stockpiles of chemical weapons still await destruction in several nations, and it is alleged that stockpiles of biological weapons are still maintained in a few nations. Although the technical knowledge and materials needed to produce CBW are relatively available, the ability to "weaponize" and target these materials remains extremely limited. The risk of their use appears to be small, but any use constitutes a threat to public health.

TYPES OF BIOLOGICAL AGENTS

There are at least seventy types of bacteria, viruses, rickettsiae, and fungi that can be weaponized, including tularemia, anthrax, Q fever, epidemic typhus, smallpox, brucellosis, Venezuelan equine encephalitis, botulinum toxin, dengue fever, Russian spring-summer encephalitis, Lassa fever,

Marburg, Ebola, Bolivian hemorrhagic fever (Machupo), and Argentinean hemorrhagic fever (Junin). Antibiotic resistant strains of anthrax, plague, tularemia, and glanders have allegedly been developed. Viruses and toxins can be genetically altered to heighten their infectiousness, permitting the development of pathogens capable of overcoming existing vaccines. It is estimated that no more than 20 to 30 percent of the diseases the aforementioned agents cause can be effectively treated.

RECENT HISTORY OF CONTROL

In 1994 U.S. president Bill Clinton issued an Executive Order asserting that the potential use of nuclear, biological and chemical weapons "by terrorist groups or rogue states" represents "an unusual and extraordinary threat to the national security, foreign policy and economy of the United States." This Order, renewed annually, makes it illegal for anyone in the United States to help anyone to acquire, design, produce, or stockpile CBW. The Order was amended in 1998 to include penalties for trafficking in equipment that could indirectly contribute to a foreign biological warfare program.

In 1995 President Clinton announced a new policy against "superterrorism"—terrorism involving weapons of mass destruction. The Departments of Defense, Energy, and State, together with the FBI and the CIA, were to oversee a wide network of military and civilian agencies, including the Centers for Disease Control and Prevention, dedicated to identifying CBW attacks and to coping with their consequences. In 1997, a $52.6 million Domestic Preparedness Program was authorized for emergency response teams in 120 selected cities, whereby police, fire departments, and public health officials were to receive special training and equipment to help them combat biological and chemical terrorism.

In 1998 President Clinton announced new initiatives to address bioterrorism. Hearings before a committee of the U.S. Senate in 1998 included witnesses who stated that such proposals were misguided because so many resources were being assigned to military rather than to medical or public health authorities. Ethical questions raised include whether such funds could be better spent on providing adequate public health measures, preventive medicine, and treatment for endemic illness to the population.

LIMITATIONS OF COUNTER-TERRORISM MEASURES

Overall, there is little evidence that specific vaccine programs or other technical defensive programs are effective or ethical preventive measures against the use or threat of use of biologic weapons. Many public health experts argue that the best defenses against use of biological weapons lie in ethical proscription of work on them by health professionals and scientists and protection of the global population against all serious infectious disease, not just diseases caused intentionally, by ameliorating poverty and inadequate nutrition, housing, and education.

As part of this effort, it is argued, industrialized countries should enable developing countries to build capacity for detection, diagnosis, and treatment of all disease by providing technical information and needed resources. Article X of the BWC, encouraging the exchange of information and materials for peaceful purposes, should be strengthened. Research organizations, professional societies, and individual scientists should pledge not to engage knowingly in research or teaching that furthers the development and use of biological weapons. Furthermore, all countries could prohibit the development of novel biological agents that do not have an unambiguously peaceful purpose, even if these activities are promoted for defensive purposes.

An important reason that a few nations, groups, or individuals may continue to develop or stockpile chemical or biological weapons, known as "the poor nation's nuclear weapons," lies in the massive stockpiles of nuclear weapons maintained by the United States and other nuclear powers. As long as these nations fail to recognize their obligations under the 1970 Nuclear Non-Proliferation Treaty to move expeditiously toward nuclear weapons abolition, biological and chemical weapons will remain a threat.

VICTOR W. SIDEL
ROBERT GOULD

(SEE ALSO: *Arms Control; Genocide; Violence*)

BIBLIOGRAPHY

Alibek, K. (1999). *Biohazard.* New York: Random House.

Carter, A.; Deutch, J.; and Zelikow, P. (1998). "Combating Catastrophic Terrorism." *Foreign Affairs* (Nov/Dec):80–94.

Cohen, H. W.; Gould, R. M.; and Sidel, V. W. "Bioterrorism Initiatives: Public Health in Reverse?" *American Journal of Public Health* 89:1629–1631.

Gould, R., and Connell, N. D. (1997). "The Public Health Effects of Biological Weapons." In *War and Public Health,* eds. B. S. Levy and V. W. Sidel. Washington, DC: American Public Health Association.

Lifton, R. J. (1999). *Destroying the World to Save It: Aum Shinrikyo, Apocalyptic Violence, and the New Global Terrorism.* New York: Henry Holt.

Lockwood, A. H. (1997). "The Public Health Effects of the Use of Chemical Weapons." In *War and Public Health,* eds. B. S. Levy and V. W. Sidel. Washington, DC: American Public Health Association.

Piller, C., and Yamamoto, K. R. (1990). "The U.S. Biological Defense Research Program in the 1980s: A Critique." In *Preventing a Biological Arms Race,* ed. Susan Wright. Cambridge, MA: MIT Press.

Sidel, V. W; Nass, M.; and Ensign, T. (1998). "The Anthrax Dilemma." *Medicine and Global Survival* 5:97–104.

Tucker, J. B. (1997). "National Health and Medical Services Response to Incidents of Chemical and Biological Terrorism." *Journal of the American Medical Association* 278:389–395.

TERTIARY PREVENTION

Tertiary prevention generally consists of the prevention of disease progression and attendant suffering after it is clinically obvious and a diagnosis established. This activity also includes the rehabilitation of disabling conditions. Examples include eliminating offending allergens from asthmatic patients; routine screening for and management of early renal, eye, and foot problems among diabetics; and preventing reoccurrence of heart attack with anticlotting medications and physical modalities to regain function among stroke patients. For many common chronic illnesses, protocols to promote tertiary preventive interventions have been developed, often called "disease management." Disease treatments are not usually included, but the boundary with tertiary prevention is not always clear.

ROBERT B. WALLACE

(SEE ALSO: *Chronic Illness; Clinical Preventive Services; Prevention; Prevention Research; Preventive Medicine; Primary Prevention; Secondary Prevention*)

TESTICULAR SELF-EXAMINATION

Although testicular cancer is rare, it is the most common solid tumor in young men. It is also one of the most highly curable cancers, especially when detected early. Testicular self-examination has not been extensively studied, but most physicians recommend that men eighteen to thirty-five years old perform it monthly. Testicular self-examination is best performed after a warm shower when the scrotal skin is looser. The fingertips are used to slowly palpate the entire surface of each testicle for lumps. A tumor is usually painless when squeezed and feels like a rock emanating from within the testicle. This should not be confused with the epididymis, which is a comma-shaped structure that runs alongside each testicle and contains tubes that carry sperm. Most scrotal abnormalities detected by healthy men do not turn out to be cancer, but they must be checked by a primary-care physician or a urologist.

MARK S. LITWIN

(SEE ALSO: *Cancer; Self-Care Behavior*)

TETANUS

Tetanus, an acute infectious noncontagious disease caused by *Clostridium tetani*, is characterized by a prolonged illness associated with severe complications, including death. In industrialized countries, tetanus primarily affects elderly adults, while in developing countries, neonatal tetanus predominates and is a substantial major contributor to infant mortality. Elimination of tetanus, especially neonatal tetanus, through vaccination is a global public health priority.

CLINICAL DESCRIPTION

Tetanus (lockjaw) is an acute neurologic disease that occurs when *C. tetani* spores infect a site of injury and produce a neurotoxin. Wounds accompanied by tissue injury and necrosis produce the anaerobic conditions necessary for bacterial replication and toxin production. The diagnosis is usually established clinically and supported by the epidemiologic setting. Major symptoms are spasm of the muscles of mastication (trismus or lockjaw) and generalized hyperreflexia, which produces painful and uncontrollable muscular contractions. Generalized spasms can occur, often induced by external sensory stimuli. The incubation period ranges from two days to two months, with an average of ten days. The course of illness may last several weeks (often requiring intubation) and subsides gradually in survivors.

The case fatality rate ranges between 10 and 90 percent. Survival is correlated with longer incubation periods and access to medical care. Shorter incubation periods are usually associated with heavily contaminated wounds, more serious disease, and worse outcomes. A wound history can be established in approximately 80 percent of tetanus patients in the United States; however, absence of a wound does not rule out tetanus. Laboratory confirmation of tetanus is difficult and may not be definitive. Culture of the wound may rarely yield *C. tetani*; serology is often not helpful because disease can be caused by quantities of toxin insufficient to induce an immune response.

Neonatal tetanus (NT) is caused by unsanitary conditions during childbirth, specifically contamination of the umbilical stump. Neonatal tetanus can be prevented by education about the need for clean deliveries and immunization of women of childbearing age (including pregnant women).

EPIDEMIOLOGY

Clostridium tetani is a normal inhabitant of soil and of animal and human intestines and occurs worldwide. Cases increase during warmer months in temperate climates, most likely because of increased outdoor activity. In the United States, an average of forty-six tetanus cases per year were reported to the Centers for Disease Control and Prevention (CDC) from 1990 to 1999, as compared to an average of sixty-seven cases in the 1980s.

In developing countries, neonatal tetanus is a leading cause of neonatal mortality, accounting for over 250,000 deaths annually.. Neonatal tetanus has been called "the silent killer," since infants often die before their birth is recorded.

CONTROL MEASURES

In the United States, five doses of tetanus toxoid are recommended at 2, 4, 6, and 18 months and between 4 and 6 years of age, most often administered with diphtheria toxoid and acellular pertussis vaccine (DTaP). Subsequent booster shots for tetanus, combined with diphtheria toxoid, are recommended every ten years. Less than one percent of tetanus cases recently reported in the United States were in persons with up-to-date immunizations.

There is no herd immunity for tetanus since *C. tetani* is not transmitted from person to person. Although tetanus is a highly preventable disease, all individuals remain at risk if they do not acquire and maintain immunity through vaccination and periodic boosters.

ELIZABETH FAIR
ROLAND SUTTER

(SEE ALSO: *Communicable Disease Control; Immunizations*)

BIBLIOGRAPHY

American Academy of Pediatrics (2000). "Tetanus." In *Red Book 2000: Report of the Committee on Infectious Diseases,* 25th edition, ed. L. K. Pickering. Elk Grove Village, IL: Author.

American Public Health Association (2000). "Tetanus." In *Control of Communicable Diseases Manual,* 17th edition, ed. A. S. Benenson. Washington, DC: Author.

Bardenheier, B.; Prevots, D. R.; Khetsuriani, N.; and Wharton, M. (1998). "Tetanus Surveillance: United States, 1995–1997." In *Centers for Disease Control Surveillance Summaries* 47(SS-2):1–13.

Wassilak, S. G. F.; Orenstein, W. A.; and Sutter, R. W. (1999). "Tetanus Toxoid." In *Vaccines,* 3rd edition, eds. S. A. Plotkin and W. A. Orenstein. Philadelphia, PA: W. B. Saunders.

TETRACHLOROETHYLENE

Tetrachloroethylene is a dry-cleaning agent and industrial degreaser that often goes under the name perchloroethylene (PERC). The National Institute of Occupational Safety and Health estimates that 650,000 U.S. workers are exposed to PERC annually. PERC enters the environment through evaporation or through transport into groundwater and drinking water supplies. Through widespread use it has become a frequent drinking water contaminant, and it is present in approximately half of the nation's Superfund sites.

PERC has a low odor threshold and its smell is that associated with a dry-cleaning establishment. High levels of PERC released in workplace accidents can produce loss of consciousness and death. There is some evidence that longer-term exposures to lower levels at the workplace can lead to kidney and liver damage, cancer, neurological impairment, including changes in memory and learning, and to problems with visual perception. Reproductive and developmental effects have been suggested.

Whether any of these effects occur at the much lower levels present in the general environment is controversial. There is increased pressure to regulate PERC because of particular concern for children living in apartment buildings above dry-cleaning establishments, and because as a chlorinated compound it can be a precursor of dioxins.

BERNARD D. GOLDSTEIN

(SEE ALSO: *Dioxins; Toxicology*)

BIBLIOGRAPHY

New York State Department of Health (1997). *Tetrachloroethylene (PERC) in Indoor and Outdoor Air: Fact Sheet.* Albany, NY: Author.

U.S. Health Department of Health and Human Services (1997). *Toxicological Profile for Tetrachloroethylene.* Washington, DC: Public Health Service, Agency for Toxic Substances and Disease Registry.

THEORIES OF HEALTH AND ILLNESS

Theories about health and illness deal with the ideas people use to explain how to maintain a healthy state and why they become ill. Ideas about illness causation may include such ideas as breach of taboo, soul loss, germs, upset in the hot-cold balance of the body, or a weakening of the body's immune system. Theories of illness causation derive from the underlying cognitive orientation of a cultural group, and therapeutic practice usually follows the same cultural logic.

Anthropologists often divide theories of illness into two broad categories: personalistic and naturalistic. In a personalistic system, illness is believed to be caused by the intervention of a sensate agent who may be a supernatural being (a deity or dead ancestor) or a human being with special powers (a witch or a sorcerer). The sick person's illness is considered to be a direct result of the malign influence of these agents. In naturalistic causation, illness is explained in impersonal terms. When the body is in balance with the natural environment, a state of health prevails. However, when that balance is disturbed, illness results. Often, people invoke both types of causation in explaining an episode of illness, and treatment may entail two corresponding types of therapy.

According to personalistic theories of illness, illness may be linked to transgressions of a moral and spiritual nature. If someone has violated a social norm or breached a religious taboo, he or she may invoke the wrath of a deity, and sickness—as a form of divine punishment—may result. Possession by evil spirits is also thought to be a cause of illness in many cultures. This may be due to inappropriate behavior on the part of the patient—failure to carry out the proper rituals of respect for a dead ancestor, for example—or it may be simply due to bad luck. Sometimes, one person's envy of another's good fortune is believed to exert a malign influence through the "evil eye," which can result in illness or other calamities. Witches and sorcerers are malevolent human beings who manipulate secret rituals and charms to bring calamity upon their enemies. Recovery from an illness arising from personalistic causes usually involves the use of ritual and symbolism, most often by practitioners who are specially trained in these arts.

Naturalistic theories of disease causation tend to view health as a state of harmony between a human being and his or her environment; when this balance is upset, illness will result. The humoral system is a naturalistic approach to illness whose roots are over two thousand years old. Humoral concepts of health and illness are widely found in India, southeast Asia, China, and, in a somewhat different form, in Latin and South America. Maintaining humoral balance involves attention to appropriate diet and activity, including regulating one's diet according to the seasons. Illnesses may be categorized into those due to excess heat and those due to excess cold. Treatment of an illness of overheat would involve measures such as giving cooling foods and application of cool compresses.

In India, the ancient system of Ayurveda is based on naturalistic ideas of illness causation. Therapy in Ayurveda includes a vast pharmacopeia of preparations made from herbs and minerals, and dietary advice also forms part of every prescription. Ayurveda is actively practised in India today and has shaped the way Indians think about their bodies in health and in illness.

An important set of theories about health and illness, often called "vitalist" theories, is widespread in China, South Asia, and Southeast Asia. When vital forces within the body flow in a harmonious pattern, a positive state of health is maintained. Illness results when this smooth flow of energy is disrupted, and therapeutic measures are aimed at restoring a normal flow of energy in the body. In China this vital force is known as "chi"; in India it is called "prana." In China the ancient art of acupuncture is based on this understanding of the body. Acupuncture needles are inserted at various points along the "meridians," or energy orientations, of the body. The stimulation of the needles helps to restore a proper flow of energy within the body. In India, yoga (particularly hatha yoga, the physical form of yoga) is used therapeutically to restore a balanced energy flow through body and mind.

Biomedicine (modern traditional medicine) is founded on a naturalistic set of theories about the body, and these theories are continually evolving. One of the core theories of contemporary biomedicine, the germ theory of disease, is of relatively recent origin. According to an older biomedical concept, the miasma theory of disease, poisonous emanations from rotting vegetation or carcasses were believed to cause disease. By the mid-1800s, controversy still raged as to whether miasma or a waterborne pathogen was the cause for cholera. The "body-as-machine" metaphor has been a powerful way of conceptualizing the body within biomedicine, and a core assumption of the value system of biomedicine is that diagnosis and treatment should be based on scientific data. However, treatment approaches are often not rigorously analyzed scientifically before being employed therapeutically. For example, angina pectoris has been treated in a variety of ways, including with the use of xanthines, khellin, vitamin E ligation of the internal mammary artery, and implantation of this artery. These treatments were used for many years before controlled trials finally showed that the efficacy of these treatments were no better than placebo alone (Helman). Ritual and symbolism play important roles in the healing process in biomedicine, as they do in other healing systems. Taking a prescribed medication, for example, has a symbolic as well as a pharmacological effect. Symbolically, taking the medication may indicate to others that the person is unwell and is deserving of concern and sympathy. Surgical treatments such as coronary bypass surgery employ complex equipment and are performed in specialized settings. These settings and equipment all have powerful symbolic associations as well as technical functions. Rituals are patterned forms of behavior that have symbolic significance, that often help to provide a context of meaning in a strange or frightening situation. Both patients who undergo the surgery and surgeons who perform the surgery are involved in rituals that serve to order a life-changing event (i.e., major surgery). The processes of obtaining informed consent, getting a patient prepped for surgery, and complex stages of post-operative care all have ritual as well as technical functions.

Alternative therapies (also called complementary therapies) have been rapidly gaining in popularity worldwide. These therapies are diverse, ranging from traditional treatments adapted from their lands of origin, such as acupuncture and shiatsu, to newly developed forms of therapy such as therapeutic touch. Many alternative therapies have underlying theories of illness causation that are quite different from that of biomedicine. In therapies such as acupuncture, reiki, and shiatsu the concept of vital energy, or chi, is the basis for the practice.

Successful therapy is that which regulates and harmonizes energy flows. In iridology, particular areas on the iris of the eye are thought to correspond to specific body organs, and a diagnosis of malfunction of the organs can be made by an examination of the iris. Conceptually, this theory of illness links to an ancient philosophical system of "homologies" that makes connections between the cosmic and the terrestrial; between the outer environment and the inner; and between the external body and the internal body.

All theories of health and illness serve to create a context of meaning within which the patient can make sense of his or her bodily experience. A meaningful context for illness usually reflects core cultural values, and allows the patient to bring order to the chaotic world of serious illness and to regain some sense of control in a frightening situation.

KAREN TROLLOPE-KUMAR

(SEE ALSO: *Anthropology in Public Health; Black Magic and Evil Eye; Cultural Factors; Ethnicity and Health; Folk Medicine; Lay Concepts of Health and Illness; Miasma Theory*)

BIBLIOGRAPHY

Good, B. (1994). *Medicine, Rationality and Experience: An Anthropological Perspective.* Cambridge, UK: Cambridge University Press.

Hahn, R. A. (1999). *Anthropology in Public Health.* New York: Oxford University Press.

Helman, C. (1990). *Culture, Health and Illness.* Oxford: Butterworth-Heineman.

THEORY OF PLANNED BEHAVIOR

The theory of planned behavior (TPB), outlined by Icek Ajzen in 1988, is an extension of the theory of reasoned action in that it identifies the importance of assessing the amount of control an individual has over behaviors and attitudes (perceived behavioral control). The TPB takes into account that all behavior is not under volitional control and that behaviors are located at some point along a continuum that extends from total control to a complete lack of control. Control factors include both internal factors (such as skills, abilities, information, and emotions) and external factors (such as situation or environmental factors). The components of the model, as they relate to behavioral intention, include attitude toward the behavior, subjective norms, and perceived behavioral control.

DONALD E. MORISKY

(SEE ALSO: *Attitudes; Behavioral Change; Health Belief Model; Social Cognitive Theory; Theory of Reasoned Action*)

BIBLIOGRAPHY

Ajzen, I. (1988). *Attitudes, Personality, and Behavior.* Chicago: The Dorsey Press.

THEORY OF REASONED ACTION

The theory of reasoned action (TRA) was developed by Martin Fishbein and Icek Ajzen in 1975 to examine the relationship between attitudes and behavior. TRA looks at behavioral intentions rather than attitudes as the main predictors of behavior. According to this theory, attitudes toward a behavior (or more precisely, attitudes toward the expected outcome or result of a behavior) and subjective norms (the influence other people have on a person's attitudes and behavior) are the major predictors of behavioral intention. TRA works most successfully when applied to behaviors that are under a person's volitional control. The health-education implications of this theory allow one to identify how and where to target strategies for changing behavior (e.g., prevention of sexually-transmitted diseases and health fitness behaviors).

DONALD E. MORISKY

(SEE ALSO: *Attitudes; Behavioral Change; Health Belief Model; Social Cognitive Theory; Theory of Planned Behavior*)

BIBLIOGRAPHY

Ajzen, I., and Fishbein, M. (1975). *Belief, Attitude, Intention, and Behavior: An Introduction to Theory and Research.* Reading, MA: Addison-Wesley.

—— (1980). *Understanding Attitudes and Predicting Social Behavior.* Englewood Cliffs, NJ: Prentice-Hall.

THREE MILE ISLAND

The most serious nuclear reactor accident to date in the United States occurred at 4 A.M. on March 28, 1979, at the Three Mile Island nuclear power plant outside Middletown, Pennsylvania. Operator errors in dealing with a pump that had shut down caused the Unit 2 pressurized-water reactor to lose coolant and overheat. The temperature of the reactor core then rose to the point at which some of the zirconium-alloy fuel cladding failed, fuel itself partially melted, and cladding reacted with steam to produce bubbles of vapor and hydrogen, which then escaped into the reactor building, along with fission products from the reactor core. As a result of the failure to close a backup valve that could be operated manually, coolant was not restored to the reactor core until more than six hours after the accident, by which time enough hydrogen had accumulated in the building to pose the treat of a low-level explosion. The building had been designed to seal automatically in the event of a pressure rise, but no rise occurred, and four hours were allowed to elapse before the building was sealed, during which time radioactive gases escaped into the atmosphere.

Within three hours after the first sign of trouble, elevated radiation levels were detected by monitors in the reactor auxiliary building. A site emergency was declared, and officials enlisted the aid of local, state, and federal emergency personnel. The presence of a large hydrogen bubble in the reactor vessel prompted widespread fear that the reactor might explode, a concern that experts failed to allay although they knew it to be a misapprehension. Adding to the fear, dosimeter readings made in a helicopter three hundred feet above the auxiliary building's ventilation stack were misinterpreted by officials to signify elevated ground levels of radiation, prompting the governor of Pennsylvania to recommend the evacuation of all pregnant women and preschool children residing within five miles of the plant, who then complied.

Although large amounts of radiation were released, the resulting exposure of the public was relatively slight, resulting mainly from xenon-133 that was present in the gaseous plume. The largest dose of radiation any member of the public may have received is estimated to have been smaller than his or her annual dose from natural background irradiation, and the average dose to those living within fifty miles of the reactor is estimated to have been 40 to 50 times smaller than that. Because of the small magnitude of the doses that were received, no demonstrable injuries from the radiation were expected, nor have any actually been observed. Nevertheless, the legacy of fear and resentment left by the accident has adversely affected the well-being of those living nearby, and it has heightened negative attitudes toward nuclear energy.

ARTHUR C. UPTON

(SEE ALSO: *Energy; Environmental Determinants of Health; Nuclear Power*)

BIBLIOGRAPHY

Baum, A.; Gatchel, R.; and Schaeffer, M. (1983). "Emotional, Behavioral, and Psychological Effects of Chronic Stress at Three Mile Island." *Journal of Consulting and Clinical Psychology* 51:565–572.

Kemeny, J .G. (1979). *The President's Commission on the Accident at Three Mile Island.* New York: Pergamon Press.

Moss, T. H., and Sills, D. L., eds. (1981). "The Three Mile Island Nuclear Accident: Lessons and Implications." In *Annals of the New York Academy of Sciences* 365. New York: New York Academy of Sciences.

THRESHOLD

A threshold is the exposure level or dose of an agent above which toxicity or adverse health effects can occur, and below which toxicity or adverse health effects are unlikely. For example, taking aspirin is therapeutic and not dangerous up to a contain dose, but above that dose it can cause nausea, brain damage, bleeding, and, eventually, death. Sulfuric acid is not dangerous when only small amounts of it get on a person's skin, but if the amount gets too high, it burns. Thresholds for toxicity exist because, up to a certain point, the body can repair damage and detoxify chemicals to which it is exposed. If the exposures get too high, however, the detoxification and repair mechanisms are overwhelmed and toxicity starts to occur.

Thresholds for toxicity can be different in different people, with some people likely to be sensitive to smaller levels of exposures than others. In other words, toxicity thresholds are distributed differently within a population. For example, some people can breathe a lot of paint stripper without feeling ill, while others get sick from it quite easily. So while it may be easy to demonstrate a chemical's threshold for toxicity in identical laboratory animals, a threshold for toxicity in a diverse human population may be very difficult to determine.

The concept of a threshold for toxicity has played an important role in chemical regulation. Until recently, chemicals that cause cancer were assumed to have no threshold for their effects, while chemicals that cause other kinds of health effects were assumed to have thresholds. It is now known that some cancer-causing chemicals have thresholds and some other toxic agents do not, and this knowledge is slowly making its way into regulatory guidelines.

An example of a nonregulatory guideline that is based on toxicity thresholds is the threshold limit value (TLV). TLVs were derived as chemical exposure levels that are permissible in the workplaces—if workplace exposures stay below the TLVs, workers are unlikely to be adversely affected. TLVs were established first in 1968 by a nongovernmental organization known as the American Conference of Governmental Industrial Hygienists (ACGIH) based on available scientific information and best professional judgment. The ACGIH TLV Committee periodically reevaluates and updates the TLVs, based on professional judgment and new scientific information, but it uses no explicit risk-based or feasibility-based methodology. When the Occupational Safety and Health Act was enacted in 1970, the new Occupational Safety and Health Administration adopted existing TLVs as workplace permissible exposure limits (PELs).

GAIL CHARNLEY

(SEE ALSO: *Carcinogen; Exposure Assessment; Herbicides; National Institute for Occupational Safety and Health; Occupational Safety and Health Administration; Pesticides; Regulatory Authority; Risk Assessment, Risk Management; Toxicology*)

BIBLIOGRAPHY

Aldridge, W. N. (1986). "The Biological Basis and Measurement of Thresholds." *Annual Review of Pharmacology and Toxicology* 26:39–58.

—— (1995). "Defining Thresholds in Occupational and Environmental Toxicology." *Toxicology Letters* 77:109–118.

American Conference of Governmental Industrial Hygienists (ACGIH) (2001). *Documentation of the Threshold Limit Values and Biological Exposure Indices*, 7th edition. Cincinnati, OH: Author.

Ottoboni, M. A. (1997). *The Dose Makes the Poison: A Plain Language Guide to Toxicology*, 2nd edition. New York: Van Nostrand Reinhold Co.

THYROID DISORDERS

Thyroid disorders fall into two general categories: (1) dysfunction of thyroid hormone production; and (2) development of thyroid enlargements, called goiters, which include generalized enlargement of the gland and benign and malignant nodules. Thyroid dysfunction results either from increased or decreased secretion of thyroid hormones, called hyperthyroidism or hypothyroidism, respectively.

NORMAL THYROID FUNCTION

The principal role of the thyroid gland is to manufacture, store, and secrete the thyroid hormones, l-thyroxine and l-triiodothyronine. A critical and unique component of these hormones is their iodine content: 4 atoms of iodine per molecule for l-thyroxine (T4) and 3 atoms per molecule for l-triiodothyronine (T3). Iodine is a trace element in the crust of the earth, and the thyroid has evolved mechanisms to concentrate iodine from the blood plasma and retain it for the manufacture of the thyroid hormones. Once made, the hormones are stored within a protein molecule, called thyroglobulin, within tiny follicles that are lined with thyroid cells. In a controlled manner, thyroglobulin is taken back into the thyroid cells, degraded by enzymes and the thyroid hormone that is released is secreted into the circulating blood.

Function of the thyroid gland uniquely and absolutely requires thyroid-stimulating hormone (TSH; also known as thyrotroptin), which is secreted by specific cells in the anterior pituitary gland. Secretion of TSH is also negatively controlled by the blood concentrations of thyroid hormones. In this classic negative feedback system, excessive serum concentrations of thyroid hormones decrease secretion of TSH, and decreased serum thyroid hormones increase serum TSH. In the normal individual, the serum concentrations both of TSH and thyroid hormones are within the normal range.

THYROID DYSFUNCTION

Thyroid hormones regulate the rate of metabolism, heat production, and oxygen consumption of the entire organism, as well as the concentration of specific proteins in different organs and tissues. In general, symptoms of thyroid dysfunction are related to changes in the rate of metabolism and heat production, though changes in specific proteins may also have a profound impact in the body. For example, since thyroid hormones regulate the production of growth hormone, growth-hormone concentration decreases in the setting of hypothyroidism, resulting in cessation of growth in hypothyroid children.

Hyperthyroidism. In hyperthyroidism, also called thyrotoxicosis, excessive concentrations of thyroid hormones circulate through the body, affecting most tissues and organs, and producing a hypermetabolic state. In this setting, patients complain of fatigue and the feeling that their body temperature is too warm; they have increased sensitivity to external heat and a rapid heartbeat (called palpitations); and they have increased and inappropriate perspiration, nervousness, excess energy, tremors, and an increased frequency of bowel movements. On examination, patients have warm, moist skin, tremor, heat radiating from their skin; rapid heartbeat, and an abnormal thyroid examination. These symptoms reflect an increase in heat production and metabolic rate. Such patients are at increased risk for dangerous, abnormal rhythms of the heart (atrial fibrillation), muscle weakness, and loss of calcium from the bones.

In the United States, the incidence of hyperthyroidism is about 0.5 to 1.0 percent in adult populations, and in patients older than 70 years it approaches 1 to 2 percent. The most common cause of hyperthyroidism is Graves' disease, an autoimmune disorder that may occur in multiple generations, particularly in women. The inheritance appears to be a susceptibility to develop the autoimmune disorder, and its expression is likely influenced by environmental factors. In this disorder, antibodies that appear in the circulation bind to the protein receptor of TSH on the surface of thyroid cells. Once bound, the antibody, called thyroid-stimulating immunoglobulin, simulates the stimulatory action of TSH. Unlike TSH, however, the antibody is not negatively regulated by thyroid hormones, and it provides continuous stimulation of the thyroid leading to overproduction and secretion of excessive amounts of thyroid hormones.

Another cause of hyperthyroidism, particularly in middle-aged or older individuals, is benign thyroid tumors that produce thyroid hormones—even in the absence of TSH—called Plummer's disease or toxic thyroid adenoma. The TSH-independence of the thyroid tissue in these tumors, which may be single or multiple, is likely due to mutations in the TSH receptor protein or other proteins involved in transmission of the TSH signal into the cell.

A third common cause of hyperthyroidism is thyroiditis, caused either by an aberration of the immune system in patients with chronic autoimmune thyroiditis, or by a viral infection. In these disorders, the thyroid is not hyperfunctioning; rather, the structure of the thyroid is disturbed by inflammation and the hormones essentially leak out of the gland and enter the circulation in an unregulated manner. The latter conditions are self-limited and the hyperthyroidism persists only as long as previously manufactured and stored thyroid hormone remains in the thyroid. Other relatively rare causes of hyperthyroidism are pituitary tumors that secrete TSH in an unregulated manner and very high concentrations of the normal placental hormone, chorionic gonadotropin, that may occur in a small minority of pregnancies or in tumors called choriocarcinoma.

The treatments employed for hyperthyroidism are dependent on their cause. For example, the hyperthyroidism that occurs during pregnancy due to excessive chorionic gonadotropin resolves after pregnancy is over. Hyperthyroidism due to TSH-secreting tumors of the pituitary are treated by removal of those tumors, and the hyperthyroidism associated with thyroiditis is self-limited and persists only as long as previously manufactured thyroid hormones persist in the thyroid gland.

For the common causes—Graves' disease and functioning thyroid tumors—available treatments include use of antithyroid drugs (methimizole and propylthiouracil), radioactive iodine (I-131), and surgery. The antithyroid drugs decrease production of thyroid hormone and restore patients to a normal metabolic state. The natural history of Graves' disease includes remission in 25 percent of patients in North America (35–50 percent in Europe; 50–60 percent in Japan), so that control of the disease with antithyroid drugs looking forward to a possible remission is a reasonable approach for many patients. For those who do not enter remission, destructive treatment is usually recommended and accomplished by surgery (subtotal thyroidectomy), or by administration of radioactive iodine. The latter has been in use since the 1940s and is safe and effective. It has none of the immediate side effects or long-term risks that are usually attributed to radiation. Functioning thyroid tumors that are associated with hyperthyroidism do not resolve spontaneously and are therefore usually treated by surgery or radioactive iodine administration.

Hypothyroidism. In hypothyroidism, serum concentrations of thyroid hormones are decreased, resulting in a hypometabolic state. In this setting, patients complain of fatigue and sleepiness and the feeling that their body temperature is low, and they have increased sensitivity to the cold and the feeling that mental function is slow. Appetite remains normal but body weight may increase modestly. Cramping pain in the muscles and constipation are common. On examination, skin is dry and cool and the hair may be brittle. Patients have a slow heart rate, hoarse voice, and slowed mental function. Swelling around the eyes occurs and the reflexes are abnormal. Such patients also have raised concentrations of cholesterol in the blood plasma and are at increased risk for heart disease.

The incidence of hypothyroidism in the United States is 1 to 2 percent in patients under fifty years of age and then increases with age. In women who are older than seventy years of age, moderate to severe hypothyroidism occurs in 2 to 4 percent, and a milder form of hypothyroidism, sometimes called subclinical hypothyroidism, occurs in about 10 percent. Hypothyroidism occurs in males at an incidence that is about 25 percent that of females. Congenital hypothyroidism occurs in 1 in 3,500 births and can be determined by hormone measurements in one drop of blood. If treated soon after birth, affected children appear to develop quite normally. However, in untreated infants, brain development is severely impaired, resulting in cretinism.

A common cause of hypothyroidism is Hashimoto's disease, an autoimmune disorder of the thyroid that is closely related to Graves' disease. Both disorders occur in multiple generations in the same family, particularly in women, and involve an immune response within the thyroid gland and the appearance of antibodies in the blood plasma. In Hashimoto's disease, antibodies that can be easily measured are directed against thyroglobulin and another thyroid protein, thyroid peroxidase. The immune inflammation of the thyroid is painless, and involves gradual replacement of thyroid tissue with lymphocytes and fibrous (scar) tissue.

Other causes of hypothyroidism include surgical removal of the gland in the course of treatment of thyroid nodules, goiter, and cancer; destruction of the thyroid by radioactive iodine (I-131), which occurs commonly after the use of the isotope for the treatment of Graves' disease; and hyperthyroidism due to hyperfunctioning thyroid nodules. Diseases of the hypothalamus and pituitary that result in insufficient TSH for normal thyroid function can also cause hypothyroidism. Finally, areas in the world that still suffer from iodine deficiency have a high incidence of hypothyroidism and goiter. The diagnosis of hypothyroidism can be easily confirmed by measurements of thyroid hormones and TSH.

Treatment of hypothyroidism is straightforward in comparison to treatment of hyperthyroidism. No matter what the cause, the ramifications of the disease result from deficiency of thyroid hormone. Thus, simple, once-a-day treatment with thyroid hormone restores the body's thyroid hormone to normal, relieves all symptoms and signs of disease, and prevents the long-term sequelae of hypothyroidism. Most physicians prescribe synthetic l-thyroxine to accomplish this goal.

Goiters and Nodules. Goiter is an enlargement of the thyroid gland. When all of the thyroid tissue is enlarged, called a diffuse goiter, the cause may be manifold, including Graves' or Hashimoto's disease, congenital goiter, and iodine deficiency in those areas of the world where iodine intake is particularly low. Goiter is therefore a reflection of a disease process and may occur with or without thyroid dysfunction. Once the cause of goiter is determined, specific treatment can be prescribed.

Goiter is frequently caused by lumps or nodules in the thyroid, which may be cysts, inflammation, or benign or malignant tumors. The physician can feel single or multiple nodules in 4 to 7 percent of the adult population in the United States. Nodules are found at a much higher frequency by applying ultrasound (sonography) or computerized tomography to the thyroid area. Similar to other thyroid diseases, most patients are female. Current estimates are that the annual incidence of thyroid nodules discovered by examination is about 0.1 percent of the adult population. However, the annual incidence of thyroid cancer is about 0.004 percent. Therefore, only about one in twenty newly discovered thyroid nodules are likely to be malignant.

Upon discovery of a thyroid nodules(s), the physician's main concern should be to determine whether the nodule is benign or malignant. The cornerstone for this determination is the fine-needle aspiration biopsy, a procedure in which a very fine needle is inserted directly through the skin into the nodule and, with gentle suction, cells from the nodule are aspirated, placed on glass slides, stained, and evaluated by microscopy. The biopsy, done with or without direct visualization by sonography, is a simple, safe, and relatively painless office procedure. The sensitivity for detection of thyroid cancer is about 85 percent and the specificty is about 92 percent. Cytology results in a diagnosis in 85 percent of samples, with 75 percent being benign, 5 percent being malignant and 20 percent suspicious for malignancy. The remaining samples are nondiagnostic or unsatisfactory samples. The experience of the operator and cytologist has a large influence on these results.

When the aspiration biopsy demonstrates thyroid cancer, patients are usually referred for total thyroidectomy and are also frequently treated with radioactive iodine (I-131) as well as l-thyroxine at doses that at least maintain normal thyroid function. The nature of most thyroid cancers, and the success of these treatments, usually result in a lifetime cure rate that is greater than 90 percent.

Treatments for benign thyroid nodules vary according to their cause, size, location, and rate of growth. Some nodules may require no treatment at all, whereas others may require surgical excision because they cause pressure on vital structures within the neck such as the windpipe (trachea), food tube (esophagus), or blood vessels.

MARTIN I. SURKS

(SEE ALSO: *Goiter; Hyperthyroidism; Hypothyroidism; Iodine; Thyroid Function Tests*)

BIBLIOGRAPHY

Brennan, M. D. (1999). "Lymphocytic Thyroiditis: Hashimoto's Disease." In *Atlas of Clinical Endocrinology, Vol. I: Thyroid Diseases,* ed. M. I. Surks. Philadelphia, PA: Current Medicine.

Burman, K. D.; Becker, K. L.; Cytryn, A. S.; and Goodglick, T. A. (1999). "Graves' Disease." In *Atlas of Clinical Endocrinology, Vol. I: Thyroid Diseases,* ed. M. I. Surks. Philadelphia, PA: Current Medicine.

Gharib, H. (1999). "Nontoxic Diffuse and Nodular Goiter." In *Atlas of Clinical Endocrinology, Vol. I: Thyroid Diseases,* ed. M. I. Surks. Philadelphia, PA: Current Medicine.

Hupart, K. H. (1999). "Thyroiditis." In *Atlas of Clinical Endocrinology, Vol. I: Thyroid Diseases,* ed. M. I. Surks. Philadelphia, PA: Current Medicine.

Kaptein, E. M., and Nelson, J. C. (1999). "Serum Thyroid Hormones and Thyroid-Stimulating Hormone." In *Atlas of Clinical Endocrinology, Vol, I: Thyroid Diseases,* ed. M. I. Surks. Philadelphia, PA: Current Medicine.

Medeiros-Netos, G. (1999). "Congenital and Iodine-Deficiency Goiters." In *Atlas of Clinical Endocrinology, Vol. I: Thyroid Diseases,* ed. M. I. Surks. Philadelphia, PA: Current Medicine.

Morris, J. C. (1999). "Hyperthyroidism from Toxic Nodules and Other Causes." In *Atlas of Clinical Endocrinology, Vol. I: Thyroid Diseases,* ed. M. I. Surks. Philadelphia, PA: Current Medicine.

Shapiro, L. E. (1999). "Hypothyroidism." In *Atlas of Clinical Endocrinology, Vol. I: Thyroid Diseases,* ed. M. I. Surks. Philadelphia, PA: Current Medicine.

Singer, P. A. (1999). "Thyroid Dysfunction in the Elderly." In *Atlas of Clinical Endocrinology, Vol. I: Thyroid Diseases,* ed. M. I. Surks. Philadelphia, PA: Current Medicine.

Wartofsky, L. (1999). "Hyperthyroidism." In *Atlas of Clinical Endocrinology, Vol. I: Thyroid Diseases,* ed. M. I. Surks. Philadelphia, PA: Current Medicine.

THYROID FUNCTION TESTS

The key tests to determine thyroid function are serum measurements of free thyroid hormones and thyroid-stimulating hormone (TSH). Thyroid hormones have a negative feedback on TSH secretion from the anterior pituitary. In hyperthyroidism, free thyroid hormones are increased above the normal range and TSH levels are markedly decreased. In hypothyroidism, free thyroid hormones are decreased and TSH concentrations are increased when the cause is disease of the thyroid gland; when caused by a deficiency of TSH, free thyroid hormones are decreased but TSH is usually low. Radioactive iodine studies of the thyroid gland, which used to be the mainstay of testing, have been supplanted by these blood tests.

MARTIN I. SURKS

(SEE ALSO: *Goiter; Hyperthyroidism; Hypothyroidism; Iodine; Thyroid Disorders*)

BIBLIOGRAPHY

Kaptein, E. M., and Nelson, J. C. (1999). "Serum Thyroid Hormones and Thyroid-Stimulating Hormone." In *Atlas of Clinical Endocrinology, Vol. I: Thyroid Diseases,* ed. M. I. Surks. Philadelphia, PA: Current Medicine.

TIME SERIES

A "time series" is an epidemiological research design in which a single population group of defined size is studied over a period during which preventive or therapeutic interventions take place, with measurements of factors and variables of interest at specified time intervals. The aim is to detect trends such as variations in incidence rates of disease or other health-related phenomena in response to particular interventions. It may be a simple pre-test/post-test design, or an interrupted time series, in which several measurements are made both before and after an intervention; the latter is regarded as the more valid of these methods.

JOHN M. LAST

(SEE ALSO: *Cohort Study; Epidemiology; Observational Studies*)

TITLE V

Title V of the U.S. Social Security Act of 1935 authorized a federal program to provide health care for poor women and children, particularly for those with special health care needs. Framed upon the principles of the short-lived 1912 Children's Bureau and the Shepperd-Towner Act of 1921, Title V addressed a major national health policy need—to provide minimum health care services for the nation's poorest and most fragile citizens.

Today, the Title V-initiated Maternal and Child Health Bureau operates within the U.S. Health Resources and Services Administration (HRSA). Proven programs, infant mortality reduction initiatives, and an expanded planning capacity keep Title V a vital resource for poor women and children.

JAMES F. QUILTY, JR.

(SEE ALSO: *Child Health Services; Health Resources and Services Administration; Maternal and Child Health; Maternal and Child Health Block Grant; Poverty*)

TOBACCO CONTROL

Tobacco use is the leading preventable cause of death in developed countries, and by the year 2030 is projected to be so for the entire world. The situation is particularly tragic given that the harm caused by tobacco use has been known by the medical and public health communities, as well as by the tobacco industry, for nearly half a century, and that the means to reduce tobacco use are well known and relatively inexpensive and cost-effective.

THE HARM CAUSED BY TOBACCO USE

In the United States, cigarette smoking is responsible for over one in five deaths (over 400,000 deaths a year), with an annual loss of over 5 million years of life. Globally, about 3 to 4 million people die every year as a result of tobacco use, primarily in the developed world. The World Health Organization (WHO) projects that if current trends in tobacco use continue through to 2030, approximately 10 million people around the world will die each year, the majority in developing countries, which can ill afford the health costs of tobacco-related illness and the associated loss of productivity.

It is estimated that one out of two lifelong smokers will have their lives shortened as a result of their addiction to tobacco products. On average, a death caused by smoking robs about twelve years of life from the smoker, compared to the life expectancy of a person who has never smoked. While there is a substantial lag time from the beginning of tobacco use to the usual manifestation of symptoms, the death and disease caused by smoking is not limited to the older age groups. Cigarette smoking is a major killer of those in middle age (ages forty-five to sixty-four) and it is estimated that 80 percent of coronary heart disease deaths in this age group are caused by cigarette smoking.

Tobacco use causes a panoply of diseases, affecting nearly all vital organ systems. Diseases of the pulmonary and cardiovascular systems predominate, with heart, cancer, and respiratory diseases being most common. In the United States each year, smoking causes 155,000 cancer deaths, 122,000 cardiovascular deaths, and 72,000 chronic lung disease deaths, along with 81,000 deaths from other causes. Among all diseases, smokers are now most likely to die of lung cancer (123,000 deaths a year). This is true for both men and women, with lung cancer recently surpassing breast cancer as the leading cause of cancer death among U.S. women. The magnitude of the lung cancer burden is particularly tragic given that, in the beginning of the twentieth century, lung cancer was a relatively rare disease, and that nearly 90 percent of lung cancer today has been caused by cigarette smoking.

In addition to cigarette smoking, other forms of tobacco use also cause disease. Pipe and cigar smoking increases the risk of lip, oral, and lung cancer, and smokeless (spit) tobacco causes oral cancer, as well as other oral lesions. Other tobacco products, popular throughout the world, are also harmful and can cause death and disease. Most notably, *kreteks*, popular in Indonesia, and *bidis*, popular in India, have been shown to cause cancer, heart, and lung diseases. The use of these novel tobacco products is beginning to spread from their original location, and, unfortunately, are becoming popular among children, particularly in the United States.

Not only does smoking cause disease in the smoker, but nonsmokers also are adversely effected by exposure to secondhand smoke. In 1986, a report by the U.S. Surgeon General concluded that exposure to secondhand smoke causes disease, including cancer, in otherwise healthy adults. In 1992, the U.S. Environmental Protection Agency documented the effects of secondhand smoke on respiratory outcomes, especially among children, and concluded that secondhand smoke was a potent carcinogen.

THE MAGNITUDE OF THE USE OF TOBACCO PRODUCTS

In the United States, tobacco products have been used for hundreds of years. Early consumption of tobacco products was predominantly ceremonial use by Native Americans, followed by more widespread use of tobacco for pipes, hand-rolled cigarettes, cigars, and chewing. Cigarette smoking as we know it today—as a highly addicting and habituated behavior—is a function of the twentieth century. The introduction of blended tobacco that allowed for inhalation, the invention of the safety match, the ability to mass produce cigarettes, coupled with sophisticated distribution systems and unprecedented marketing efforts led to the rapid adoption of cigarette smoking during the first half of the twentieth century, peaking in the mid-1960s. Annual per capita cigarette consumption increased from 54 cigarettes in 1900 to a high of 4,345 cigarettes in 1963. The release of a landmark report by the Surgeon General in 1964, which detailed the health effects of smoking, has led to a series of social and behavioral changes associated with a nearly 50 percent decline in annual per capita consumption, to a level of 2,136 cigarettes in 1999.

In addition to the reduction in per capita cigarette consumption, the United States has also experienced a reduction in adult smoking prevalence, decreasing from about 43 percent in 1965 to 24 percent in 1998, meaning there are tens of millions of fewer smokers than if earlier rates of smoking had continued. The reduction in the proportion of the adult population who smoke has not been as great as the reduction in per capita consumption, indicating that those who continue to smoke are also smoking fewer cigarettes.

While the U.S. reduction in adult smoking rates has been substantial when compared to the level of smoking in 1964, there has been relatively little progress in the 1990s, when adult smoking rates appeared to have plateaued at about 25 percent. In addition, the progress that has been achieved since 1964 has not been experienced equally by all U.S. population groups. Smoking rates appear to vary by race and ethnicity, level of education, age, poverty status, and region of the country. Contrary to other parts of the world, there is a relatively small difference in smoking rates based on gender. In 1998, there was a nearly threefold difference in the likelihood of smoking based on race and ethnicity, with the highest smoking rates occurring among American-Indian and Alaska Native populations (40.0%), and the lowest occurring among Asian and Pacific Islander groups (13.7%). A similar differential is seen in relation to level of education, with high school drop outs at least three times more likely to smoke than college graduates (36.8% vs. 11.3%, respectively), and the difference between the two groups appear to be increasing. Additionally, state of residence seems very important, with the lowest smoking rates in Utah (13.9%) and the highest in Nevada (31.5%). Lastly, smoking rates vary by age and poverty level, but not as greatly as for race and ethnicity, educational level, or state of residence. For example, those sixty-five years of age and older, and those whose income is at or above the poverty level, are less likely to smoke than those under sixty-five years of age and those living in poverty.

The 1994 Surgeon Generals Report *Preventing Tobacco Use among Young People* focused intense interest on smoking among young people. This report emphasized the fact that smoking onset, and nicotine addiction, almost always begin in the teen years, and it provided an early warning of an increase in the use of tobacco products among young people. In fact, after more than a decade of relatively stable youth smoking rates in the 1980s, cigarette smoking began increasing among high school students in the early 1990s, peaking in 1997.

One of the most interesting observations about youth-smoking rates is the difference in likelihood of smoking between black and white youth. In the late 1970s, there was virtually no difference between smoking rates based on race. However, over the subsequent two decades, white youth continued relatively high smoking rates, while smoking rates among black youth plummeted. Unfortunately, this difference between black and white youth in high school is beginning to erode, and there is no difference in cigarette smoking rates between black and white middle school students.

While cigarette smoking rates among young people may have peaked, there is a disturbing increase in the use of alternative or novel tobacco products, notably in cigars, bidis, and kreteks. Because of the harm caused by all tobacco products, it is important to monitor total tobacco consumption. When this is done, tobacco use rates typically are in the 30 to 40 percent range for all demographic subgroups, and actually exceeds 50 percent for white, high school boys.

Broadly speaking, other developed countries are experiencing changes in smoking rates similar to that observed in the United States. These changes can be characterized by gradual declines in adult smoking, contrasted with increases in the early and mid-1990s among young people. The situation in the developing world, however, is quite different and somewhat difficult to characterize due to less systematic attention to monitoring patterns of tobacco use over time in a manner that allows for inter-country comparisons. However, it can be said that global tobacco consumption is increasing, with over one billion smokers, but with large differences in tobacco use by gender, type of product consumed, and intensity of tobacco use. For example, in many countries in the Far East, the majority of men smoke, but relatively few women do. In India, relatively few women smoke, but smokeless tobacco use is common. In many countries, smoking intensity (the number of cigarettes smoked per day) is much lower than in developed countries. However, all of these parameters are likely to change as the multinational tobacco companies increase marketing and promotion efforts in developing countries.

In an effort to systemize and standardize the collection of tobacco data, the World Health Organization (WHO), in collaboration with the Centers for Disease Control and Prevention (CDC), have developed the Global Youth Tobacco Survey (GYTS), which is an effort to collect in-depth data on tobacco use patterns and attitudes from adolescents throughout the world. By the end of 2001, over seventy countries are expected to have collected standardized data on tobacco use among young people as part of the GYTS project. Clearly, more is needed to standardize the global collection of tobacco data, not just tobacco-use rates, but country-specific data on the effect of tobacco use on public health, the presence of tobacco-control legislation, and the cost of cigarettes. Accordingly, the American Cancer Society, in collaboration with WHO and CDC, has recently published *Tobacco Control Country Profiles*, which is a summary of the existing tobacco-related data for each country of the world.

EFFORTS TO REDUCE TOBACCO USE

The reduction of cigarette smoking in the United States during the final third of the twentieth century has been counted as one of the ten greatest public health achievements of the century. Unfortunately, the achievement is only half completed, and the progress that has been achieved in reducing tobacco use has come too late for millions of smokers. The CDC estimates that since the time of the first Surgeon General's Report, in 1964, 10 million Americans have died as a result of smoking. Additional analysis suggests that, if current trends continue, another 25 million Americans alive today, including 5 million children, will be killed by cigarette smoking, Thus, while progress in the United States and other developed countries has been significant, the past and future public health burden caused by tobacco continues to be unacceptable.

To accelerate efforts to reduce tobacco use, the United States has proposed specific objectives for the year 2010, including the bold objective of reducing tobacco use by one-half, to no more than 12 percent for all population groups. While this is an extremely ambitious objective in the face of demographic trends, it is felt that it can be achieved if the nation, states, and communities simply implement what is known to work in preventing and reducing tobacco use.

To assist in this effort, the U.S. Department of Health and Human Services (USDHHS) has prepared a series of publications reviewing the evidence on the effectiveness of tobacco control interventions. In 1999, the CDC published *Best Practices for Comprehensive Tobacco Control Programs* to assist states in the development, implementation and evaluation of comprehensive tobacco-control programs. *Best Practices* provides the research and scientific evidence in support of nine programmatic elements that have been shown to be effective in reducing tobacco use. In 2000, *Reducing Tobacco Use: A Report of the Surgeon General* was released. This publication took a broader view of tobacco control, reviewing the evidence for programmatic work and assessing the effectiveness of economic and regulatory strategies to reduce tobacco use. Most recently, the Task Force on Community Preventive Services established rules of evidence to rigorously review the published literature on a variety of tobacco-control strategies, including efforts to reduce exposure to environmental tobacco smoke, increasing tobacco-use cessation, and preventing initiation. Additional reviews will be forthcoming on pricing, minors' access to tobacco products, and media campaigns.

While these several documents were developed for slightly different purposes, together they provide a complete picture of the evidence for tobacco control, and the Surgeon General has concluded that if the evidence-based interventions that already exist were applied, the *Healthy People 2010* objective of reducing tobacco use in half could be achieved. If smoking rates are reduced in half, millions of lives will be saved, and the expenditure of billions of dollars on treating diseases caused by smoking can be averted. Preliminary evidence from California is already demonstrating that sustained implementation of effective tobacco-control interventions not only reduces smoking rates, but can save lives and dollars.

There are many important components in successfully reducing tobacco use. Most practitioners and scholars recommend comprehensive approaches, where the different program elements work in concert to reinforce a specific tobacco-control message. These program components should strive to reduce both the demand and the supply of tobacco products, although a recent review of the evidence strongly recommends that "demand" reduction strategies are more effective than those attempting to influence the "supply" of tobacco products. The most influential supply-side intervention is control of smuggling.

Many interventions have been found to influence reduction in tobacco use (e.g., increasing the price of tobacco products, treating nicotine addiction, restricting indoor smoking), while others have been shown to increase the use of tobacco products (e.g., tobacco advertising campaigns targeted to young people, decreases in the price of tobacco products), other actions have little evidence, simply because they have yet to be tried or adequately evaluated (e.g., product regulation, plain packaging, limits on tar and nicotine levels).

Of the strategies not yet tested, regulation of tobacco products may be one of the most important to consider. Tobacco products are currently subject to minimal regulation, and they are expressly exempted from regulation by a number of federal laws designed to protect consumers, such as the Consumer Product Safety Act.

Many people consider the Food and Drug Administration (FDA) the logical U.S. agency to regulate tobacco products. However, up until recently, the FDA had not considered such regulations. This perspective changed dramatically in February 1994, when FDA commissioner David Kessler announced his intent to investigate the role of nicotine in tobacco products and whether the regulations of these products should come under FDA authority. Following a thorough investigation, the FDA did determine that nicotine was a drug that causes addiction, and that cigarettes were medical devices, intended to deliver nicotine in a manner to affect the structure and function of the body—the critical threshold for FDA to assert jurisdiction. During the last half of the 1990s, the FDA went forward with its rule-making authority, asserted jurisdiction over tobacco products, with an initial focus on the sale and marketing of tobacco products to young people. The tobacco industry, along with advertising groups, challenged the FDA's authority to regulate tobacco, with the case going all the way to the Supreme Court. In

March 2000, the Supreme Court ruled five to four against the FDA asserting its jurisdiction over tobacco, citing the fact that Congress had not provided such authority.

Part of meaningful product regulation includes restrictions on the promotion and marketing of tobacco products. The evidence is clear that money spent by the tobacco industry to market and promote tobacco products contributes to continued usage by improving the appeal, access, and affordability of tobacco products. In 1999, the U.S. cigarette companies reported spending $8.24 billion on marketing and promoting cigarettes, the most ever spent—and a 22 percent increase from expenditures in the preceding year. This amounts to an annual marketing expenditure of approximately $165 per smoker, or over forty cents for every pack sold. The magnitude of this expenditure is presumably in response to the rapid decline in per capita consumption, which decreased 10.3 percent between 1998 and 1999, following a 4.2 percent decline between 1997 and 1998.

Implementing comprehensive tobacco-control programs that fully integrate all available approaches to tobacco control, including educational, clinical, and regulatory approaches, will result in significant gains in longevity and quality if life.

MICHAEL ERIKSON

(SEE ALSO: *Addiction and Habituation; Adolescent Smoking; Advertising of Unhealthy Products; Counter-Marketing of Tobacco; Environmental Tobacco Smoke; Gateway Drug Theory; Mass Media and Tobacco Control; Office on Smoking and Health; Smoking Behavior; Smoking Cessation; Smuggling Tobacco; Taxation on Tobacco; Tobacco Sales to Youth, Regulation of; Workplace Smoking Policies and Programs*)

BIBLIOGRAPHY

American Cancer Society (1999). *Cancer Facts and Figures–1999*. Atlanta, GA: Author.

Centers for Disease Control and Prevention (1996). "Projected Smoking-Related Deaths among Youth—United States, 1996." *Morbidity and Mortality Weekly Report* 45:971–974.

—— (1997). "Smoking-Attributable Mortality and Years of Potential Life Lost—United States, 1984." *Morbidity and Mortality Weekly Report* 46:444–451.

—— (1999). *Best Practices for Comprehensive Tobacco Control Programs–August 1999*. Atlanta, GA: Author.

—— (2000). "State-Specific Prevalence of Current Cigarette Smoking among Adults and the Proportion of Adults Who Work in a Smoke-Free Environment—United States, 1999." *Morbidity and Mortality Weekly Report* 49:978–982.

Corrao, M. A.; Guindon, G. E.; Sharma, N.; and Shokoohi, D. F., eds. (2000). *Tobacco Control Country Profiles*. Atlanta, GA: American Cancer Society.

Environmental Protection Agency (1992). *Respiratory Health Effects of Passive Smoking: Lung Cancer and Other Disorders*. Washington, DC: Author.

Jha, P., and Chaloupka, F. J., eds. (2000). *Tobacco Control in Developing Countries*. New York: Oxford University Press.

Peto, R.; Lopez, A. D.; Boreham, J. et al. (1994). *Mortality from Smoking in Developed Countries, 1950–2000*. New York: Oxford University Press.

U.S. Department of Health and Human Services (1986). *The Health Consequences of Involuntary Smoking: A Report of the Surgeon General*. Rockville, MD: Author.

—— (1994). *Preventing Tobacco Use among Young People: A Report of the Surgeon General*. Atlanta, GA: Author.

—— (1998). *Tobacco Use among U.S. Racial/Ethnic Minority Groups–African Americans, American Indians and Alaska Natives, Asian Americans and Pacific Islanders, and Hispanics: A Report of the Surgeon General*. Atlanta, GA: Author.

—— (2000). *Reducing Tobacco Use: A Report of the Surgeon General*. Atlanta, GA: Author.

—— (2000). *Healthy People 2010* (conference edition). Washington, DC: Author.

U.S. Public Health Service (1964). *Smoking and Health. Report of the Advisory Committee to the Surgeon General of the Public Health Service*. Washington, DC: Author.

Warren, C. W.; Riley, L.; Asma, S. et al. (2000). "Tobacco Use by Youth: A Surveillance Report from the Global Youth Tobacco Survey Project." *Bulletin of the World Health Organization* 78:868–876.

TOBACCO CONTROL ADVOCACY AND POLICIES—CANADA

Canada is recognized as a world leader in tobacco control. In the 1970s and early 1980s, Canada had the world's highest per capita tobacco consumption, but by 1992, adult per capita consumption was 40 percent lower than in 1982. Government data indicate that the smoking rate fell from 50 percent of adults in 1965 to 25 percent in 1999.

In 1964, tobacco manufacturers adopted a voluntary code with modest advertising restrictions, later amended to prohibit direct television and radio advertising starting in 1978. Effective in 1989, the federal Tobacco Products Control Act (TPCA) included a phased-in tobacco advertising ban. In practice, however, tobacco manufacturers shifted marketing expenditures to sponsorship advertising. Following a tobacco industry constitutional challenge, in 1995 the Supreme Court of Canada invalidated key parts of the TPCA. A replacement law, the Tobacco Act, was adopted in 1997. This act contains significant advertising restrictions and, effective October 1, 2003, a total ban on sponsorship advertising. Since 1989, federal law has prohibited free distribution of tobacco products, and has banned incentive promotions (e.g., contests, gifts, rebates, and frequent purchaser programs).

Health warnings on cigarette packages first appeared in Canada in 1972, with a single voluntary statement placed by manufacturers in small print on the package. In 1989, federal legislation required one of four rotated warnings to cover 20 percent of the package front and back. In 1994, one of eight rotated warnings had to cover about the top 35 percent of the package front and back. The warnings appeared in black and white instead of in package colors as in previous warnings. As of 2001, sixteen rotated warnings are required, covering the top 50 percent of the package front and back. The warnings include color photographs of the health effects of smoking. Further, sixteen rotated interior messages are required, including messages with cessation advice. Toxic emission reporting on the side panel has become more detailed over time, with yields for tar, nicotine, carbon monoxide, formaldehyde, benzene, and hydrogen cyanide required.

Significantly, increased tobacco taxes in the 1980s and early 1990s were important in reducing smoking. However, in 1994 there was a dramatic tobacco tax rollback by the federal government and five provinces in response to large-scale smuggling. In Ontario and Quebec, the retail price of cigarettes was effectively cut in half, adversely impacting smoking trends. Roughly 90 percent of

cigarette contraband was originally manufactured in Canada, exported to the United States, and then smuggled back into Canada. In 1999, alleging conspiracy, the Canadian Government initiated attempts to recover damages from some manufacturers due to smuggling.

Beginning with Ottawa in 1977, hundreds of municipalities, and most provinces, have implemented laws restricting where smoking is permitted. Vancouver has been a leader in this area: a 1986 smoking bylaw addressed smoking in private workplaces, and, in 1995, restaurants were required to be smoke-free. The 1988 federal Nonsmokers' Health Act restricts smoking in federally regulated workplaces—about 10 percent of Canadian workplaces. Smoking was banned on all domestic flights of Canadian airlines in 1989, and all international flights in 1994.

Since 1994, federal law prohibits tobacco sales to persons under age 18 (a minimum national age of 16 had been in place since 1908). Vending machines are prohibited except in bars. "Selfservice" retail displays are banned, as are mail order sales. Six provinces (British Columbia, Ontario, New Brunswick, Nova Scotia, Prince Edward Island, and Newfoundland) have 19 as the minimum age, and Ontario and Nova Scotia have banned vending machines altogether. Several provinces had prohibited tobacco sales to minors starting in the 1890s.

By 2000, four provinces had prohibited tobacco sales in pharmacies, and some now require that tobacco retailers display signs with a health message. Since 1994, Ontario has prohibited smoking on school grounds. Since 1994, the federal government has imposed a profit surtax on tobacco manufacturers. In 1998, British Columbia required public disclosure of ingredients by brand, a world first, and in 1994 the House of Commons Standing Committee on Health recommended implementation of plain packaging.

Lawsuits to recover tobacco-related medicare costs from the tobacco industry were filed by British Columbia (1998, re-filed 2000) and Ontario (2000). About ten individual and class action lawsuits have been filed against the industry since 1988.

Efforts to adopt tobacco control legislation have been marked by strong, well-funded opposition by tobacco manufacturers and allied groups.

Health organizations, typically working in coalitions, have actively lobbied governments to enact measures. At the national level, prominent organizations include Health Canada, the Canadian Cancer Society, the Non-Smokers' Rights Association, Physicians for a Smoke-Free Canada, and the Canadian Council for Tobacco Control.

Rob Cunningham

(SEE ALSO: *Smoking: Indoor Restrictions; Smuggling Tobacco; Tobacco Control; Tobacco Control Advocacy and Policies–U.S.; Tobacco Control Advocacy and Policies in Developing Countries*)

BIBLIOGRAPHY

Cunningham, R. (1996). *Smoke & Mirrors: The Canadian Tobacco War.* Ottawa: International Development Research Centre.

Grossman, M., and Price, P. (1992). *Tobacco Smoking and the Law in Canada.* Toronto: Butterworths.

TOBACCO CONTROL ADVOCACY AND POLICIES— U.S.

At its simplest level, advocacy involves writing or speaking in an effort to convince others to take some type of action. Tobacco control advocacy is aimed at reducing the harm caused by tobacco use by changing the underlying political, economic, and social conditions that encourage tobacco use. In this effort, groups of citizens, or advocates, band together to promote policies and practices that protect people from exposure to cigarette smoke, prevent young people from starting tobacco use, and create an environment supportive of quitting smoking. Typically, science, politics, and activism are combined to generate public support for these goals.

Leaders of the highly profitable tobacco industry view tobacco control advocacy as a threat to their business. Tobacco companies have spent billions of dollars lobbying federal, state, and local lawmakers to vote against policies promoted by tobacco control advocates. The industry also conducts expensive campaigns to convince smokers, business owners, and the general public to resist adoption of tobacco control policies.

Tobacco control advocates often work with far fewer resources than the tobacco industry. Tobacco control advocacy represents a substantial extension of earlier public health efforts that focused on educating smokers directly about quitting and on teaching school children about the dangers of smoking. Advocacy efforts now focus on change at the community level—on improving the environment in which people make decisions to use tobacco or not. This often requires public awareness, understanding, activation, and sometimes outrage. Ultimately, advocacy changes the behavior of individuals by targeting institutional policies and practices.

Advocates often organize their efforts by joining forces in local or state coalitions. They strategically use mass media to publicize the changes needed to protect people from tobacco's harmful effects and to expose the tobacco industry's aggressive marketing and lobbying efforts. Both tobacco control advocates and their opponents try to shape the debate by framing the issue or message to succinctly illustrate their views (e.g., describing tobacco use as a "pediatric disease" or as an "individual freedom").

Tobacco control advocates promote a variety of public and private policies at the federal, state, and local levels. States and communities vary greatly in the number and types of laws passed and in how well they are enforced. The following are examples of the major types of policies promoted by tobacco control advocates.

INCREASING PRICE THROUGH TAXATION

State and local governments have the authority to increase taxes paid by people who buy tobacco products, which increases the price an individual pays for these products. In theory at least, the more tobacco costs, the less tobacco people use. As of 2000, the federal tax on cigarettes was 24 cents per pack. All fifty states also impose cigarette taxes—ranging from 2.5 cents a pack in Virginia to one dollar per pack in Alaska and Hawaii. Several states increased tobacco taxes in the 1980s and 1990s. For example, California passed a law in 1988 increasing the state's cigarette tax by 25 cents per pack; and the tax proceeds were mostly used to finance tobacco-related education and research programs, media campaigns, and health services.

RESTRICTING TOBACCO MARKETING

Tobacco is one of the most heavily advertised products in the world. A federal law passed in 1969 prohibits tobacco advertising on television and radio, and state and local ordinances passed in the 1980s and 1990s restricted some forms of tobacco marketing. Additionally, in 1998, the tobacco industry agreed to end all outdoor advertising and promotional giveaways as a part of the Master Settlement Agreement with state attorneys general in forty-six states. However, cigarette advertising continues to be prominent in magazines, in stores that sell tobacco products, and through industry sponsorship of car races, concerts, art exhibits, and other events.

ESTABLISHING SMOKE-FREE WORKPLACES AND PUBLIC SPACES

Smoke-free environments protect nonsmokers from breathing toxic tobacco smoke and help smokers reduce or quit smoking. Since the 1970s, thousands of employers have restricted smoking in their work spaces and hundreds of local governments have passed ordinances banning tobacco use in schools, restaurants, theatres, libraries, shopping malls, and other public places.

RESTRICTING YOUTH ACCESS TO TOBACCO

Most tobacco users begin smoking as preteens or teenagers and become addicted during the first few years of tobacco use. All states have laws prohibiting tobacco sales to those under 18 years of age, but these laws are often unenforced, making it easy for underage people to get cigarettes. Policies to restrict youth access to tobacco include increasing enforcement of laws prohibiting underage tobacco sales, banning or limiting access to vending machines, posting warning signs where youths attempt to purchase tobacco products, and establishing a minimum age for clerks who sell tobacco. The Synar Amendment, a federal law adopted in 1994, encourages states to enforce youth access laws by threatening to reduce federal funding for mental health programs to any state that does not demonstrate effective enforcement.

Increasingly, lawsuits are being brought against tobacco companies to hold them accountable for their actions. This is an effective strategy that was bolstered in the 1990s by the increased availability of internal tobacco industry documents revealing a long standing practice of targeting underage users and potential users. Although tobacco control advocacy started with small groups at the community level, it has developed into a subdiscipline within public health, and many organizations made tobacco control a priority.

TRACY ENRIGHT PATTERSON
DAVID G. ALTMAN

(SEE ALSO: *Adolescent Smoking; Counter-Marketing of Tobacco; Enforcement of Retail Sales of Tobacco; Health Promotion and Education; Mass Media and Tobacco Control; State Programs in Tobacco Control; Smoking Behavior; Smoking Cessation; Taxation on Tobacco; Tobacco Control; Tobacco Sales to Youth, Regulation of; Workplace Smoking Policies and Programs*)

BIBLIOGRAPHY

Altman, D.; Balcazar, F.; Fawcett, S.; Seekins, T.; and Young, J. (1994). *Public Health Advocacy: Creating Community Change to Improve Health.* Palo Alto, CA: Stanford Center for Research in Disease Prevention.

Chapman, S., and Lupton, D. (1994). *The Fight for Public Health: Principles and Practice of Media Advocacy.* London: BMJ Publishing Group.

Fishman, J.; Allison, H.; Knowles, S.; Fishburn, B.; Woollery, T.; Marx, W.; Shelton, D.; Husten, C.; and Eriksen, M. (1999). "State Laws on Tobacco Control—United States, 1998." *Morbidity and Mortality Weekly Report* 48(SS03):21–62.

Institute of Medicine (1994). *Growing Up Tobacco Free: Preventing Nicotine Addiction in Children and Youths.* Washington, DC: National Academy of Sciences Press.

Jacobson, P., and Wasserman, J. (1997). *Tobacco Control Laws: Implementation and Enforcement.* Santa Monica, CA: RAND.

U.S. Department of Health and Human Services (1994). *Preventing Tobacco Use Among Young People: A Report of the Surgeon General.* Atlanta, GA: Author.

Wallack, L.; Dorfman, L.; Jernigan, D.; and Themba, M. (1993). *Media Advocacy and Public Health: Power for Prevention.* Thousand Oaks, CA: Sage Publications.

TOBACCO CONTROL ADVOCACY AND POLICIES IN DEVELOPING COUNTRIES

There were approximately 1.1 billion smokers in the world in 2000, a figure predicted to exceed 1.6 billion by the year 2025. Smoking causes one in ten deaths globally, and by 2030 it will be closer to one in six. By 2020, it is predicted that 70 percent of people who die from smoking-related causes will live in developing countries. In addition, the age at which people first try smoking in developing countries is decreasing. Between 82,000 and 99,000 young people start smoking every day, over 80 percent of whom live in developing countries. While many developing countries have low rates of smoking among females, these rates are also on the rise. Aggressive marketing by the tobacco industry has fueled this trend.

During the last two decades of the twentieth century, governments responded to the smoking epidemic with diverse tobacco control (TC) policies. These measures have faced many domestic and global challenges, including a lack of funds and competition with other pressing problems. Serious challenges to TC policies also come from transnational tobacco companies (TTCs).

ELEMENTS OF TOBACCO CONTROL POLICIES

Tobacco control policies may address both the supply and demand side of the tobacco equation. Supply-side controls include limiting tobacco sales and imports, as well as policies to support alternative crops or livelihoods. Demand-side controls include taxation, bans (partial or total) on advertising and other forms of tobacco marketing, restrictions on where people smoke, prohibiting tobacco sale to minors, health warnings, restrictions on the ingredients in tobacco products, and the provision of accessible nicotine replacement therapies. Policies vary considerably across nations.

Many demand-side measures aim to reduce smoking prevalence and discourage young people from starting. Taxation has been shown to be an effective tool. Between 1979 and 1991, there was an inverse relationship between the real tobacco price index and teen smoking in Canada. In South Africa, cigarette taxes are now 47 percent of the price of a package. Such policies, however, face severe opposition from the tobacco industry. Mexico, for example, reduced taxes on cigarettes in the late 1980s under pressure from tobacco companies.

Banning tobacco advertising is another policy tool. China has laws that ban tobacco advertising in the print media and on radio and television, as well as advertising directed at adolescents—though these laws are unevenly enforced. South Africa also bans direct advertising of cigarettes on television, and recently banned tobacco sponsorships for sporting and cultural events. Other countries lag behind. In Senegal, advertising through sponsorships of sporting and cultural events is common. Under Mexico's partial ban, companies are discouraged from associating smoking with civic, religious, or sports activities, and are not allowed to use models younger than twenty-five years old. Tobacco advertising is permitted on television in the evening, however.

Policies to control environmental tobacco smoke (ETS) are also becoming more common in developing countries. Doctors, nurses, and teachers smoke in the workplace in Senegal, and in Mexico few restrictions exist on smoking in public places other than in poorly ventilated public buildings. In South Africa, however, smoking is restricted in government buildings, airports, and restaurants. Enforcement of clean air policies and associated penalties is often minimal. In China, smoking is restricted in most public places, on public transportation, and on domestic airline flights—but the fine for infractions is less than the cost of a package of imported cigarettes.

Warning labels on cigarette packages tend to be worded much less strongly in developing countries. Statements such as "This product may be harmful to your health" or "Smoking is hazardous to your health" are used. This is in stark contrast to Canada's use of graphic images of the impact of smoking on health, introduced in January 2001.

Despite successes, country-specific, comprehensive TC policies are still uncommon and their ineffective implementation is alarming. In countries such as Senegal and China, TC policies of the 1980s and 1990s have become progressively weaker due to poor enforcement.

CHALLENGES, AND A ROLE FOR CIVIL SOCIETY

Limited funding and large disparities in the willingness of the public and policy makers to develop and enforce policies pose a challenge to the success of TC policies. Barriers also include low literacy rates, multiple languages within a country, and high rates of smoking among health professionals—especially doctors, who exert a significant influence over communities' attitudes and behaviors. The heavy dependence of some economies on tobacco is also a threat. In Malawi and Zimbabwe, governments fear that a decrease in tobacco consumption would eventually lead to higher unemployment and lower foreign capital. Many challenges are easier to overcome where strong political support, popular support, and relevant research findings exist, as South Africa has proven. Effective advocacy organizations also contribute to the development of TC policies.

Advocacy groups are sometimes invited to participate in the development of TC policies. Unfortunately, civil society in developing countries may be weak or focused on other pressing issues, such as democracy, the environment, or primary health care. Nevertheless, organizations such as ASH Thailand (Action on Smoking and Health) have played an active role in the development and implementation of TC policies and serves as models for others. Unfortunately, tobacco companies encourage groups to lobby governments against new TC policies, for lenient legislation, or for free trade in tobacco.

For instance, in the 1980s, American-based TTCs began to pressure Asian countries to open their markets through a group called the United States Cigarette Exporting Association (USCEA). In 1985, despite a tobacco import ban, USCEA began advertising in Thailand. The following year, the Thai Anti-Smoking Campaign Project started to pressure the government until, in 1989, all tobacco advertising was banned. When negotiations between USCEA and the Thai government broke down later that year, the association asked the U.S. trade representative to use the U.S. Trade Act to pressure the Thai government to open the cigarette market, prompting a strong reaction from Thai and international anti-smoking groups and advocates. Finally, in 1990, the General Agreement on Trade and Tariffs (GATT, the forerunner of the WTO) ruled that Thailand could not continue to ban imports of cigarettes, but that it could continue to enforce its ban on tobacco advertising provided the law was applied equally to domestic and foreign products. Thailand's partial success in fighting American-based tobacco companies is indicative of the difficulties in fighting TTCs' destructive use of its power.

TOBACCO CONTROL POLICIES IN A GLOBAL CONTEXT

Globalization comprises two general trends. The first is economic globalization by way of global trade liberalization. The second trend is toward a transnational sharing of cultural, political, and social values, which has been factored by electronic communications and the media. Both trends present distinct challenges and opportunities to effective TC policies.

Economic globalization reduces trade barriers between countries, including tariffs, subsidies, and import restrictions. Tobacco control researchers, advocates, and health officials are concerned that these agreements open the door to TTCs to flood the markets of developing countries with their cigarettes, and thus hinder a nation's ability to control tobacco use. Using homogenizing cultural images, TTCs also exploit social and cultural globalization in their marketing (e.g., Philip Morris's Marlboro man and ads focused on women suggesting that smoking is modern and emancipated).

Given political commitment and organized efforts, it is possible to successfully fight the efforts of the tobacco companies. The effectiveness of cross-national coalitions of advocacy and research groups will continue to be crucial (e.g., the International Non-Governmental Coalition Against Tobacco, GLOBALink), as will the efforts of organizations such as the United Nations.

INTERNATIONAL ORGANIZATIONS AND TOBACCO CONTROL POLICIES

The World Bank no longer lends money to countries for tobacco-related projects and has recently laid out its approach to tobacco control, which focuses on demand-side strategies including taxation, non-price measures, and cessation therapies.

In 1998, the WHO created the Tobacco Free Initiative (TFI), which aims to reduce smoking prevalence and tobacco consumption globally. TFI is also developing the Framework Convention for Tobacco Control (FCTC), which, if signed by all WHO member countries, will provide a legal instrument as the basis of global and national TC policies in the face of transnational threats. Scheduled to be completed by May 2003, the FCTC will enable effective regional and global cooperation regarding TC concerns such as smuggling and advertising.

The health, economic productivity, and quality of life of the citizens in developing countries is under threat by increased tobacco consumption. Yet, despite many efforts, research, policy, and enforcement remain inadequate. Future success will largely depend on a strong research base to support policy development, as well as effective advocacy and coalition building to bridge the gap between research and policy.

LINDA WAVERLEY BRIGDEN
MONTASSER KAMAL

(SEE ALSO: *Counter-Marketing of Tobacco; Environmental Tobacco Smoke; International Development of Public Health; Smoking Behavior; Smoking Cessation; Smuggling Tobacco; Taxation of Tobacco; Tobacco Control*)

BIBLIOGRAPHY

Aftab, M.; Kolben, D.; and Lurie, P. (1999). "International Cigarette Labeling Practices." *Tobacco Control* 8(4):368–372.

Cunningham, R. (1996). *Smoke and Mirrors: The Canadian Tobacco War*. Ottawa: IDRC Books.

Ernster, V.; Kaufman, N.; Nichter, M.; Samet J.; and Yoon, S. (2000). "Women and Tobacco: Moving from Policy to Action." *Bulletin of the World Health Organization* 78(7):891–901.

Global Analysis Project Team (2000). "Political Economy of Tobacco Control in Low-Income and Middle-Income Countries: Lessons from Thailand and Zimbabwe." *Bulletin of the World Health Organization* 78(7):913–919.

Hammond, R. (1998). *Addicted to Profit: Big Tobacco's Expanding Global Reach*. Washington, DC: Essential Action.

Health Canada (2000). "New Tobacco Regulations Become Law." News Release, June 28, 2000.

Joossens, L. (2000). "From Public Health to International Law: Possible Protocols for Inclusion in the Framework Convention on Tobacco Control." *Bulletin of the World Health Organization* 78(7):930–937.

Ong, E. K., and Glantz, S. A. (2000). "Tobacco Industry Efforts Subverting International Agency for Research on Cancer's Secondhand Smoke Study." *The Lancet* 355:1253–1259.

Saloojee, Y., and Dagli, E. (2000). "Tobacco Industry Tactics for Resisting Public Policy on Health." *Bulletin of the World Health Organization* 78(7):902–910.

Taylor, A., and Bettcher, D. (2000). "WHO Framework Convention on Tobacco Control: A Global 'Good' for Public Health." *Bulletin of the World Health Organization* 78(7):920–929.

Townsend, J. (1998). "The Role of Taxation Policy in Tobacco Control." In *The Economic of Tobacco Control: Towards an Optimal Policy Mix*, eds. I. Aberdian, R. van der Merwe, N. Wilkins, and P. Jha. Cape Town: Applied Fiscal Research Centre, University of Cape Town.

Vateesatokit, B.; Hughes, B.; and Ritthphakdee, B. (2000). "Thailand: Winning Battles, But the War's Far from Over." *Tobacco Control* 9:122–127.

World Bank (1999). *Curbing the Epidemic: Governments and the Economics of Tobacco Control*. Washington, DC: The World Bank.

Yach, D., and Bettcher, D. (2000). "Globalization of Tobacco Industry Influence and New Global Responses." *Tobacco Control* 9:206–216.

TOBACCO SALES TO YOUTH, REGULATION OF

Governments often use regulatory powers to protect the health of citizens. In 1854 Dr. John Snow investigated the source of a cholera outbreak. Based on his evidence, local authorities closed the contaminated Broad Street water pump. A century later, epidemiological studies began to implicate tobacco as an agent of chronic illness. As evidence and public concern increases, authorities are being compelled to control tobacco. Comparable to closing the contaminated water supply at Broad Street, governments seek to restrict the supply of tobacco from prospective young smokers. One strategy is to control retail outlets by licensing tobacco vendors, ensuring customers meet the minimum age requirement, usually eighteen, at the point of purchase, and monitoring vending machines. Some state legislation also allows punishment of the underage customer, but this has been criticized as "blaming the victim."

RONALD A. DOVELL

(SEE ALSO: *Enabling Factors; Tobacco Control*)

TOTAL SUSPENDED PARTICLES (TSP)

Total suspended particles (TSP) is an archaic regulatory measure of the mass concentration of particulate matter (PM) in community air. It was defined by the (unintended) size-selectivity of the inlet to the filter that collected the particles. Unfortunately, the size cut varied with wind speed and direction and was from 20 to 50 µm (microns) in aerodynamic diameter. Under windy conditions the mass tended to be dominated by large wind-blown soil particles of relatively low toxicity.

In 1987 the EPA revised the National Ambient Air Quality Standard (NAAQS) for PM, and changed the PM pollution index to PM10, an index of the PM that can enter the thorax and cause or exacerbate lower respiratory tract diseases, such as chronic bronchitis, asthma, pneumonia, lung cancer, and emphysema. This switch to a more health-related index stimulated studies of the associations between ambient air PM and mortality, morbidity, and cardiopulmonary function indices. Some of the studies also used measures of the fine PM concentrations in the air, as indexed by PM2.5 and/or sulfate, and were able to show that annual mortality rates were more closely associated with fine particles than with the larger PM10.

In 1997, in its next revision of the PM NAAQS, the EPA supplemented its regulations on PM10 with new regulations on PM2.5. The cut points are not perfectly sharp for any of these PM size indicators; some particles larger than the cut-point are collected and some particles smaller than the cut point are not retained.

The terms "fine" and "coarse" were originally intended to apply to the two major atmospheric particle distributions which overlap in the size range between 1 and 3 microns. Now, "fine" has been defined by EPA as PM2.5 and "coarse" as PM10–2.5. However, PM2.5 may contain, in addition to the fine-particle mode, some of the smaller sized "coarse" particles. Conversely, under high relative humidity conditions, the larger particles in the accumulation mode extend into the 1 to 3 micron range.

The chemical complexity of airborne particles requires that the composition and sources of a large number of primary and secondary components be considered. Major components of fine particles are $SO_4 =$, H^+, NO_3^-, NH_4^+, organic compounds, trace elements (including metals that volatize at combustion temperatures), elemental carbon, and water. Major sources of these fine mode substances are fossil fuel combustion by electric utilities, industry, and motor vehicles; vegetation burning; and the smelting or other processing of metals.

Background emission sources (geogenic and biogenic) include: (1) windblown dust from erosion and reentrainment; (2) long-range transport of dust (including Sahara desert dust over Florida); (3) sea salt; (4) particles formed from the oxidation of sulfur compounds emitted from oceans and wetlands; and the oxidation of NOx from natural forest fires and lightning; and (5) the oxidation of hydrocarbons (such as terpenes) emitted by vegetation.

Major components of coarse particles are aluminosilicates and other oxides of crustal elements (e.g., Fe, Ca, etc.) in soil dust; fugitive dust from roads, industry, agriculture, construction and demolition; fly ash from combustion of oil and coal; and additional contributions from plant and animal material.

Since fine and coarse particles have distinctly different sources, both natural and anthropogenic, different control strategies are needed.

MORTON LIPPMANN

(SEE ALSO: *Airborne Particles; Ambient Air Quality [Air Pollution]; Environmental Protection Agency; Hazardous Air Pollutants; Inhalable Particles [Sulfates]; National Ambient Air Quality Standards; Smog [Air Pollution]*)

BIBLIOGRAPHY

Lippmann, M., ed. (2000). *Environmental Toxicants,* 2nd edition. New York: Wiley.

U.S. Environmental Protection Agency (2001). *Air Quality Criteria for Particulate Matter.* EPA 600/p.99/002. Washington, DC: Author.

TOXIC SUBSTANCES CONTROL ACT

During the early part of the twentieth century there was a tremendous increase in the development of new synthetic chemicals, as well as a rise in industrial uses for older ones. By 1976 it was estimated that there were 60,000 chemical substances in commercial use in the United States. A need was identified for a comprehensive framework for the prevention of risks that might be posed by these chemicals. In response to this need, Congress enacted the Toxic Substances Control Act (TSCA) in 1976 (see Figure 1). The TSCA addressed three major policy goals:

- Those who manufacture and process chemical substances and mixtures should develop adequate data with respect to the effect of chemical substances and mixtures on health and the environment.

- The government should have adequate authority to regulate chemical substances and mixtures that present "an unreasonable risk of injury to health or the environment, and to take action with respect to chemical substances and mixtures that are imminent hazards."

- Government's authority over chemical substances and mixtures should be exercised "in such a manner as not to impede unduly or create unnecessary economic barriers to technological innovation" while assuring that such substances and mixtures do not present "an unreasonable risk of injury to health or the environment."

Further, Congress made clear its intent that the government "shall consider the environmental, economic, and social impact of any action the administrator takes or proposes to take."

In addition to general provisions related to chemicals and substances, the TSCA contained specific requirements to regulate polychlorinated biphenyls (PCBs). Over the years, TSCA was amended to specifically regulate asbestos (1986), Radon (1988), and lead (1992).

The TSCA contains a number of major provisions that provide the EPA with tools for assessment and control of chemicals used in commerce or proposed to be added to commerce. TSCA authorized a number of activities under the EPA Administration including the authority to issue chemical test rules (section 4); a requirement for a Premanufactive Notification PNM) to be filed at least 90 days prior to manufacture or processing of a new chemical (section 5); authority to regulate chemical risks (section 6); a requirement to report chemical data and information on adverse health and environmental effects (section 8); requirements related to export and import of chemicals (sections 12–13); and protection by EPA of confidential business information (section 14). These provisions broadly direct the EPA to assure that the public will be protected from "unreasonable risks" to health and the environment. Although the statute did not clearly define "unreasonable risk," since its enactment (through administrative and judicial actions) this has come to be interpreted as including aspects of both risk analysis, which analyzes the severity and magnitude of health and environmental effects, and economic analysis, which looks at the economic benefits of the use of the substance as well as the availability and costs of switching to alternatives. In the cases of PCBs, asbestos, radon, and lead, Congress saw fit to identify that unreasonable risks did indeed exist and gave the EPA very specific direction for how to address those risks.

Several aspects of TSCA's chemical regulatory regime have been studied extensively by the National Academy of Sciences, the Congressional Office of Technology Assessment, the General Accounting Office, and the EPA itself.

Generally, the regulation of existing chemicals under TSCA has been modest. The General Accounting Office concluded in 1994 that the EPA regulates few chemicals under TSCA section 6, listing only five (polychlorinated biphenyls, chlorofluorocarbons, dioxin, asbestos, and hexavalent chromium), and noting that the

Figure 1

Toxic Substances Control Act

Title/Section	Purpose	Activities
Title I	**Control of Toxic Substances**	
4	Chemical testing	Test rules must show that the chemical "may present an unreasonable risk" or that "substantial" exposure may exist.
5	New chemical notices	Premanufacture Notification (PMN) must be filed at least 90 days prior to manufacture or processing of a new chemical. No test data are required at this stage. If the chemical will pose an unreasonable risk, EPA must act. If it "may" pose an unreasonable risk, EPA can impose temporary controls or restrictions until data are developed.
6	Regulation of hazardous chemical substances and mixtures	EPA can take action against chemicals that pose an unreasonable risk to health or the environment. Actions include banning or restricting production, processing, distribution, use and requiring warning labels.
6(e)	Regulation of polychlorinated biphenyls	Phased out the manufacture and certain uses of PCBs, as well as PCB import and export.
8	Industry reporting of chemical data	Directs manufacturers and processors to maintain records and provide data to the EPA as required. Such data can include chemical identity, categories of use, production levels, by-products, existing data on adverse health and environmental effects, and the number of workers exposed.
9	TSCA's relationship to other laws	Requires that EPA make referrals to other agencies when it determines there is an unreasonable risk under a statute administered by that other agency. The other agency must move to promulgate a regulation or publish a notice of why no action is needed. Directs the EPA to use other laws it administers to protect against unreasonable risks, unless it determines that it is in the public's interest to regulate under TSCA.
12/13	Chemical export and import provisions	Require notices to other nations when controlled chemicals are exported. Controls import of chemicals into US commerce.
14	Disclosure of chemical data	Authorizes EPA to release chemical information obtained under TSCA. Protects confidential business information from disclosure.
Title II	Asbestos Hazard Emergency Response	Measurement, assessment and monitoring of asbestos hazards in buildings. Operations and maintenance of buildings to prevent asbestos hazards. Response measures. Laboratory accreditation. State asbestos programs. Worker protection.
Title III	Indoor Radon Abatement	Radon construction standards. State radon programs. Public information. Radon in schools.
Title IV	Lead Exposure Reduction	Identification of dangerous levels of lead in homes. Training and certification of lead inspectors and abatement workers for homes. Methods for lead abatement and measurement. State lead programs. Public information.

SOURCE: Toxic Substance Control Act.

act itself required the regulation of one of the five, PCBs. In only two cases, for PCBs and asbestos, did the EPA take a comprehensive approach to the regulation of chemicals, and in one of these cases—asbestos—the rule was essentially overturned by the courts. In 1994, the GAO found that of 23,971 premanufacture notices for new chemicals (PMNs) that had been reviewed, action to reduce risks was taken on only about 10 percent. No test data are required as part of a PMN submission. If the EPA determines that the chemical will pose an unreasonable risk, it must act within 90 days. There is also the option of imposing temporary controls or restrictions. Finally, the GAO found that the EPA had formally referred only four chemicals to other agencies for control under their statutes—4,4-methylene dianiline; 1,3-butadiene; glycol ethers; and dioxin in bleached wood pulp and papers used for food packaging.

Various studies have indicated that the informational provisions of TSCA have fallen short of expectations. The GAO pointed to the breadth of the confidential information protections and the significant costs to the EPA in assessing claims made by manufacturers under the law. Likewise, gathering of new information about chemicals under section 4 has been judged unproductive. Few test rules have been promulgated under Section 4, which requires that the EPA determine that a chemical "may present an unreasonable risk" or that "substantial" exposure may exist to justify imposition of a test rule. In recent years, industry has begun to voluntarily develop "screening level" test data for the high volume chemicals in U.S. commerce (those produced at least one million pounds per year).

LYNN R. GOLDMAN

(SEE ALSO: *Asbestos; Chlorofluorocarbons; Dioxins; Environmental Determinants of Health; Environmental Movement; Environmental Protection Agency; Exposure Assessment; Lead; PCBs; Radon; Risk Assessment, Risk Management; Toxicology; Toxic Torts*)

BIBLIOGRAPHY

Congress of the United States, Office of Technology Assessment (1995). *Screening and Testing of Chemicals of Commerce. Background Paper.* Washington, DC: Author.

National Research Council, Commission on Life Sciences (1984). *Toxicology Testing: Strategies to Determine Needs and Priorities.* Washington, DC: National Academy Press.

U.S. Environmental Protection Agency, Office of Prevention Pesticides and Toxic Substances (1998). *Chemical Hazard Data Availability Study: What Do We Really Know about the Safety of High Production Volume Chemicals? EPA's 1998 Baseline of Hazard Information That Is Readily Available to the Public.* Washington, DC.: Author.

U.S. General Accounting Office (1994). *Toxic Substances Control Act: Legislative Changes Could Make the Act More Effective.* Washington, DC: Author.

TOXIC TORTS

In law, a tort is a wrongful act that causes harm and for which a court will provide a remedy. For example, a pedestrian injured by a careless driver may file a "tort action" (lawsuit) to recover compensation from the driver. A *toxic* tort is one in which the wrongful act consists of exposure to a toxic substance. This could occur in a variety of ways, such as an accidental release (e.g., a chemical spill or explosion), workplace exposure (e.g., to solvent fumes or asbestos), or harmful effects from medications or other consumer products.

Tort compensation, or damages, may be recovered for a variety of losses, including medical expenses, lost earnings, and pain and suffering. By shifting these costs from the victim to the wrongdoer, the tort system seeks to accomplish certain policy goals, including deterrence of harmful conduct and, where relevant, the promotion of public health and safety.

The injury in a toxic tort case may be "acute" (immediate)—fatal poisoning or burns to the skin are acute injuries. Classically, however, the injury involved in toxic tort litigation is a serious latent disease, such as cancer or birth defects, that may not develop until many years after the toxic exposure. In cases involving latent disease, there is virtually always a dispute over causation. The plaintiff has the difficult burden of proving that the disease resulted from the particular exposure, which may have occurred ten or twenty years earlier, rather than from some other cause (e.g., genetic inheritance, smoking, lack of exercise, diet, some other toxic exposure, or simply from "unknown causes").

Asbestos is one exception where medical science can positively trace the substance that caused a patient's cancer or other serious disease. As a result, huge tort recoveries have virtually closed down asbestos manufacturing in this country.

The potential for toxic tort liability can affect new products as well. A manufacturer may decide against the development and marketing of a dangerous product if tests show that the risk of injury—and therefore of tort liability—is too high. Sometimes, however, the specter of toxic tort litigation deters the manufacture of beneficial products, such as vaccines and other pharmaceuticals. In the 1980s and 1990s, numerous toxic tort suits alleged that the controversial drug Bendectin, prescribed for morning sickness during pregnancy, caused birth defects. Scientific evidence presented by the manufacturer persuaded the courts that Bendectin does not cause birth defects. Nevertheless, the manufacturer stopped producing Bendectin, reportedly due to the high cost of defending itself in repetitious litigation.

Courts can grant a variety of remedies in toxic tort cases that can benefit public health. For example, where toxic wastes leach from a disposal facility and contaminate a public water supply, a court can require the facility's owner to clean up the contamination, pay for an alternative safe water supply, and pay for medical care of anyone who develops disease from the contamination. Moreover, the desire to avoid tort liability may persuade facilities to exercise greater care to prevent the escape of toxic wastes.

Toxic tort lawsuits are sometimes initiated soon after a toxic exposure—especially a mass exposure—even though the plaintiffs have no physical symptoms of disease. Plaintiffs have argued, without much success, that they should receive present compensation because the exposure increases their risk of developing cancer in the future, and also for the emotional distress caused by their fear of future cancer. Courts have been more receptive to the argument that exposure victims should be compensated for the expense of periodic medical monitoring. Courts have reasoned that monitoring awards will foster early detection and treatment, which would help eliminate or mitigate future disease.

RUSSELLYN S. CARRUTH

(SEE ALSO: *Asbestos; Public Health and the Law; Toxic Substances Control Act*)

BIBLIOGRAPHY

Boston, G. W., and Madden, M. S. (1994). *Law of Environmental and Toxic Torts.* New York: West Publishing Co.

Eggen, J. M. (1995). *Toxic Torts in a Nutshell.* New York: West Publishing Co.

Hensler, D. et al. (1985). *Asbestos in the Courts: The Challenge of Mass Toxic Torts.* Santa Monica, CA: Rand Corporation.

TOXICOLOGY

Toxicology is the science of poisons. Understanding the potential for toxicity of agents found in nature has been a necessity for human survival. Learning to use natural toxins for purposes such as hunting and warfare was as much a part of human adaptation of the environment as was the taming of fire. One of the first known examples of the unwanted toxicity of a manufactured product was the lead poisoning that occurred in Roman times as a result of lead plumbing and lead dishware. Today, the emphasis of toxicology is on detecting and preventing the unwanted effects of chemical and physical agents, although concerns about the intentional misuse of chemicals, including chemical warfare, will persist for the foreseeable future.

As a science, toxicology is at the interface between chemistry and biology. There are three "laws" of toxicology. The oldest, that "the dose makes the poison," is attributed to Paracelsus, a fifteenth-century German physician. The concept that all chemical agents are toxic at some dose is central to a respect for the inherent hazard of all chemicals. The second "law" of toxicology, that the biologic actions of chemicals are specific to each chemical, has been attributed to Ambroise Paré, a sixteenth-century French surgeon who recognized that toxic agents have different effects dependent upon their inherent nature. Understanding the specific action of chemicals, known as hazard identification, depends upon recognizing the structural determinants of the activity of chemicals, and the biological niches in which chemicals interact. Very subtle changes in chemical structure can make an enormous difference in biological effects. The third "law" is that humans are animals. Protection against the toxicity of chemicals today would be impossible without the ability to study the effects of toxic agents in laboratory animals. As a corollary, animal rights activists advocating a ban on all animal research present a major threat to environmental protection and public health.

Toxicologists generally consider two types of dose-response relationships. One has a threshold below which no effect is expected. For example, one drop of fuming sulfuric acid will burn a hole in skin, yet this same drop in a bathtub full of water dilutes the sulfuric acid to a level at which no effects will occur. This theoretical threshold (experimentally known as a "no-observed-effect level") is presumed to exist for all agents, except for those that produce their effects through mutation, most notably many cancer-causing agents. A mutation can theoretically occur through a single chemical molecule producing a specific change in the chemical structure of a DNA molecule, thereby altering the genetic code from that of a normal cell to that of a mutated cell. As a further simplification, two molecules have twice as much chance as causing this effect. This can be described as a linear one-hit relationship between the dose of a mutational agent and the likelihood that the mutation will occur. The theoretical risk for any one molecule causing a mutation is infinitely small—there are about 1 trillion molecules of benzene, a known cause of leukemia, in every breath taken in an average American city, yet very few people develop leukemia. There are also many defense mechanisms within cells, as well as DNA repair mechanisms, that can impact on the likelihood of chemical exposures causing cancer.

Extrapolation of data from laboratory animals to humans, and from high to low doses, is central to modern toxicology. In addition to understanding dose-response relationships, knowledge about differences among species in the uptake, metabolism, and disposition of chemicals is also of importance. There is a strong similarity among mammalian species. Where differences do exist, attention to the kinetics of the processes that determine how an external exposure level is translated to the dose of a chemical at a target organ provides information of value to cross-species extrapolation.

A major challenge in modern toxicology is to prevent unwanted effects of otherwise valuable chemicals, including therapeutic agents. Understanding chemical mutagenesis and carcinogenesis has permitted the development of bacterial mutagenesis assays, such as the Ames test. These and other short-term assays for toxic effects are routinely used during the development phase of new chemicals to screen out potential toxic agents. Before marketing, additional testing is often required, depending in part on the use of the chemical. For new pharmaceutical agents, extensive toxicity and efficacy data are required, including studies in humans. Such agents are expected, at anticipated human dose levels, to have a biological effect of benefit to the consumer. In contrast, the developers of consumer chemicals, such as a new paint, hope that no biological effects will occur at usual doses to humans.

There are intermediate agents, such as insecticides and herbicides, for which a biological effect is intended at usual doses—for these agents, protection of humans depends, in large part, on our different biology. Accordingly, premarket testing is usually less rigorous for consumer chemicals than for therapeutic agents, and there is more dependence on structure-activity relationships (SAR). SAR, in essence, is a comparative analysis of aspects of chemical structure in relation to the existing toxicological database—a useful, but not completely effective, approach. In the United States, the Toxic Substances Control Act requires premanufacturing notification of new chemicals to the U.S. Environmental Protection Agency, which has the option of asking for additional testing. Such tests might include a battery of shorter-term and longer-term tests for acute and chronic diseases, including cancer. The recognition of the dangers inherent in compounds that bioaccumulate or otherwise persist in the environment has led to tests to identify and exclude such compounds from commerce.

Long-term animal assays, usually two-year studies in male and female rats and mice, are the mainstay of thorough safety assessment of chemicals, particularly those for which there is a concern about cancer or other chronic effects. The basic approach is to first perform a multiple-dose ninety-day study to choose the maximum tolerated dose (MTD). This dose is then used for a two-year study. Sole reliance on standard safety-assessment approaches carries a small but finite risk of missing a potentially toxic agent, a risk which is lessened if studies assessing the mechanism of toxicity of the chemical are also performed. A major goal of toxicological research is a better understanding of the processes by which chemical agents produce adverse biological effects, which will lead to the development of better safety-assessment tests.

The pathways of chemicals into and through the body are usually considered under the headings of absorption, distribution, metabolism, and excretion. Absorption, the process by which an external dose is converted to an internal dose, occurs by ingestion, inhalation, or through the skin. Distribution of a chemical depends in part on the pathway of entry and on specific chemical and biological factors; for example, only certain types of chemicals are able to penetrate the blood-brain barrier and enter the central nervous system.

Much emphasis has been placed on understanding chemical metabolism, as this is central both to the impact and to the detoxification of chemicals. The activity of many of the metabolic enzymes can vary greatly among individuals due to genetic and environmental factors, including types of food. Further, metabolic rates may vary within a given individual at different times due to induction of metabolic enzymes by these same environmental factors. Studies of resistance to cancer chemotherapeutic agents have led to an understanding of mechanisms by which toxic agents can be rapidly transported out of an otherwise susceptible cell, including specific transporter proteins, which can also be induced in response to environmental factors.

The major metabolic organ is the liver, but all organs have some level of metabolic enzymes. Certain chemicals, such as benzene, are harmless until they are metabolized by the body to form toxic chemical intermediates. Further, not all chemicals are metabolized; some pass through the body unchanged, while others react directly with biological targets.

Major excretory pathways are through urination, defecation, and exhalation. Lactation is also a means of excretion, particularly of fat-soluble chemicals, to the potential detriment of the infant.

Differential sensitivity to chemicals is an important subject to toxicologists for which modern molecular biology is providing new insights, particularly through the understanding of the human genome. For most human disease, genetics will determine what is necessary, but the environment, defined broadly, will determine what is sufficient. A reasonable estimate is that over two-thirds of human disease is environmentally determined. Many of the genetic and environmental factors responsible for disease operate at the level of modifying the absorption, distribution, metabolism, or excretion of exogenous chemicals, including food constituents.

Susceptibility to toxic agents is also conferred by factors such as age, gender, and concomitant conditions. Children, the elderly, and those with preexisting disease tend to be more susceptible to environmental toxins than are healthy adults. For example, the greater respiratory ventilation per unit of body mass in children accounts for the tragic finding of death due to carbon monoxide poisoning in the children, but not the adults, in a snowbound car.

So-called safety factors have traditionally been used in establishing public health and regulatory guidelines and standards based on toxicological data. These are based on no-observed-effect levels in animals, which are then reduced by a factor of ten to provide assurance that the animal data is protective of humans. In general, a tenfold factor is used to account for the possibility that humans are more sensitive than the animal species from which the data are obtained. Another tenfold factor is based on the greater diversity in susceptibility factors among humans than in inbred laboratory animals. The resultant hundredfold safety level has been used on a relatively routine basis for establishing acceptable daily intake (ADI) levels by the Food and Drug Administration, as well as for other regulatory standards. Additional factors of ten can be added based upon the toxic endpoint involved, or in order to protect children. Conversely, when there is a sufficiently robust database on humans, such as for certain air pollutants, routine factors of ten are not used, and scientific judgment contributes to the determination of an appropriate margin of safety.

The effect of toxic agents on ecosystems has become increasingly recognized as being important to human health. Traditionally, ecotoxicology (in relation to human health) has focused on contamination of the food chain, including the biomagnification and bioaccumulation of toxic agents within foods. The recognition of the role of ecosystems in overall planetary health, including feedback loops affecting climate, desertification, and crop yield, as well as the importance of the natural world and its animal and plant components to human well-being, has led to additional emphasis on understanding the toxicity of chemical and physical agents to components of nature.

BERNARD D. GOLDSTEIN

(SEE ALSO: *Ames Test; Benzene; Carcinogenesis; Ecosystems; Environmental Determinants of Health;*

Environmental Protection Agency; Ethics of Public Health; Genes; Genetics and Health; Lead; Maximum Tolerated Dose; One-Hit Model; Risk Assessment, Risk Management; Safety Assessment; Safety Factors; Threshold)

BIBLIOGRAPHY

Goldstein, B. D., and Henifin, M. S. (2000). "Reference Guide on Toxicology." In *Reference Manual on Scientific Evidence*, 2nd edition. Washington, DC: Federal Judicial Center.

Klaassen, C. D., ed. (1996). *Casarett and Doull's Toxicology: The Basic Science of Poisons*, 5th edition. New York: McGraw-Hill.

Lippman, M., ed. (1999). *Environmental Toxicants: Human Exposures and Their Health Effects*, 2nd edition. New York: John Wiley.

TOXOPLASMOSIS

Toxoplasmosis is an infection caused by a single-celled protozoan parasite named *Toxoplasma gondii* found throughout the world in humans, mammals, and birds. Cats, the definitive host for *T. gondii*, usually become infected by eating infected prey, and are the only animal that sheds the organism (as oocysts) in their feces. Animals other than cats are usually infected by ingesting oocysts in the soil or by eating infected animals.

Humans can become infected with *T. gondii* by one of three main routes: (1) by eating raw or inadequately cooked meat that contains *T. gondii* cysts (bradyzoites) or by eating uncooked foods that have come in contact with infected meat via, for example, cutting boards or cooking utensils; (2) by inadvertently ingesting oocysts that cats have passed in their feces either from a cat litter box or from soil (for example, from gardening) or by eating unwashed fruits and vegetables; (3) a newly infected woman can transmit the infection to her fetus.

Toxoplasmosis in adults usually does not cause symptoms, or causes only mild, nonspecific symptoms such as fever and swelling of the lymph glands. Therefore, the diagnosis is usually made by testing for antibodies that are produced in reaction to *T. gondii* infection. However, serious illness can occur when a newly infected woman passes the infection to her unborn fetus. Such an infection can lead to an infant with mental retardation, blindness, or other neurologic disorders. An estimated 400 to 4,000 congenital infections with *T. gondii* occur in the United States each year. Serious illnesses, including infection of the brain, can also occur in persons who have either old (latent) or new *T. gondii* infections when they do not have normal immune system function. Such persons include those with human immunodeficiency virus (HIV) infection or congenital immune illnesses, persons taking drugs that decrease immune system function, and persons with some types of cancer.

Effective means of preventing toxoplasmosis are as follows: (1) cook meat fully (internal temperature of 160° F) before eating it; (2) peel or wash fruits and vegetables before eating them; (3) wash hands, kitchen tools, counters, and sinks with soap and water after they have touched raw meat or unwashed fruits or vegetables; (4) clean the cat litter box every day so *T. gondii* oocysts do not have time to become infectious (one to five days); (5) wear gloves and wash hands after changing cat litter (pregnant women should not change cat litter if at all possible); (6) keep cats indoors so they do not become infected by eating prey; (7) feed cats only commercially prepared cat food, never undercooked or raw meat; and (8) wear gloves when gardening and wash hands after contact with soil and sand with which cats may have had contact.

JEFFREY L. JONES

(SEE ALSO: *Communicable Disease Control*)

BIBLIOGRAPHY

Centers for Disease Control and Prevention (1999). "1999 USPHS/IDSA Guidelines for the Prevention of Opportunistic Infections in Persons Infected with Human Immunodeficiency Virus: U.S. Public Health Service (USPHS) and Infectious Disease Society of America (IDSA)." *Morbidity and Mortality Weekly Report* 48(RR-10):7–9.

—— (2000). "CDC Recommendations Regarding Selected Conditions Affecting Women's Health: Preventing Congenital Toxoplasmosis." *Morbidity and Mortality Weekly Report* 49(RR-2):57–76.

Dubey, J. P. (1994). "Toxoplasmosis." *Journal of the American Veterinary Medical Association* 205:1593–1598.

Frenkel, J. K., and Fishback, J. L. (2000). "Toxoplasmosis." In *Hunter's Tropical Medicine and Emerging Infectious Diseases,* 8th edition, ed. G. T. Strickland. Philadelphia, PA: W. B. Saunders Company.

TRACHOMA

Trachoma is a virulent form of conjunctivitis caused by *Chlamydia trachomatis*, a bacterial organism transmitted by flies that crawl into the eyes of small children. Direct transmission of the organism from fingers, damp towels, and other objects also occurs. Characteristically, reinfection is frequent in endemic regions; this leads to severe scarring and contractures, especially of the upper eyelid, and also causes blood vessels to invade the cornea, rendering it opaque. These effects of recurrent infection make trachoma a leading cause of blindness in those parts of the world where the condition is prevalent. These are predominantly poor, rural areas in hot, dry countries such as some nations in the Middle East and in arid regions of North Africa, India, Pakistan, and inland Australia.

Trachoma is responsible for about 6 million out of a total of 20 million cases of blindness worldwide, and it causes impaired vision in about 140 million people. Determined efforts have greatly reduced the incidence of new cases in the last two decades of the twentieth century, however. It is rare in industrially developed nations with good hygiene and effective fly control measures—such as screened windows. Trachoma is an exclusively human infection, so if vulnerable populations can be protected from exposure (e.g., if flies can be reduced or eliminated), transmission will cease and the infection can be prevented. These tactics have worked well in many regions, including among Australian Aborigines, where the prevalence was very high until control programs were established.

Control was achieved in Australia by an aggressive campaign led by Dr. Ida Mann, who devoted her life to this cause. Her methods comprised topical application of antiseptic and antibiotic eyedrops, disinfection and face washing, education about personal hygiene, and fly control programs. Initially this was a mass campaign, and it was reduced to individual case management as endemic conjunctivitis was brought under control. The same tactics have worked in the Middle East (e.g., among nomadic Bedouin populations in Saudi Arabia), and they are working well in endemic regions of India and Pakistan. The World Health Organization, with strong support from several foundations and nongovernmental organizations devoted to prevention of blindness, aspires to eliminate trachoma by 2020.

JOHN M. LAST

(SEE ALSO: *Vision Disorders*)

TRADE UNIONS

See Labor Unions

TRADITIONAL HEALTH BELIEFS, PRACTICES

The beliefs and traditions of community members have a profound effect on the health of the community. Traditional beliefs regarding specific health behaviors such as smoking can influence policy, for example, on whether or not funds will be spent on antismoking legislation or on some other matter such as highway infrastructure. These beliefs also influence the types of food, recreational activities, and health services available in a community. Traditional health-related beliefs and practices among different ethnic groups fall into three groups: (1) beliefs that result in no harmful health effects, (2) beliefs that may produce beneficial health outcomes, and (3) beliefs and traditions which have serious, harmful health outcomes.

HARMLESS BELIEFS

Societies and cultures throughout the world are replete with traditional health beliefs and practices surrounding fertility. For example, pregnant women in many Asian cultures are advised that if they eat blackberries their baby will have black spots, or that if they eat a twin banana they will give birth to twins. Such ethnocentric beliefs have their foundation in folklore and traditional practices. The Vietnamese traditionally believe that disease is caused by an imbalance of the humoral forces of yin and yang. When ill, Vietnamese commonly use herbal medicines and a set of indigenous folk practices referred to as "southern medicine" in an effort to restore the yin/yang balance. These practices, from the Western viewpoint, were once thought to pose barriers to health. Recent investigations, however, revealed that certain beliefs and practices predicted neither lack of access to, nor underutilization of, health services. In fact, individuals should not be discouraged from placing faith in such beliefs, as they may result in positive health outcomes.

POSITIVE HEALTH OUTCOMES

The popular Western belief, "an ounce of prevention is worth a pound of cure," aptly illustrates the value of prevention—the planning for and taking action to prevent or forestall the occurrence of an undesirable event. Prevention is more desirable than intervention, which is the taking of action during an event. Preventive activities include immunization for childhood diseases, the use of protective clothing or sunscreen to prevent skin cancer, health-education and health-promotion programs, the use of automotive passenger restraints and bicycle helmets, chlorination of a community's water supply, and safe-housing projects.

Cigarette smoking, the largest preventable cause of death and disability in developed countries (and a rapidly growing health problem in developing countries), is a classic example of a behavior for which an ounce of prevention is truly worth a pound of cure. Despite thousands of conclusive studies establishing cigarette smoking as a cause of cancer, and despite the resulting coughing, odor, facial wrinkles, skin discoloration, ostracism, and increasingly socially unacceptable nature of this behavior, smoking rates remain high in certain population groups. Between 1993 and 1995, 47 percent of both black males and white males with less than twelve years of education were smokers. Among U.S. youths, in the late 1990s, more than one-third of high school seniors reported having smoked during the preceding two weeks. Unfortunately, because the debilitating effects of smoking are not visibly present for many

years following initiation of the behavior, most individuals are not willing to do the "ounce of prevention" part of the adage. A different story emerges for those who do quit smoking. Smokers who have quit for up to five years soon regain positive health benefits, such as less coughing, better breathing, and life expectancies equivalent to individuals of the same age who have never smoked. An additional benefit to society is purely economic: for every dollar invested in a smoking cessation program, society gets back ten dollars in terms of decreased rates of tobacco-related morbidity and mortality (or a cost savings of over $50 billion per year at current rates of investment).

NEGATIVE OUTCOMES

On the other side of the scale are health beliefs and practices that result in physical harm or negative health outcomes. Female circumcision, or female genital mutilation (FMG), is a graphic illustration of a traditional practice with a negative health outcome. The traditional belief is that the practice of FMG ensures virginity and family honor, secures fertility, promotes the economic and social future of daughters, and perpetuates a "religious tradition." FMG is also believed to preserve group identity, help maintain cleanliness and health, and further marriage goals, including enhancement of sexual pleasure for men. As of 2001, the practice was outlawed in the United Kingdom, Sweden, Belgium, the United States, Canada, Switzerland, France, Denmark, and in some African nations, such as Egypt, Kenya, and Senegal. The practice of FMG is justified by proponents who assert it "attenuates sexual desires in girls and protects their morals." Complications occurring immediately after the practice, and in ensuing years, range from disability to premature death. The practice is also believed to play a significant role in facilitating the transmission of human immunodeficiency virus (HIV) infection through numerous mechanisms.

DONALD E. MORISKY

(SEE ALSO: *Acculturation; Assimilation; Barefoot Doctors; Cross-Cultural Communication, Competence; Cultural Anthropology; Cultural Appropriateness; Cultural Factors; Cultural Norms; Folk Medicine; Lay Concepts of Health and Illness*)

BIBLIOGRAPHY

Brady, M. (1999). "Female Genital Mutilation: Complications and Risk of HIV Transmission." *AIDS Patient Care and Studies* 13(12):709–716.

Eke, N., and Nkanginieme, K. E. (1999). "Female Genital Mutilation: A Global Bug That Should Not Cross the Millennium Bridge." *World Journal of Surgery* (10):1082–1086.

Jenkins, C. N.; Le, T.; McPhee, S. J.; Stewart, S.; and Ha, N. T. (1996). "Health Care Access and Preventive Care Among Vietnamese Immigrants: Do Traditional Beliefs and Practices Pose Barriers?" *Social Science and Medicine* 43(7):1049–1056.

U.S. Department of Health and Human Services (1999). *Health, United States, 1999.* Hyattsville, MD: National Center for Health Statistics.

TRAFFIC SAFETY

See Reckless Driving

TRAINING FOR PUBLIC HEALTH

Preparation for a career in public health usually requires formal training at the graduate level, typically resulting in a Master of Public Health (M.P.H.) degree. Career options for a person with an M.P.H. are varied, and there are many types of organizations that employ public health professionals. Historically, these have included mainly federal, state, and local health departments, but contemporary public health practice has broadened to include many other employment settings, such as community-based organizations, health care facilities, insurance agencies, foundations, voluntary health agencies, and various business and industry settings.

All of these career options, regardless of employer, share an emphasis on populations rather than on individual clients or patients, and a broadly shared mission to promote health and prevent disease and disability. Major public health job titles, for example, include epidemiologists, biostatisticians, health-services administrators, health policy analysts, environmental health scientists, industrial hygienists, occupational health and safety specialists, biomedical and laboratory technicians, health educators, evaluation researchers, and health-services researchers. In addition, many people combine clinical training with public health training for jobs such as preventive medicine physicians, public health nurses, and public health nutritionists.

The M.P.H. degree is the most recognized professional degree in public health, although other degree titles are occasionally used. The M.P.H. degree usually takes between one and two years of full-time study, with the shorter course of study limited to individuals who enter with a prior professional degree, such as medicine or dentistry, or who have many years of public health work experience. The longer course of study is typical for students who enter the M.P.H. program directly from a baccalaureate program and without work experience.

The M.P.H. degree usually requires a set of public health core courses, a set of courses that provide skill development in a specialty area, a practicum or internship, and a final integrative project or experience. The public health core—the knowledge considered essential for all public health professionals regardless of their job titles—provides basic competencies in biostatistics, epidemiology, health-services administration, environmental health, and the social and behavioral sciences. The specialty courses build in-depth skills in one of these areas or in other recognized areas of public health practice, such as maternal and child health, international health, and public health nutrition. The particular specialties that a school or program offers beyond the public health core depends in large part on available faculty expertise. A practice experience, usually carried out in an agency setting, gives the student an opportunity to apply skills and knowledge learned in the coursework. A final integrative assignment, such as a thesis or a major essay, allows the student to demonstrate that he or she has mastered the content and is ready for practice. With some minor variations across schools and specialty areas, these four components are common to nearly all M.P.H. degree programs.

There are undergraduate training programs in selected areas of public health practice, such as community health education, health administration, and environmental health. Only a few undergraduate programs are offered in schools of public health, but many are available in baccalaureate- and master's-level colleges and universities. Although baccalaureate training is sometimes acceptable for entry-level public health positions, leadership positions usually require at least a masters degree. Doctoral training—leading to the Doctor of Public Health (D.P.H.) degree, which is the primary professional doctorate in public health, or to the Doctor of Philosophy (Ph.D.) degree, which is a highly specialized research degree—is offered in all U.S. schools of public health and in some of the larger programs outside schools of public health.

Public health, as a recognized profession, emerged in the early and mid-1800s with the onset of the Industrial Revolution. In response to the debilitating social and environmental conditions associated with the Industrial Revolution, public health emerged as a field of practice devoted to reducing disease and maintaining the health of the population. Drawing on the talents of physicians, nurses, engineers, chemists, lawyers, and statisticians, early public health efforts sought to solve community health problems. With the breakthrough of bacteriology in the late 1800s, public health became a science-based field, and the need for formal training was firmly established. However, it was not until the early part of the 1900s that a consensus emerged about a specific body of knowledge needed to achieve the goals of public health.

Elizabeth Fee, a noted public health historian and the author of *The History of Education in Public Health: Health that Mocks the Doctors Rules*, recounts the development of the public health profession as part of a "deliberate plan and strategy," not a haphazard, incremental set of events. She points to a conference in 1914 in the offices of the General Education Board of the Rockefeller Foundation as a "critical event in shaping the future structure of the public health profession." This meeting, which involved university leaders, early public health practitioners, and foundation representatives, set about "defining the necessary knowledge base for public health practice and designing the educational system needed to train a new profession." The Welch-Rose Report of 1915, written by two participants at that conference, would

become the major reference document for the early design of schools of public health.

Formally organized and independent schools of public health emerged in this nation shortly afterwards, largely modeled after the Johns Hopkins University School of Hygiene and Public Health, which was the first of several schools of public health to be endowed by the Rockefeller Foundation. In the 1920s, Johns Hopkins, Yale, Columbia, and Harvard all established schools of public health. In the following decade, the Universities of Michigan, Minnesota, North Carolina, and California at Berkeley established full-fledged schools. However, a variety of other public health training programs emerged in other institutions of higher education, where offerings included short intensive courses, certificates, diplomas, or multi-year degree programs.

At about this same time, the American Public Health Association, then and now the major professional public health organization in the United States, launched a series of activities intended to standardize the formal training that was needed for public health practice. In 1946, the APHA established a formal accreditation process to publicly recognize those universities that met these standards. This action responded in part to the urgings of the Association of Schools of Public Health, a new organization established by the leading schools of public health, and in part to recommendations of the U.S. Surgeon General. The Surgeon General sought from APHA an authoritative list of educational institutions where post-World War II funds for public health training could best be invested. Ten schools of public health were initially accredited, one of them a Canadian institution.

By 1974 the APHA sought to transfer the accreditation responsibility to a new independent group, and in collaboration with the Association of Schools of Public Health, incorporated the Council on Education for Public Health (CEPH). In addition to schools of public health, CEPH began in the late 1970s to accredit graduate community health education programs and graduate community health/preventive medicine programs. These programs are usually smaller and more narrow in the scope of offerings than a school of public health, but they, too, prepare public health

Table 1

Schools and Programs Accredited by the Council on Education for Public Health, October 2000

Schools of Public Health

University of Alabama at Birmingham	Loma Linda University	Saint Louis University
Boston University	University of Massachusetts, Amherst	San Diego State University
University of California, Berkeley	University of Michigan	University of South Carolina
University of California, Los Angeles	University of Minnesota	University of South Florida
Columbia University	State University of New York, Albany	University of Texas, Houston
Emory University	University of North Carolina, Chapel Hill	Tulane University
George Washington University	Ohio State University	University of Washington
Harvard University	University of Oklahoma	Yale University
University of Illinois at Chicago	University of Pittsburgh	
University of Iowa	University of Puerto Rico	
Johns Hopkins University		

Community Health Education Programs

California State University, Long Beach	New Mexico State University	Southern Connecticut State University
California State University, Northridge	New York University	Temple University
East Stroudsburg University	University of North Carolina at Greensboro	University of Wisconsin at La Crosse
University of Illinois, Urbana-Champaign	University of Northern Colorado	
Indiana University at Bloomington	San Jose State University	

Community Health/Preventive Medicine Programs

Arizona State University and Northern Arizona University and University of Arizona	Morehouse School of Medicine	University of Tennessee, Knoxville
	UMDNJ Robert Wood Johnson Medical and Rutgers, the State University	University of Texas Medical Branch, Galveston
California State University, Fresno	University of New Mexico	Tufts University
University of Colorado Health Sciences Center	Northern Illinois University	Uniformed Services University of the Health Sciences
University of Connecticut	North Texas Health Science Center and University of North Texas	University of Utah
East Tennessee State University		Virginia Commonwealth University
Eastern Virginia Medical School and Old Dominion University	Northwestern University Medical School	West Virginia University
Florida A & M University	Nova Southeastern University	Medical College of Wisconsin
Florida International University	Oregon Health Sciences University and Oregon State University and Portland State University	
Hunter College, City University of New York		
University of Kansas and Wichita State University	University of Rochester	
University of Miami	University of Southern California	
	University of Southern Mississippi	

SOURCE: Council on Education for Public Health, Washington, DC.

practitioners at the master's level, usually award-ing the M.P.H.

Schools of public health are usually independent schools or colleges, organizationally similar to other professional schools, such as law, medicine, and engineering schools. In contrast, public health programs usually are located within some other organizational unit, such as schools of medicine, allied health, education, health, physical education, recreation and dance, public administration and policy, human ecology, pharmacy, or health and human services. Both schools and programs are located almost exclusively in the nation's large research universities. They are often a part of an academic health center, which serves as an umbrella organizational structure for schools of the health professions and medical care facilities that may be owned or operated by the university. The health professions schools typically include medicine, dentistry, nursing, pharmacy, veterinary medicine, allied health, and public health. The alignment of the health professions training programs in an academic health center facilitates communication and collaboration across disciplines, a hallmark of education in public health.

The most notable difference in the public health professional preparation landscape now and when CEPH was established in 1974 is the sheer number of institutions of higher education offering graduate training in public health. While there were 10 accredited schools in 1946 and 18 accredited schools in 1974, by October 2000, CEPH had accredited 72 schools and programs. These included 29 schools, 13 community health education programs, and 30 community health/preventive medicine programs. A list of accredited schools and programs is presented in Table 1 and an updated list is available through CEPH's web site (http://www.ceph.org).

The growth in public health training capacity during the past pales in comparison to the growth that appears to be on the immediate horizon. In 2000, projections based on the number of institutions that were formal applicants for accreditation or in some stage of planning and development, and that expect to seek CEPH accreditation in the future, indicated that the number of schools and programs accredited between 1974 and 1999 was likely to more than double between 2000 and 2010.

In addition to the great expansion in the number and type of institutions providing public health training, many innovations have occurred in public health training. Among these are: (1) collaborative organizations in which two or more universities jointly sponsor and operate a single, geographically dispersed M.P.H. program or school; (2) the rapid development and deployment of nontraditional, technology-based ways of delivering education, especially through interactive video and web-based distance learning options; (3) the emergence of new public health specializations in areas such as public health genetics, clinical investigations, and informatics; and (4) new and nontraditional partnerships among multiple universities and among public health practice agencies to deliver training opportunities for the public health workforce.

PATRICIA P. EVANS

(SEE ALSO: *American Public Health Association; Association of Schools of Public Health; Careers in Public Health; Council on Education for Public Health; Public Health Practice Program Office*)

BIBLIOGRAPHY

Fee, E., and Acheson, R. M. (1991). *A History of Education in Public Health: Health that Mocks the Doctor's Rules.* New York: Oxford University Press.

National Association of County and City Health Officials (1996). *Exploring Public Health Career Paths: An Overview of Public Health Career Opportunities.* Washington, DC: Author.

National Health Council (1998). *270 Ways to Put Your Talent to Work in the Health Field.* Washington, DC: Author.

TRANSIENT ISCHEMIC ATTACKS

Transient Ischemic Attacks (TIAs) are transient neurological deficits, such as temporary blindness of one eye (amaurosis fugax), hemiparesis, or aphasia. Most typically, these symptoms last for periods of minutes or even hours, and they may persist for up to twenty-four hours. TIAs frequently result from platelet aggregates forming and then dislodging to embolize peripherally, or from significant atherosclerotic disease of extracranial carotid arteries, especially at the carotid bifurcation.

Because TIAs due to extracranial carotid stenosis (constriction) were recognized to be harbingers of larger and even devastatingly severe strokes, efforts to eliminate these offending lesions resulted in widespread carotid endarterectomies (CEA) being performed in the expectation of averting strokes. To scientifically assess the value of CEAs, three large-scale prospective randomized studies were undertaken, and the results were published in 1991. In patients with TIAs in the carotid distribution, and showing significant extracranial disease (greater than 70% diameter stenosis at the carotid bifurcation), carotid endarterectomy in competent surgical hands was shown to reduce stroke recurrence significantly. In these patients, control of risk factors for atherosclerosis should also be instituted, such as those for hypertension, smoking, diabetes mellitus, elevated cholesterol, stress, and, perhaps, sedentary lifestyle. In nonsurgical candidates, in addition to risk factor reduction, aspirin and other antiplatelet drugs can prevent subsequent strokes.

FRANK YATSU

(SEE ALSO: *Atherosclerosos; Cardiovascular Disease; Stroke*)

TRANSMISSIBLE SPONGIFORM ENCEPHALOPATHY

Bovine spongiform encepalopathy (BSE) is a transmissible, degenerative neurological disease of cattle that causes neither fever nor inflammation in the organs. Cattle infected with BSE experience a progressive degeneration of the nervous system. Symptoms include nervousness or aggression; abnormal posture, loss of coordination, and difficulty in standing; excessive itching or licking; decreased milk production; and loss of body weight despite continued appetite. The average age of symptom onset is five years, and death usually results within four months. The common name, "mad cow disease," is related to abnormal motor control and aggressiveness, which are also symptoms of rabies, which afflicts "mad dogs." Between 1986 and 2000, more than 170,000 cases of BSE were identified in cattle in the United Kingdom. The epidemic peaked in 1992–1993 at almost 1,000 cases per week.

The cause of BSE in British cattle was probably the use of commercial cattle feed containing meat and bone meal (MBM) derived from the rendered carcasses of sheep infected with scrapie, a degenerative disease of sheep. MBM is manufactured by rendering (melting) out the fat, and then drying the protein portion of by-products from the meat processing industry. Using MBM as a protein source in animal feed has been common for several decades. Apparently, the pre-1970 rendering methods, which included fat removal with solvents followed by a steam treatment, eliminated the infective agent in the rendered material before it was used in cattle feed. A change to "low temperature rendering" in the 1970s may have allowed the infective agent to remain in the protein portion that was dried and used as animal feed.

Natural transmission of BSE in cattle occurs when they eat infective material. The required oral dose for BSE transmission is small—five hundred to one thousand milligrams of BSE-infected brain tissue for calves. The BSE agent has been found only in the brain, spinal cord, retina, and the small intestines of cattle.

BSE and scrapie are transmissible spongiform encephalopathies, or TSEs. TSEs appear to be caused by an unconventional infectious agent known as a "prion" (proteinaceous infectious particle), an agent that contains no DNA or RNA. A prion is a normal protein (PrP) present on or in nerve cell membranes that can assume an abnormal (infective) physical shape referred to as PrP^{sc}. One PrP^{sc} molecule can induce normal PrP molecules to change shape into PrP^{sc}.

Mutations in the PrP gene may make the conversion of normal PrP to disease-causing PrP^{sc} more likely. There are at least twenty mutations in the PrP gene sequence resulting in "spontaneous" PrP^{sc} formation. Once a few PrP^{sc} molecules are formed, they rapidly convert other normal molecules to the infective form. Ingested PrP^{sc} can travel to the central nervous system where it converts normal PrP to PrP^{sc}.

The nerve cell attempts to break down the prion; however, PrP^{sc} is very resistant to the enzymes that normally break proteins down. The cell can be cleaved into fragments, which fill up and kill the cell (leaving holes known as "spongiform" damage). These fragments aggregate and precipitate the formation of plaques.

Creutzfeldt-Jakob disease (CJD) is a human TSE that occurs primarily in those over sixty-five years of age. It produces rapidly progressing neurological symptoms and dementia. In 1995, a new form of CJD, variant, or new variant, CJD (vCJD), was recognized. Patients have behavioral and psychiatric disturbances (e.g., depression, personality change), failure of muscular coordination, and memory impairment. The original ten cases occurred in people under forty-two years of age and were fatal within thirteen months. The hypothesized cause was consumption of BSE-infected food materials. As of March 2001, ninety-five cases of vCJD had been identified in the United Kingdom, with a few isolated cases occurring in France and Ireland.

TSEs occur more often in specific subgroups of populations (certain breeds of sheep, cattle, mink, and human families) suggesting a genetic component. Some gene combinations are very resistant, while some are particularly susceptible to the disease. In addition, a TSE in a specific species can exist in several strains, with each producing specific symptoms, times of onset and progression, and lesions in the brain that are distinctly different from those produced by other strains. Recent evidence indicates that the TSE strain occurring in vCJD is not different from the strain responsible for BSE in cattle. If the TSE strain that causes BSE also causes vCJD, the question arises of whether there is likely to be an epidemic of vCJD. The chances of such an epidemic are reduced by the fact that the incubation period for CJD is relatively long in humans, and because much of the population is likely genetically resistant to the PrP^{sc} that causes the disease. Further, while the infective dose in humans is not known, the dietary consumption of known infective tissues (brain, spinal cord, etc.) is low. However, it may be years before the full impact of this disease on the human population is known. As of 2001, no cases of BSE in cattle had been identified in the United States and no products had been imported that appear to pose potential risk to either human or animal health.

M. SUSAN BREWER

(SEE ALSO: *Bovine Spongiform Encephalopathy; Epidemics; Prions; Veterinary Public Health*)

BIBLIOGRAPHY

Blanchfield, R. (1996). *Bovine Spongiform Encephalopathy.* IFST. Available at http://www.easynet.co.uk/ifst/ Position Statement.

Bruce, M.; Will, R. G.; Ironside, J. W.; McConnell, I.; Drummond, D.; Suttie, A.; McCardle, L.; Chree, A.; Hope, J.; Birkett, C.; Cousens, S.; Fraser, H.; and Bostock, C. J. (1997). "Transmissions to Mice Indicate that New Variant CJD Is Caused By the BSE Agent." *Nature* 389:498–501.

Hill, A. F.; Desbruslais, M.; Joiner, S.; Sidle, K. C. L.; Gowland, I.; Collinge, J.; Doey, L. J.; and Lantos, P. (1997). "The Same Prion Strain Causes vCJD and BSE." *Nature* 389:448–450.

United Kingdom Minister of Agriculture, Fisheries and Food (1997). *Spongiform Encephalopathy Advisory Committee. SEAC Meeting Public Summary.* Surrey, UK: MAFF.

—— (1998). *Bovine Spongiform Encephalopathy: Number of Cases of BSE Reported.* Available at http://www. oie.org/indemne/bse_a.htm#ru.

Prusiner, S. B. (1995). "Prion Diseases." *Scientific American* 272(1):48–57.

TRANSTHEORETICAL MODEL OF STAGES OF CHANGE

The transtheoretical model of intentional behavior change describes change as a process that unfolds over time and progresses through six stages: precontemplation (not ready to take action); contemplation (getting ready); preparation (ready); action (overt change); maintenance (sustained change); and termination (no risk of relapse). Progress requires the application of specific change processes such as consciousness raising (education and feedback) at the precontemplation stage and reinforcement and helping relationships during action. Tailoring public health programs to each stage of change can dramatically increase recruitment, retention, and progress and impacts on entire populations at risk for chronic disease and premature death.

JAMES O. PROCHASKA

(SEE ALSO: *Behavioral Change; Communication for Health; Enabling Factors; Health Promotion and Education; Predisposing Factors*)

TRAVEL HEALTH PRECAUTIONS

Millions of persons travel abroad each year, often to lesser-developed areas of the world. The risk of illness or injury while traveling is determined by many factors, including the health status of the traveler, geographic destination, duration of stay, activities engaged in while traveling, and preventive measures taken—including pretravel immunizations.

The most common causes of death of U.S. citizens abroad are due to cardiovascular disease (49%) and unintentional injury (22%), the latter being primarily from motor vehicle accidents and drowning. Death from infection or homicide (including terrorism) is uncommon. (Figure 1 details the percentages of all causes of death of travelers.)

The most common medical problem encountered by travelers to developing countries is traveler's diarrhea, with attack rates ranging from twenty to fifty percent. The cause is usually bacterial, most often enterotoxigenic *Escherichia coli*, though the etiology is unknown in twenty to fifty

Figure 1

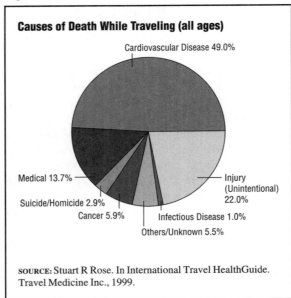

Causes of Death While Traveling (all ages)

Cardiovascular Disease 49.0%

Injury
(Unintentional)
22.0%

Medical 13.7%

Suicide/Homicide 2.9%

Cancer 5.9%

Infectious Disease 1.0%

Others/Unknown 5.5%

SOURCE: Stuart R Rose. In International Travel HealthGuide.
Travel Medicine Inc., 1999.

percent of cases. Travelers are advised to avoid undercooked foods and untreated water. Self-treatment involving oral rehydration, loperamide (Imodium), and bismuth subsalicylate (Pepto-Bismol) is frequently recommended for those afflicted. Antiobiotics started at the onset of bacterial diarrhea may reduce the duration of symptoms. However, prompt medical attention is required in the case of bloody diarrhea, severe abdominal pain, dehydration, or fever above 101°F.

Assessment of immunization needs should begin at least two months before traveling. Basic immunizations for tetanus, diphtheria, mumps, measles, rubella, varicella, influenza, and pneumococcal infection may need to be updated. Immunization for diseases prevalent in certain geographic areas (most commonly these include cholera, hepatitis A, hepatitis B, Japanese encephalitis, meningococcal meningitis, poliomyelitis, rabies, and typhoid fever) should be looked into, as well as those that are required for entry in certain countries. Proof of yellow fever vaccination may be necessary for entry upon arrival from an endemic area, either directly or earlier in the trip, and Saudi Arabia requires meningitis vaccination during the Hajj pilgrimage to Mecca.

Malaria, found in subtropical areas, is prevented with oral antimalarial medication, along with the use of insect repellents and mosquito netting. Other travel health risks include altitude sickness (above 8,000 ft.), jet lag, venomous bites and stings, intestinal parasites, tuberculosis, and human immunodeficiency virus (HIV) infection.

JEFFREY W. YATSU

BIBLIOGRAPHY

Centers for Disease Control and Prevention (2000). *CDC Health Information for International Travel 1999–2000.* Available at http://www.cdc.gov/travel.html.

Rose, S. R. (1999). *International Travel HealthGuide,* 1999 edition. Northampton, MA: Travel Medicine.

Thompson, R. F. (2000). *Travel and Routine Immunizations,* Milwaukee, WI: Shoreland.

TRICHINOSIS

Trichinosis is a disease caused by the invasion of the human body by the larval stage of the parasitic nematode worm *Trichinella spiralis.* Characteristically, humans are infected by eating poorly cooked pork, but infection sometimes follows eating the flesh of other carnivores such as bears or herbivores such as horses. The several varieties of trichinella all have the same life cycle—infection occurs when the larvae, encysted in muscle tissue ("red meat"), are ingested. The cyst wall is dissolved by gastric juices and the larvae are released into the intestine, where they undergo several developmental stages before reaching sexual maturity. Female adult worms may live for some years, continuing to produce newborn larvae that migrate through the intestinal wall and invade many organs and tissues, including the heart, brain, eye, and muscle tissue.

Heavy infection can be lethal or have devastating clinical effects such as seizures, heart attack, or blindness if the brain, heart, or eyes are affected. Light and moderate infection (when only a few cysts are ingested) causes muscle pains, skin rashes, diarrhea, and other symptoms that may be so vague that the condition escapes detection. Sometimes it comes to light only years later when calcium deposits around dead cysts show up on an X-ray. As infection occurs only by ingesting meat containing live larvae, person-to-person transmission is not possible.

Control relies on prevention. Abattoirs must be regularly and rigorously inspected and all suspect meat must be condemned; hunters need to be aware that carnivorous game animals may be infected, and must therefore ensure that meat is thoroughly cooked for long enough to kill any cysts that it may contain.

JOHN M. LAST

TRIGLYCERIDES

"Triglycerides" is the chemical name for fat. Chemically, triglycerides have a three-carbon backbone (glycerol) to which are attached fatty acids, which are strings of carbon and hydrogen atoms, most of which will eventually be oxidized to carbon dioxide and water, producing energy in the process. When not being actively oxidized or metabolized, triglycerides are stored in adipose, or fatty tissue, for oxidation at a later time. High levels of triglycerides in the blood have been associated with increased risk for heart attacks and strokes. Triglycerides may be increased by heredity, abdominal obesity, resistance to insulin, diabetes, and certain medications. They may be decreased by weight loss, control of glucose in diabetes, decreased simple sugar intake in the diet, and increased activity.

DONALD A. SMITH

(SEE ALSO: *Atherosclerosis; Blood Lipids; Cholesterol Test; Genetics and Health; HDL Cholesterol; Hyperlipidemia; LDL Cholesterol; Nutrition; VLDL Cholesterol*)

TROPICAL INFECTIOUS DISEASES

The tropics are usually defined as that part of the equatorial world bounded by the tropics of Cancer and Capricorn. Defining a tropical infectious disease is not as straightforward. Almost all infectious diseases can be found in the tropics; there are a great number that occur predominantly in the tropics; and there are a few, such as sleeping sickness, that are only found in the tropics. Before discussing some of the more prevalent tropical infections of today, it is worth taking a brief look at the history of a few of these infections.

BACKGROUND

Many of the infections that we now consider tropical used to be found throughout the more temperate climates of North America and Europe. For example, yellow fever epidemics swept through American cities from the 1600s through 1905, killing thousands of people. Cholera devastated the cities of America and Europe before the days of sewers. The Plague, known as the "Black Death," decimated the populations of medieval Europe. In the early part of the twentieth century, it was estimated that there were between 5 million and 7 million cases of malaria a year in the United States between Florida and Connecticut. Malaria was a disease familiar to the British of the sixteenth century and is even described by Shakespeare in *Henry V* (II. i. 123). Hookworm was the most common cause of anemia in the American south at beginning of the twentieth century and was only controlled after a massive public health campaign. Good sanitation, hygiene, and vector-control methods, as well as a rise in the standard of living, were responsible for the virtual eradication of these diseases from North America and Europe. The fact that so many of these infections are now considered "tropical" and are found mainly in poorer, developing countries is more a result of economics than it is of climate. There are several countries with high rates of "tropical" infections that do not have tropical climates (for example, Iran and Afghanistan).

The original designation of certain diseases as being tropical can be dated back to the 1898 publication of Sir Patrick Manson's *Tropical Diseases: A Manual of the Diseases of Warm Climates.* This volume identified twelve tropical infectious diseases, as well as a few other noninfectious diseases such as pellagra. The book was aimed at British physicians working in the warmer climates of many of the British colonies. Since then, the list of tropical infections has expanded to include well over one hundred infections. There is no list in existence that definitely identifies which infections are classified as tropical; most lists include a combination of those infections that are found exclusively in the tropics as well the large number that, though also found in more temperate climates, are predominantly a problem of developing countries with warmer climates. A discussion of tropical infectious diseases is essentially a discussion of the infectious diseases of the developing world.

As is true of all infectious diseases, the causative pathogens include viruses, bacteria, parasites, and fungi. Table 1 is a list of some tropical infections, divided by pathogen. Some infections, such as measles, human immunodeficiency virus (HIV), and tuberculosis, though found throughout the world, are included in the list as they cause such severe morbidity and mortality in tropical countries.

It is estimated that infections cause over 13 million deaths a year in developing countries, accounting for approximately 50 percent of all deaths. Only six diseases cause over 90 percent of the deaths attributed to infections: pneumonia, tuberculosis, diarrheal diseases, malaria, measles, and HIV/AIDS (human immunodeficiency virus/acquired immunodeficiency syndrome). Of these, only pneumonia is also a leading cause of death in developed countries. The others are found in developed countries but are now controlled either through vaccination programs (as with measles) or with effective medications and public health programs. Unfortunately, lack of effective health infrastructures, poor economies, and lack of access to affordable medications mean that these infections will continue to be the cause of significant morbidity and mortality in developing countries.

Approximately 2 billion people, one-third of the world's population, have latent tuberculosis (TB) infection. Of these, 8 million people a year will develop active infection and 2 million people a year will die from the infection. The rates of infection and subsequent death are increasing worldwide, with new outbreaks occurring in regions such as Eastern Europe for the first time in over forty years. In regions with high rates of HIV, the spread of tuberculosis is greatly accelerated, as are the death rates attributable to tuberculosis. The emergence of strains that are resistant to first-line drugs used in the treatment of TB means that it is becoming more difficult, and more expensive, to successfully treat the infection.

A variety of bacteria and viruses, such as cholera, rotavirus, and typhoid fever, may result in diarrheal illness. The burden of disease caused by

Table 1

Examples of Tropical Infectious Diseases by Pathogen

Bacteria	Parasites
tuberculosis	malaria
leprosy	amebiasis
cholera	giardiasis
tetanus	trypanosomiasis
plague	leishmaniasis
leptospirosis	ascariasis
shigella	strongyloides
campylobacter	schistosomiasis
typhoid fever	taeniasis
syphilis	echinococcosis
chlamydia	lymphatic filariasis
gonococcus	loiasis
anthrax	onchocerciasis
melioidosis	cryptosporidiosis
	dracunculiasis
	hookworm
	trichinosis

Viruses	Fungi
HIV	histoplasmosis
measles	sporotrichosis
poliomyelitis	cryptococcosis
viral hepatitis	coccidioidomycosis
viral diarrhea	blastomycosis
rabies	paracoccidiodomycosis
Yellow fever	
Dengue fever	
viral hemorrhagic fevers	
(e.g. Ebola, Lassa)	
arboviruses	

SOURCE: Courtesy of author.

these illnesses is huge—with an estimated 1.5 billion bouts of diarrhea a year and 2 million deaths a year, mainly in children under the age of five. The morbidity associated with diarrheal illnesses is the result of repeated episodes of dehydrating and malnourishing infections in children during their formative years. One study done in Brazil showed that such children lost over five centimeters of growth when compared to a healthy group.

Malaria, a parasitic disease caused by *Plasmodium* spp., is spread by the bite of the *Anopheles* mosquito and infects 300 to 500 million people a year, killing 1 to 3 million. The most vulnerable groups are children under five and pregnant women. Over 90 percent of lethal cases of malaria occur in sub-Saharan Africa. The deterioration in public health systems, the movement of peoples as a result of wars and civil unrest, and worsening economies in malaria-endemic countries have resulted in an increase in the rates of malaria infection. Global warming has led to an expansion of the normal range of the mosquito habitat, and thus to an expansion of the regions where infection is a risk. Increasing resistance to drugs used to treat malaria has also meant further spread of the disease and higher mortality rates.

Measles is a viral infection for which there is a very effective vaccine, which unfortunately is often not available in developing countries, partly because of difficulty maintaining the cold chain. Measles accounts for almost 1 million childhood deaths a year, especially among malnourished individuals. Survivors of the infection may have resulting disabilities such as brain damage, blindness, or deafness.

The human immunodeficiency virus was first recognized in the early 1980s. By the year 2000, over 33 million people were infected, with sub-Saharan Africa being one of the worst affected regions. There is no cure. Medications that control the infection are expensive and therefore inaccessible to the majority of infected individuals.

Other tropical infections that cause significant morbidity and mortality include leprosy, leishmaniasis, schistosomiasis, filariasis, and onchocerciasis. Although the mortality associated with these infections is not as great as those described above, they can lead to severe disfigurement and disability as well as a large economic cost and negative social impact. For example, leprosy, a bacterial infection caused by *Mycobacterium leprae* that affects more than 500,000 people a year, can result in significant disfigurement to the tissues of the face and extremities, often leading to severe disability. It is found in Africa, Latin America, and Southeast Asia. Early diagnosis and appropriate medication cure the infection and prevent disability.

Leishmaniasis, a parasitic infection spread by the bite of sand flies, is another infection that can result in severe disfigurement and disability. It causes a spectrum of clinical manifestations ranging from discrete cutaneous ulcers to disseminated visceral involvement, which causes death. It is estimated that 12 million people worldwide are infected. The most severe and lethal form of leishmaniasis, visceral leishmaniasis (also known as kala azar), is increasing in frequency in countries that also have high rates of HIV.

Lymphatic filariasis, caused by blood-borne parasites spread by biting arthropods, is one of the leading causes of long-term disability in the world. Infection with these parasitic worms can result in impairment of lymphatic drainage with resultant marked enlargement of limbs and genitals, a condition sometimes called elephantiasis. Onchocerciasis, another filarial infection afflicting almost 18 million people, can cause visual impairment and blindness.

The increasing movements of people and goods worldwide are facilitating the spread of infectious diseases. It was estimated that by the late 1990s there were over 1.4 billion airline passengers annually. It is inevitable that along with the movement of people, there will be movement of diseases. There have been well-documented cases of diseases such as tuberculosis, poliomyelitis, meningococcal meningitis, malaria, and influenza being brought to Western countries by travelers. An Asian ship that emptied contaminated ballast water off the shores of Peru in 1991 was responsible for the subsequent cholera outbreak of more than 1 million cases in South America, an area that had been cholera free for over one hundred years.

PREVENTION AND TREATMENT

Many tropical infections are preventable by means of simple, inexpensive, and currently available methods. For example, 25 percent of malaria deaths can be prevented by the use of insecticide-impregnated bednets. Comprehensive childhood vaccination programs would virtually eliminate infection with the measles virus. Clean water and good sanitation and hygiene would significantly reduce the burden of diarrheal illness as well as other water-associated infections such as schistosomiasis. Unfortunately, many of these prevention strategies are not being implemented for a variety of reasons. Some governments do not make health care a priority, and the cost of these programs is often beyond the means of some of the worst affected countries—due to poor and/or deteriorating health infrastructures, programs often cannot be undertaken. Armed conflict also often leads to an interruption or deterioration of health services.

Inexpensive and effective medications are available to treat most tropical infectious diseases. However, cost remains a significant barrier, and these medications remain unavailable to the vast majority of the world's population. Contributing to this problem are global patent protection laws that prohibit the manufacture and distribution of inexpensive copies of expensive medications patented by multinational pharmaceutical companies. Also, treatment of many of these diseases, such as tuberculosis and malaria, is now complicated by the emergence of resistance to first-line, traditional medications. Unfortunately, and perhaps understandably for the pharmaceutical industry, financial incentives to develop new products are lacking for a marketplace in which the world's poorest reside. Without the development of new drugs and vaccines, it is possible that we may not be able to effectively treat resistant tropical infectious diseases, relegating a significant proportion of the world's population to suffer or die needlessly.

The list of infections that we need to be concerned about is not static. New and reemerging infectious diseases have become a worldwide problem, the most important of which is HIV. From its initial identification in the early 1980s, HIV has become a leading cause of death in a significant number of developing countries. Other examples of new infections include hantavirus, cryptosporidium, and Ebola virus. Dengue fever, an arbovirus almost eradicated from the Americas by 1980, has made a major comeback in Central and South America as well as in Southeast Asia. Well-developed surveillance systems, accurate diagnostic tools, and an effective public health response are needed in order to identify and contain new infections as they occur.

In summary, many of the infections that we currently consider tropical were once endemic in the more temperate climates of developed countries but were successfully eradicated with a combination of public health, good sanitation and hygiene, and accessible medications. However, prevention and treatment of these infections is being hampered by war, poverty, and, perhaps most importantly, by the lack of political will on both a local and global level.

MARTHA FULFORD
JAY KEYSTONE

(SEE ALSO: *Communicable Disease Control; Contagion; Vector-Borne Diseases; Waterborne Diseases*)

BIBLIOGRAPHY

Bosman, M., and Mwinga, A. (2000). "Tropical Diseases and the 10/90 Gap." *Lancet* 356 (Supp. 1): 563.

Cook, G. C. (1997). "Tropical Medicine As a Formal Discipline is Dead and Should Be Buried." *Transactions of the Royal Society of Tropical Medicine and Hygiene* 91:372–374.

Cox, F. E. G., ed. (1996). *Illustrated History of Tropical Diseases.* London: The Wellcome Trust.

Desowitz, R. S. (1997). "Who Gave Pinta to the Santa Maria." *Torrid Diseases in a Temperate World?* New York: W. W. Norton and Company.

Epstein, P. R. (2000). "Is Global Warming Harmful to Health?" *Scientific American* 283(2):50–57.

Guerrant, R. L., and Bronwyn, B. L. (1999). "Threats to Global Health and Survival: The Growing Crises of Tropical Infectious Diseases—Our 'Unfinished Agenda'." *Clinical Infectious Diseases* 28:966–986.

Murray, H. W. et al. (2000). "Tropical Medicine." *British Medical Journal* 329:490–494.

Shears, P. (2000). "Antimicrobial Resistance in the Tropics." *Tropical Doctor* 30:114–116.

"Supplement on Tropical Medicine" (1997). *Lancet* 349: 1–32.

World Health Organization (1999). *World Health Organization Report on Infectious Diseases–Removing Obstacles to Healthy Development.* Geneva: Author.

—— (2000). *World Health Organization Report on Infectious Diseases 2000–Overcoming Antimicrobial Resistance.* Geneva: Author.

TROPICAL MEDICINE

See Tropical Infectious Diseases

TRYPANOSOMIASIS

Trypanosomiasis, also known as African sleeping sickness, is an infection endemic to sub-Saharan

Africa. It is caused by protozoan parasites called trypanosomes, which are spread by the bite of the tsetse fly. There are two subspecies of trypanosomes that infect humans, each causing a different form of the disease. *Trypanosoma brucei rhodesiense*, found in eastern and southern Africa, causes an acute illness leading to death within weeks or months. *Trypanosoma brucei gambiense*, found in western and central Africa, causes a more chronic form of the illness which may last several years. Both forms of sleeping sickness are fatal if left untreated.

It is estimated that approximately 60 million people are at risk for the disease. Accurate assessment of the extent of the disease is made difficult by the remoteness of the areas in which it is found and the variability in the tests used for diagnosis. Trypanosomiasis often occurs focally, so scattered pockets of infection will be found within an endemic region.

Following the bite of an infected tsetse fly, a scab, or chancre, often forms. After an incubation period of days to weeks, the trypanosomes enter the blood and lymphatic systems and multiply. During this stage, patients may experience headaches, fevers, sweating, rash, and malaise. Enlargement of lymph glands occurs, particularly at the back of the neck. The enlarged nodes may be the only visible sign during this phase of the infection. Eventually the trypanosomes will invade the central nervous system, giving rise to neurological symptoms. This stage, aptly called "sleeping sickness," is characterized by headache, apathy, lethargy, and somnolence. Patients may experience personality and cognitive changes, tremors, and coordination problems. They become increasingly wasted and drowsy, and eventually fall into a coma and die. This progression to death usually occurs in months with *T. b. rhodesiense* and in years with *T. b. gambiense*.

Diagnosis is made by microscopic identification of the parasite, which may be found in the chancre, lymph glands, blood, or cerebral spinal fluid, depending on the stage of the disease. There are several serologic assays available. The sensitivity and specificity of these tests are variable. They are used mainly for epidemiological surveys, but they do have some clinical utility as well.

The form of treatment depends on whether the central nervous system (CNS) is involved. If the disease has not affected the CNS, suramin or pentamidine may be used. In cases of CNS involvement, melarsoprol is the drug of choice. This is a very toxic drug which may have severe side effects, including a fatal encephalopathy. Another effective medication for the treatment of *T. b. gambiense* is eflornithine. Unfortunately, this drug is not currently readily available.

Human beings are the main hosts of *T. b. gambiense*. Control of this infection involves routine screening of at-risk populations, treatment of infected individuals, and control of exposure to tsetse flies, which often inhabit riverine areas. *T. b. rhodesiense* is found in savannah areas in antelopes, other wild game, and domestic cattle, so control of infection is more complicated and involves the coordination of medical, veterinary, agricultural, entomological, and other services.

MARTHA FULFORD
JAY KEYSTONE

(SEE ALSO: *Comunicable Disease Control; Vector-Borne Diseases*)

BIBLIOGRAPHY

Burri, C. et al. (2000). "Efficacy of New, Concise Schedule for Melarsoprol in Treatment of Sleeping Sickness Caused by *Trypanosoma brucei gambiense*: A Randomised Trial." *Lancet* 355:1419–1425.

Neva, F. A., and Brown, W. (1994). *Basic Clinical Parasitology.* Englewood Cliffs, NJ: Prentice Hall.

Smith, D. H.; Pepin, J.; and Stich, A. H. R. (1998). "Human African Trypanosomiasis: An Emerging Public Health Crisis." *British Medical Bulletin* 54:341–355.

World Health Organization (1998). "Control and Surveillance of African Trypanosomiasis." *World Health Organization Technical Report Series* 881(vi):1–114.

—— (2000). "African Trypanosomiasis." *WHO Report on Global Surveillance of Epidemic-Prone Infectious Diseases.* Geneva: Author.

T-TEST

A normal distribution plays a prominent role in tests of hypothesis that involve the mean of a population. In particular, if a random sample of observations is normally distributed, statistical inferences for the sample mean can be made by constructing a Z-test statistic that follows a standard normal distribution. However, the use of this statistic requires knowledge of the true variance of population from which the observations were sampled. Frequently, this quantity is unknown and can only be estimated using the values obtained through sampling. Specifically, an estimate of the sample variance (s^2) can be obtained as follows:

$$s^2 = \frac{1}{n-1} \sum_{i=1}^{n} (x_i - x)^2$$

where n is the total number of observations, x is the mean of the sampled observations, and x_i is the value for the *ith* observation ($i = 1, 2, \ldots n$). When the population variance is estimated using sampled data, the use of the Z-test statistic to perform hypothesis testing can lead to biased results. A solution to this problem was put forth in 1908 by William Gossett, a statistician employed by an Irish brewery who went by the pseudonym "Student." Today, the "Student's t-distribution" is routinely used to perform tests of hypothesis.

The Student's t-distribution is not a unique distribution, but rather a family of distributions whose shape is symmetric and determined by the number of sampled observations, or equivalently, the number of degrees of freedom. Like other probability distributions, the total area under the curve of a t-distribution is equal to one. The p-values for tests of hypothesis based on this distribution can typically be extracted from the published tables that appear as an appendix in most statistical texts. As the number of degrees of freedom increases, the shape of the t-distribution converges to that of the standard normal distribution.

The t-distribution can be used to compare the mean of a sampled population to some fixed, known value. This statistical test of hypothesis is referred to as a "one-sample t-test." For example, a researcher might be interested in determining whether the average family income among Chicago residents was higher or lower that the average family income in the entire United States. Suppose that we knew that the average family income in the United States was $35,000 per year. The mean income from a random sample of Chicago residents could be calculated, and a one-sample t-test could be used to determine whether their mean income level was significantly different from the national average. This one sample t-test statistic is calculated as follows:

$$t_{df} = \frac{x - \mu}{\sqrt{\frac{s^2}{n}}}$$

where x represents the mean of the sampled data, μ represents the hypothesized value of this mean, and n represents the total number of sampled measures. In the above example, μ would equal $35,000 while x would be the average income calculated using data supplied by n Chicago residents. This t-statistic has $n-1$ degrees of freedom.

In practice, the two-sample t-test is a more commonly used statistic. This statistic can evaluate whether or not there are significant differences in the means of two independently sampled populations. In addition to the assumption of independence, it is assumed that within each population the variable of interest is normally distributed with equal variances. The mathematical derivation of this test statistic is as follows:

$$t_{df} = \frac{(x_1 - x_2)}{\sqrt{\left(\frac{s_p^2}{n_1} + \frac{s_p^2}{n_2}\right)}} = \frac{(x_1 - x_2)}{\sqrt{s_p^2\left(\frac{1}{n_1} + \frac{1}{n_2}\right)}}$$

where n_1 and n_2 are the number of observations in each of the two groups; x_1 and x_2 are the means of the two groups, and s_p^2 is an estimate of the pooled sample variance. The sample variance is calculated using the formula:

$$s_p^2 = \frac{(n_1 - 1)s_1^2 + (n_2 - 1)s_2^2}{n_1 + n_2 - 2}$$

where s_1^2 and s_2^2 represent the sample variances in the two groups. The total number of degrees of freedom associated with this t-test is $n_1 + n_2 - 2$.

To illustrate the application of this test statistic, consider the situation where an investigator would like to determine whether infant birthweight was significantly different between mothers who smoked during pregnancy and those who did not. Suppose that the mean birthweight among ten infants whose mothers smoked was 5 lbs., while the mean birthweight among the same number of infants whose mothers did not smoke was 8 lbs. If the pooled sample variance based on the weight measurements taken on these twenty infants was 3 lbs., then using the above formula, the calculated t-test statistic would be approximately 3.9 with 18 degrees of freedom. The two-sided p-value associated with this test is approximately 0.0006. In other words, there is about a 6 out of 10,000 probability of observing a difference at least as large as 3 lbs. by chance alone if there was truly no association between maternal smoking and birthweight. We would therefore conclude that the observed mean difference of 3 lbs. was unlikely to be explained by chance, and consider the observed difference statistically significant.

When the variances in two groups being compared are not equal, the "modified t-test" should be used to compare the means. Instead of using a common pooled estimate of variance,

$$\text{modified } t_{df} = \frac{(x_1 - x_2)}{\sqrt{\frac{s^2_1}{n_1} + \frac{s^2_2}{n_2}}}$$

the variance for each group is used in the calculation of the t-test statistic. Specifically, where n_1 and n_2 are the number of observations in each of the two groups; x_1 and x_2 are the means of the two groups and s_1^2 and s_2^2 represent the variances of the two groups. Because the exact distribution of the modified t-test statistic is difficult to derive, it is necessary to approximate the number of degrees of freedom using the following formula:

$$d = \frac{[(s_1^2 / n_1) + (s_2^2 / n_2)]^2}{(s_1^2 / n_1)^2 / (n_1 - 1) + (s_2^2 / n_2)^2 / (n_2 - 1)}$$

This value of d is rounded down to the nearest integer. Using the calculated modified t-test statistic and the estimated number of degrees of freedom, the p-value can then obtained from the appropriate t-distribution to determine whether the two means are significantly different from each other.

Paired data is frequently collected in studies of public health. Here, each observation in the first sample is matched to a unique data point in the second sample. In the technique of self-pairing, measurements are taken on a single subject, or entity, at two distinct points in time. One example of self-pairing is the before and after experiment where each individual is examined both before and after a certain treatment has been applied. Because the data are no longer independent, the two-sample t-test can no longer be used to test the before and after means. Instead, the *paired t-test* can be used to test the hypothesis that the mean difference of the pairs is equal to zero. This test is

constructed by taking the mean difference of all observed pairs and dividing this by the standard error of all observed differences. The degrees of freedom associated with this test statistic is equal to the number of pairs less one.

Finally, the t-distribution plays a role in hypothesis tests using results obtained from multivariate regression analysis. Multivariate regression models are used to describe the association between an outcome variable and a series of independent variables. Computer programs have been developed to estimate the value of the model coefficients and their standard errors. Tests of significance about each independent variable can be performed by taking the ratio of these parameter estimates and their associated standard errors; this ratio follows a t-distribution. The number of degrees of freedom for these test statistics are determined by the number of observations and the number of independent variables in the fitted model.

PAUL J. VILLENEUVE

(SEE ALSO: *Normal Distributions; Sampling; Statistics for Public Health*)

TUBERCULIN TEST

See Mantoux Test

TUBERCULOSIS

Tuberculosis (TB), an infectious disease, has been present throughout ancient and modern history. TB rates in the United States are on the decline after a resurgence from 1985 to 1992. However, TB continues to be a major killer in much of the world. The implications of this epidemic are global, as travel and migration are now part of everyday life.

Although the cause, diagnosis, and treatment and prevention of TB are known, paradoxically, the disease continues to increase as a public health challenge. Caused by a bacterium called *Mycobacterium tuberculosis*, TB spreads via an airborne route from an infectious person coughing, sneezing, laughing, or singing. The bacteria infect mainly other individuals who have frequent and prolonged contact with a contagious TB case.

HISTORY

TB's existence dates back many centuries. There are references to TB in third-century B.C.E. Chinese and second-century B.C.E. Indian texts; Plato and Hippocrates wrote about it around 400 B.C.E. TB was commonly known as consumption in Europe, a cause of death for hundreds of thousands in the late eighteenth and nineteenth centuries. This is when TB in close groups was first observed and assumed to have a genetic cause, since it was commonly seen in families.

In 1882 Robert Koch's discovery of *Mycobacterium tuberculosis* led to the recognition of TB as an infectious disease. This discovery also led to interventions for interrupting transmission from person-to-person.

Beginning in the late 1880s, TB patients were treated in sanitoria with various modalities, including exposure to fresh air, exercise, and nourishment. About 50 percent of patients recovered or had long-term remission. However, as is known today, their "cure" was not due to the treatments administered but perhaps to self-healing mechanisms.

In the early twentieth century, public health interventions became key in controlling the spread of TB in the cities, where TB was most prevalent. For example, Herman M. Biggs, General Medical Officer of New York City, actively catalogued lists of TB patients and enforced isolation and environmental mechanisms to control TB, including the opening of a TB hospital to quarantine patients. Between 1914 and 1923, the Metropolitan Life Insurance Company conducted the "Framingham Tuberculosis Project" using community nurses to visit the homes of its clients to do assessments, teach health practices, and collect data for research and policy-making purposes. The project was in response to a high rate of TB-related mortality among Metropolitan customers. As a result, mortality rates for TB in the Metropolitan pool declined by 68 percent.

Beginning in 1921, the Bacille Calmette Guerin (BCG) vaccine was used to prevent TB. Still used in many parts of the world but not in the United States, the vaccine is not effective, except perhaps in infants. The discovery of streptomycin in 1943 brought drug treatment for TB. Between 1943 and 1952, two more TB drugs, para-amino-salicylic acid (PAS) and isoniazid (INH), were discovered. Sanitoria began to close in the early 1970s, as TB could be now be treated on an outpatient basis, as evidenced by success in the decrease in TB rates with combined drug treatment and infection-control mechanisms.

RESURGENCE

By 1985, there were 22,201 cases of TB in the United States, the lowest number recorded since national case reporting began in 1953. However, rates then began to increase, until in 1992 cases peaked at 26,673. The human immunodeficiency virus (HIV) epidemic was a major contributor, as its victims are at higher risk for developing active disease once infected with TB bacteria. Migration from countries with high rates of TB added to the number. Also, improper or inadequate drug treatment for TB has led to drug-resistant strains. Finally, medical education stressed TB to a lesser degree in academic curricula, and funding and interest in TB-control programs had dwindled with decreased cases. Most authorities feel that the latter reason was the most important.

Response to the American TB resurgence resulted in increased funding for TB control programs. This gave greater access to TB treatment through health departments. The health departments were responsible not only for treating cases, but for surveillance, outreach, case management, and treatment for those who had been exposed to infectious TB cases. Directly observed therapy short course (DOTS), the observation of the ingestion of medication, has now become the basis for the worldwide standard of TB care. DOTS includes five elements: government commitment to sustained TB-control activities; case detection and self-reporting to health services; standardized treatment regimen of six to eight months for at least all confirmed infectious cases, with directly observed treatment (DOT) for at least the initial two months; a regular, uninterrupted supply of all essential anti-TB drugs; and a standardized recording and reporting system that allows assessment of treatment results for each patient and of the TB control program overall. DOTS is presently available to 25 percent of the world's TB patients, but its acceptance is slowly increasing. There was also an increase in TB educational interventions via the public health sector and medical schools. New drug trials did not create new drugs but created variations on existing drugs and regimens. TB rates began to decrease again in 1994, and as of 1999, they were at an all-time low of 17,528 cases in the United States. Globally, there are still eight million new cases of TB annually with three million deaths. Clearly, even with the exemplary level of achievement domestically, TB cannot be controlled anywhere unless it is controlled everywhere.

THE FUTURE

Although one of the *Healthy People 2010* goals calls for TB elimination from this country, the United States is still far from that goal. Many interventions need to be continued despite falling rates. For other communicable diseases, effective vaccine development and the advent of new drug therapies has been key to disease control approaching elimination. The best course for TB elimination is to develop a vaccine and new drugs while continuing surveillance, treating TB patients who may infect others, treating those who have been infected but are not yet active cases, increasing TB awareness among health professionals, and performing targeted testing for TB infection among high-risk populations. This combination of medical and public health practice can make TB elimination a reality.

RAJITA R. BHAVARAJU
LEE B. REICHMAN

(SEE ALSO: *Communicable Disease Control; Drug Resistance; Immunizations; Isolation*)

BIBLIOGRAPHY

Centers for Disease Control and Prevention (1995). *Self-Study Modules on Tuberculosis.* Atlanta, GA: Author.

—— (2000). *Core Curriculum on Tuberculosis: What the Clinician Should Know,* 4th edition. Atlanta, GA: Author.

Daniel, T. M. (1997). *Captain of Death: The Story of Tuberculosis.* Rochester, NY: University of Rochester Press.

Dublin, L. I. (1952). *A Forty-Year Campaign against Tuberculosis: The Contribution of the Metropolitan Life Insurance Company.* New York: Metropolitan Life Insurance Company.

Reichman, L. B. and Tanne J. H. (2001). *Time Bomb: The Global Epidemic of Multidrug Resistant Tuberculosis.* New York: McGraw Hill.

TULAREMIA

Tularemia is a potentially severe and fatal bacterial zoonosis caused by a gram-negative coccobacillus, *Francisella tularensis.* Tularemia occurs only in the Northern Hemisphere, most commonly in the United States and Europe. In nature, infection occurs mostly in rodents, rabbits, and hares. Humans become infected by handling infectious animal carcasses; eating or drinking contaminated food or water; being bitten by infective ticks, flies, or mosquitoes; or by inhaling contaminated aerosols. The disease is not transmitted person-to-person. The more severe *F. tularensis* strain A occurs only in the United States and Canada, while the milder strain B occurs throughout the Northern Hemisphere.

Tularemia in humans is relatively rare, and it takes several forms, depending on the route of inoculation. The ulceroglandular form is the most common. It is characterized by an ulcer that develops where infection has penetrated the skin, accompanied by painful swelling of nearby lymph glands. Other forms include the glandular, oculoglandular, oropharyngeal, pneumonic, intestinal, and septic ("typhoidal") types. Following a usual incubation period of three to five days (sometimes longer), all forms have similar acute onsets of fever, headache, musculoskeletal pain, progressive weakness, and weight loss. Patients with tularemia pneumonia typically develop a cough with minimal or no sputum production, chest pain, and difficulty in breathing. Patients with the septic form sometimes develop complications of bleeding, respiratory failure, and shock. All forms can be cured by treatment with antibiotics such as streptomycin, gentamicin, or tetracyclines. The disease can be fatal if not treated early with appropriate antibiotics.

Tularemia is best prevented by avoiding sick or dead animals, protecting against tick and insect bites, and by sanitary practices that protect against contamination of food and water by infected animals.

DAVID T. DENNIS

(SEE ALSO: *Vector-Borne Diseases; Zoonoses*)

BIBLIOGRAPHY

Beran, G. W. (1994). *Handbook of Zoonoses, 2nd edition.* Boca Raton, FL: CRC Press.

Dennis, D. T. (1998). "Tularemia." In *Maxcy-Rosenau-Last Public Health and Preventive Medicine,* 14th edition, ed. R. B. Wallace. Stamford, CT: Appleton & Lange.

TYPHOID

Typhoid, or enteric, fever is a serious systemic disease caused by a bacillus, *Salmonella typhi.* Paratyphoid fever is closely related, though generally less severe. The enteric fevers have an incubation period of one to four weeks, followed by a slow onset and prolonged course, primarily affecting the gastrointestinal tract. There is a low fever and severe toxemia. A skin rash may occur in the early stages, and later other organs (liver, kidneys, bone marrow, brain) may be invaded. Typhoid is fatal in about 3 to 4 percent of cases, with higher proportions occurring where diagnostic and treatment facilities are inadequate. Diagnosis sometimes can be made clinically on the basis of patient history and physical examination, but usually depends on isolating the organism from feces or blood culture. Worldwide there are about 16 million cases annually, resulting in 600,000 deaths; in the United States there are usually less than 500 cases a year.

Typhoid is transmitted in feces—usually in polluted water, though sometimes in food that has been prepared under unhygienic conditions by a convalescent or chronic carrier. Humans are the only host for typhoid bacilli, but paratyphoid can be carried and transmitted by domestic animals. Cases continue to excrete the infective organisms in feces, and sometimes in urine, for varying periods, sometimes up to several months after apparent clinical recovery. A chronic (e.g., virtually permanent) carrier state occurs in a small number of cases; "Typhoid Mary" was a notorious example.

There may be other intermediaries between the human source and the victim who consumes contaminated water or food. For instance, water in a river estuary polluted with raw sewage containing typhoid bacilli may be ingested by shellfish or mussels, and these are then infective. It does not require a massive dose of viable typhoid bacilli to cause the disease. There are many well-documented cases of typhoid following ingestion of minuscule amounts of contaminated water or food. For instance, it suffices to eat a few lettuce leaves from a salad that was washed in contaminated water. For this reason, travelers to regions where typhoid is endemic must exercise extreme caution in what they eat and drink. All those who travel to places where typhoid occurs should also be offered prophylactic typhoid vaccine. In the past this has required several injections of vaccine, which often induced painful and sometimes unpleasantly toxic reactions. An oral vaccine is now available.

Cases of typhoid are treated with antibiotics, and notification to public health authorities is mandatory. It is rare in communities with efficient sanitary sewage disposal services and pure water supplies—the occurrence of even a single case indicates a breakdown of sanitation and hygiene in such communities, unless the disease was acquired elsewhere. A careful and complete epidemiological investigation of every case, including a detailed history of food and fluid intake, is therefore essential in order to identify the source of the infection so it can be controlled. Epidemics of typhoid rarely occur now, although they are always a potential threat when disasters such as earthquakes and floods disable sewage treatment plants. Until about the first quarter of the twentieth century, typhoid fever was endemic in all nations, and it caused the deaths of many famous people, including Albert, the consort of Queen Victoria; U.S. president Zachary Taylor; and English poet Rupert Brooke.

JOHN M. LAST

(SEE ALSO: *Food-Borne Diseases; Typhoid Mary; Waterborne Diseases*)

TYPHOID MARY

Mary Mallon (1870?–1938), known as Typhoid Mary, was an itinerant domestic servant and cook, probably an Irish immigrant, though possibly American-born (her origin and early life are unknown). She probably had typhoid fever in 1899 and made an apparently complete recovery. However, she was a symptomless carrier of typhoid bacilli, presumably from a nidus of infection in her gallbladder, for many years—perhaps for the rest of her life.

Between 1900 and 1907, Mallon is known to have infected twenty-two people in New York City, passing the typhoid bacillus to them in cakes she had baked. One of these persons died. The nascent clinical science of bacteriological epidemiology enabled public health authorities to trace her and eventually to apprehend her. She was held in quarantine on North Brother Island, off the Bronx coast, for three years, then released after solemnly promising never to work as a cook again. But she soon broke her promise, and returned to the only occupation at which she could survive, becoming a cook in Sloan Maternity Hospital, where she infected twenty-five more people, two of whom died.

Mallon was incarcerated again in quarantine, where she remained until her death in 1938. She was apparently a likable and pleasant woman—she was said to be "good with children"—and she was an excellent cook. Her life story has been the topic of several books and a movie.

Mallon's experience is a paradigm for some of the failings of public health, which can exert authority over people's lives in order to control some diseases but cannot necessarily correct the underlying social and economic conditions that are ultimately responsible for these diseases. A modern parallel to the story of Typhoid Mary can be seen in the experience of many sex workers infected with human immunodeficiency virus (HIV), hepatitis, and other diseases.

JOHN M. LAST

(SEE ALSO: *Carrier; Communicable Disease Control; Food-Borne Diseases; Quarantine; Typhoid*)

BIBLIOGRAPHY

Leavitt, J. W. (2000). *Typhoid Mary; Captive to the Public's Health.* Boston, MA: Beacon Books.

TYPHUS, EPIDEMIC

The word "typhus" comes from the Greek word for "cloudy" or "misty," referring to the lethargic state of mind that occurs in typhus victims. Epidemic, or louse-borne, typhus, is also known as historic typhus, European typhus, jail, war, camp, or ship fever.

Epidemic typhus is caused by *Rickettsia prowazekii*, a small gram-negative obligately intracellular bacterium. The disease starts with an abrupt onset of symptoms following a one to two week incubation period. Clinical manifestations of typhus include intense headache, chills, fever, and myalgia. A characteristic rash develops on the fourth to seventh day of disease. It first appears on the upper trunk and then becomes generalized, involving the whole body except the face, palms, and soles. As the disease progresses, particularly in untreated patients, significant alterations of mental status, from stupor to coma, are observed. In patients with severe disease, hypotension and renal failure are common. Epidemic typhus is a life-threatening illness even for young, previously healthy persons. Fatal outcomes are observed in up to 40 percent of untreated cases.

Transmission and Epidemiology. Epidemic typhus is a disease of humans. The human body louse *Pediculus humanus corporis* is responsible for transmission of the agent from human to human. Charles Nicolle (1866–1936) first experimentally established this fact, and he received the Nobel Prize in 1928 for his contributions. Lice acquire rickettsiae while feeding on people infected with *R. prowazckii*. A person infested with infected lice acquires the bacteria when the lice or the rickettsiae present in the louse feces are rubbed into bite wounds or other skin abrasions. Epidemic typhus commonly occurs in cold climates where people live in overcrowded unsanitary conditions with few opportunities to change their clothes or bathe. Such conditions often occur during war and natural disasters, which typically facilitate louse infestation. The history of typhus is, in fact, largely the history of men in battle. The disease has been credited with deciding the outcome of more battles than any general's best-laid strategy. Epidemic typhus is currently prevalent in mountainous regions of Africa, South America, and Asia.

Recovery from epidemic typhus results in nonsterile immunity, permitting the persistence of *R. prowazekii* between epidemics. Individuals who have been infected sometimes suffer a relapse in the form of Brill-Zinsser disease, which has the symptoms of classic typhus but is usually milder. In the United States, *R. prowazekii* is also transmitted by the Orchopeas howarolii fleas of flying squirrels. Persons exposed to infected fleas sporadically acquire an infection that is referred to as sylvatic typhus and is typically milder than classic epidemic typhus.

Diagnosis and Treatment. Diagnosis of epidemic typhus is based on detection of specific antibodies in patient sera. The use of clinical and epidemiological data is necessary to distinguish among classic typhus, Brill-Zinsser disease, and sylvatic typhus. Doxycycline is highly effective for treatment of typhus. Epidemic typhus also responds well to treatment with tetracycline or chloramphenicol antibiotics.

Prevention and Control. Insecticides are used to kill body lice, disinfect louse-infested clothing, and prevent the spread of epidemic typhus. Control requires significant efforts to maintain sanitary conditions and living standards, as well as health education. There is no commercial vaccine for preventing epidemic typhus. Several excellent vaccine candidates have been protective in animal models, however.

MARINA E. EREMEEVA

(SEE ALSO: *Communicable Disease Control; Rickettsial Diseases; Vector-Borne Diseases*)

BIBLIOGRAPHY

Walker, D. H., ed. (1988). *Biology of Rickettsial Diseases.* Boca Raton, FL: CRC Press.

Walker, D. H.; Raoult, D.; Brouqui, P; and Marrie, T. (1998). "Rickettsial Diseases." In *Harrison's Principles of Internal Medicine,* 14th edition, eds. A. S. Fauci et al. New York: McGraw-Hill.

World Health Organization (1997). *Epidemic Louse-Borne Typhus* (WHO Fact Sheet No. 162). Geneva: Author. Available at http://www.who.int/inf-fs/en/fact162.html.

U

ULTRASOUND

See Diagnostic Sonography

ULTRAVIOLET RADIATION

The principal adverse health effects of sunlight are caused by the ultraviolet and visible radiation it contains. Ultraviolet radiation (UVR) comprises a spectrum of electromagnetic waves of different wavelengths, subdivided for convenience into three bands, which are measured in nanometers (nm): (1) UVA ("black light"), 315 to 400 nm; (2) UVB, 280 to 315 nm; and (3) UVC (which is germicidal), 200 to 280 nm. Visible light consists of electromagnetic waves varying in wavelength from about 400 (violet) to 700 nm (red).

None of these radiations penetrates deeply into human tissue, so that the injuries they cause are confined chiefly to the skin and eyes. Reactions of the skin to UVR are common among fair-skinned people and include sunburn, skin cancers (basal cell and squamuous cell carcinomas, and to a lesser extent melanomas), aging of the skin, solar elastoses, and solar keratoses. Injuries of the eye include photokeratitis, which may result from prolonged exposure to intense sunlight ("snow blindness"); photochemical blue-light injury of the retina, from gazing directly at the sun; cortical cataract of the lens; and uveal melanoma.

The effects of UVR result chiefly from its absorption in DNA, resulting in the cross-linkage of pyriminide nucleotides, which, in turn, may cause mutations in exposed cells. Sensitivity to UVR may be decreased by DNA repair defects, by agents that inhibit the repair enzymes, and by photosensitizing agents (such as psoralens, sulfonamides, tetracyclines, and coal tar) that increase the absorption of UVR in DNA.

To prevent injury by sunlight, excessive exposure to the sun should be avoided—especially by fair-skinned individuals—and protective clothing, UVR-screening lotions or creams, and UVR-blocking sunglasses should be used when necessary. Also, although the sun is unlikely to cause a retinal burn under normal viewing conditions since bright, continuously visible light normally elicits an aversion response that acts to protect the eye against injury, one must never gaze at the sun nor look directly at a solar eclipse.

From an environmental perspective, it is noteworthy that the protective layer of ozone in the stratosphere is gradually being depleted by chlorofluorocarbons and other air pollutants, and that every 1 percent decrease in stratosphereic ozone shield is expected to raise the UVR reaching the earth sufficiently to increase the frequency of skin cancer by 2 to 6 percent. Of potentially greater significance for human health than the projected increase in cancer rates, however, are the far-reaching impacts on vegetation and crop production that may result from depletion of the ozone shield.

ARTHUR C. UPTON

BIBLIOGRAPHY

American Medical Association, Council on Scientific Affairs (1989). "Harmful Effects of Ultraviolet Radiation." *Journal of the American Medical Association* 262:380–384.

English, D. R.; Armstrong, B. K.; Kricker, A.; and Fleming, C. (1997). "Sunlight and Cancer." *Cancer Causes and Control* 8:271–283.

Henriksen, T.; Dahlback, A.; Larsen, S.; and Moan, J. (1990). "Ultraviolet Radiation and Skin Cancer. Effect of an Ozone Layer Depletion." *Photochemical Photobiology* 51:579–582.

Zabriske, N. A., and Olson, R. J. (1998). "Occupational Eye Disorders." In *Environmental and Occupational Medicine*, 3rd edition, ed. W. N. Rom. Philadelphia, PA: Lippincott-Raven.

UNCERTAINTY ANALYSIS

For any variable or quantity that requires a measurement, short of a "perfect" measurement (which does not exist), the true value cannot be obtained from any known detector or analysis. For example, the measurement of an environmental pollutant will be subject to errors in instrument design, sampling rate, and analytical methods. These errors will lead to measured concentrations that may approach a true value, but will not be 100 percent accurate due to random or systematic processes during detection. Variables or quantities that are subject to uncertainty include: (1) empirical metrics (e.g., concentrations); (2) constants (e.g., diffusion coefficients); (3) decision variables (e.g., acceptable/unacceptable limits); and (4) modeling domains or boundaries (e.g., grid size). Of these variables, the empirical metrics are usually the most uncertain, since each may have many independent variables that can individually or synergistically control the total uncertainty attached to a measurement.

There are different sources of uncertainty for a variable, including:

1. Random error, which is derived from weaknesses or imperfections in measurement techniques or independent interferences.

2. Systematic error, which is due to biases in the measurement, analytical technique, or models; these can be associated with calibration, detector malfunctions, or assumptions about processes that affect variables.

3. Unpredictability, which is due to the inability to control the stability of a system or process, such as the partitioning of a semivolatile compound between the vapor and particle phase in the atmosphere.

Other sources of less importance include the lack of an empirical basis for individual values (theoretical predictions) and dependence/correlation of variables (interdependence of controlling variables in a system). Some uncertainties in variables or systems can be reduced, either by improving the methods of measurement and analysis or by improving the formulation of a model. Some nonreducible uncertainty, however, is inherent within the physical, chemical, or biological system that is being studied and can only be quantified by statistical analyses of data collected from the system.

A number of methods are used to quantify the uncertainty of a system. Analytical uncertainty analysis involves a description of the output or response variable that is a function of the uncertainty of each input variables (independent) that affects the response variable. This technique is only useful for simple systems, however; more complex systems require sophisticated techniques to determine uncertainty and its propagation within a system, such as Monte Carlo distributional methods, Latin hypercube sampling, and the stochastic response surface method.

At times uncertainty is mistaken for variability. Variability consists of the range of values that truly can be ascribed to a variable within a system. In principle, variability is based upon the differences in a variable frequently found within a system (e.g., a population distribution or concentration pattern). It is based on the number and frequency of observations of one or more variables in the system, or on the probability of the occurrence of a specific value (e.g., concentration) in the system under consideration. In this case, the uncertainty would be the quantitative error around the measurement of a single value or all values frequently observed in the system.

PAUL J. LIOY

(SEE ALSO: *Rates; Risk Assessment, Risk Management; Sampling; Statistics for Public Health*)

BIBLIOGRAPHY

Cullen, A. C., and Frey, H. C. (1999). *Probability Techniques in Exposure Assessment.* New York: Plenum Press.

Doll, J. D., and Freeman, D. L. (1986). "Randomly Exact Methods." *Science* 234:1356–1360.

Inman, R. L., and Conover, W. J. (1980). "Small Sample Sensitivity Analysis Techniques for Computer Models with Application to Risk Assessments." In *Communications in Statistics, Part A: Theory and Methods* 17:1749–1842.

Isukapalli, S. S.; Roy, A.; and Georgopoulos, P. G. (1998). "Stochastic Response Surface Methods (SRSM) for Uncertainty Propagation: Application to Environmental and Biological Systems." *Risk Analysis* 18:351–363.

—— (2000). "Efficient Sensitivity of Uncertainty Analysis Using the Combined Stochastic Response Surface Method and Automated Differentiation: Application to Environmental and Biological Systems." *Risk Analysis* 20:591–602.

UNEMPLOYMENT AND HEALTH

The "healthy worker effect" is frequently observed in epidemiological studies in which health characteristics in a working population are compared with those in the general population. The often dramatically lower incidence of morbidity and mortality among workers is due to a number of factors, among which is the higher socioeconomic status of those with jobs as compared to the unemployed, the availability of health insurance and other forms of health coverage, and the fact that individuals who develop chronic diseases before adulthood often do not enter the workforce.

There is evidence that the loss of a job is a significant life event that can lead to unhealthy behaviors, including alcoholism. Unemployment is often a cause of stress and psychological depression, and it can lead to a disintegration of the family. Job loss can also be an indicator of physical, psychological, or behavioral problems in an individual.

Response to job loss can be seen as a public health issue requiring surveillance and intervention, particularly in situations where a downturn in the economy makes reemployment problematic. Risk analyses of regulatory activities should consider the impact of unemployment on public health.

BERNARD D. GOLDSTEIN

(SEE ALSO: *Alcohol Use and Abuse; Poverty; Social Determinants; Social Health; Uninsurance*)

BIBLIOGRAPHY

Gordon, D.; Shaw, M.; Dorling, D.; and Davey Smith, G. (1999). *Inequalities in Health: The Evidence Presented to the Independent Inquiry into Inequalities in Health.* Bristol, UK: The Policy Press.

Smith, R. (1985). "Please Never Let It Happen Again: Lessons on Unemployment from the 1930s." *British Medical Journal* 291:1191–1412.

UNICEF

With its focus on the needs and rights of the child, the United Nations Children's Fund (UNICEF) devotes as much as 80 percent of its funds to programs that can be classified under the broad umbrella of public health. Working in partnership with governments as well as health-related organizations, notably the World Health Organization (WHO), UNICEF is active in programs ranging from immunization and oral rehydration campaigns to water and sanitation projects, and from the fight against acute respiratory infections to the elimination of polio and micronutrient deficiencies. Its contribution to international public health, particularly for children and mothers, has been significant and extensive. Indeed, in the last two decades of the twentieth century, UNICEF, with its activist leadership, helped shape the agenda of international health.

THE EVOLUTION OF UNICEF

The United Nations General Assembly created the UN International Children's Emergency Fund as a temporary agency on December 11, 1946, to provide urgent relief aid to children in countries ravaged by World War II in Europe and Asia. Its assistance consisted of food, shelter, and medicine. In 1953, the General Assembly gave the fund a continuing mandate to help needy children in developing countries and dropped the words "international" and "emergency" from its name. By then, however, the acronym "UNICEF" had become so well known that the Assembly retained it.

With infant mortality as high as 150 to 200 per 1,000 live births in many parts of Asia, Latin America, and Africa, UNICEF soon turned its attention to the urgent health issues of children and mothers. Guidance for such work came from a joint WHO/UNICEF committee on health policies that involved members of the governing boards of both institutions. In recent years, the UN Population Fund (UNFPA) has also joined the committee.

In the early 1950s, infectious diseases were rampant in many parts of the world, and UNICEF became heavily involved in campaigns against those diseases that could be prevented or for which there was a ready treatment. UNICEF furnished equipment and supplies to countries for mass-disease campaigns, with WHO providing the technical support. These campaigns included malaria, yaws, tuberculosis, typhus, trachoma, and leprosy. In its efforts to reduce infant mortality, UNICEF also promoted the training of traditional birth attendants and provided equipment, medicine, and transport for maternal and child health services.

The 1960s saw UNICEF working with the WHO and many governments in extending rural health services, and with the Food and Agriculture Organization of the United Nations (FAO) in fighting child malnutrition. Planning for the development of the "whole child," instead of a more piecemeal approach, became the basis of UNICEF's broader program thrust that opened the door for its focus on education as part of preparation for life.

NOBEL PEACE PRIZE

In 1965 UNICEF was awarded the Noble Peace Prize, thus linking its services for future generations with peace building. The Prize provided a solid base from which to build its effective role in advocacy for children.

UNICEF was the first UN body to take up the issue of family planning. Though the controversial subject was presented in the context of responsible parenthood to UNICEF's executive board in

1966, after an unprecedented and acrimonious debate the deeply divided board deferred its decision by one year, and it eventually took a relatively mild stance on the issue. As UNFPA was created in 1967, the pressure for UNICEF to take up the issue head-on was eased.

By the early 1970s, UNICEF shifted its emphasis to the provision of basic services for children (including education), while it maintained a predominance of its fund allocations to health programs. Though UNICEF changed its stance from its origin as a relief agency to that of a development organization, it continued to respond to emergencies. In 1974, in response to the global economic, food, and energy crises, UNICEF declared a child emergency and launched a special program to meet the urgent needs that existed.

Also in the 1970s, communication activities in support of programs made their appearance as a regular feature of UNICEF programs. These efforts were later broadened to include all relevant elements of society for a common objective, an approach now recognized as an effective development strategy by many development agencies and often referred to as "social mobilization."

ALMA-ATA AND IYC

After two decades of development, and frustrated by the slow progress for a vast majority of the rural population, public health professionals and development specialists began looking for alternative approaches to health care. Their efforts culminated in the 1978 Alma-Ata Conference, cosponsored by WHO and UNICEF, which produced the Declaration of Alma-Ata on Primary Health Care (PHC). The declaration codified earlier efforts by health pioneers in getting health care to the rural poor, and it defined a new philosophy of health that was *for* the people and *by* the people. This represented a revolutionary redefinition of health care and involved the training and employment of lay workers to tackle specific tasks at the community level, with appropriate referrals to secondary and tertiary facilities. The declaration called for a multisectoral approach to health, based on the principles of social justice, equity, self-reliance, and the use of appropriate technology.

The year 1979 was called by the UN General Assembly the International Year of the Child (IYC), and UNICEF was designated as IYC secretariat. A network of national IYC committees carried out a broad range of country-level activities, considerably expanding UNICEF's level of political advocacy and presaging UNICEF's activism of the 1980s.

CHILD SURVIVAL AND DEVELOPMENT REVOLUTION AND GOBI

In 1982 UNICEF launched its Child Survival and Development Revolution (CSDR), which focused on four inexpensive interventions to reduce child deaths. The acronym "GOBI" represents the four program components of CSDR: growth monitoring to detect early signs of child malnutrition; oral rehydration to prevent death by dehydration as a consequence of diarrhea; breast-feeding to stop the unhealthy and often deadly effects of infant formula in poor communities; and immunization against six vaccine-preventable diseases (polio, measles, tuberculosis, whooping cough, tetanus, and diphtheria). Subsequently, UNICEF added food security, female education, and family planning to complement GOBI.

Initially, the WHO expressed caution because it viewed GOBI as vertical interventions, in contrast to the PHC approach, which called for a more horizontal approach that would strengthen health systems. UNICEF was able to reassure WHO officials that GOBI programs were meant to establish entry points for PHC, and the WHO became a partner in GOBI activities. It also joined UNICEF in sponsoring the Bamako Initiative, which aimed at making available essential drugs to African countries as part of PHC, but with cost-recovery and community management as key elements of the initiative.

The term "child survival" proved an effective tool to garner considerable extra resources for child health programs. GOBI programs involving broad-scale social mobilization and the participation of many nongovernmental organizations became dominant public health activities in most developing countries in the 1980s. The oral rehydration and immunization programs have saved millions of children's lives annually. Along with GOBI, UNICEF also started a global effort in health education with its "Facts for Life" health messages, in which WHO and UNESCO were also associated.

WORLD SUMMIT ON CHILDREN

Following the initial success of GOBI, UNICEF engaged in promoting and organizing the World Summit for Children in 1990, which brought more than seventy heads of state and representatives of more than eighty member states to New York for a two-day meeting. The summit was precedent setting, as it was the largest such gathering and the first summit on social issues. It produced a declaration, a plan of action, and a set of goals to be achieved by the year 2000, most of which were in the public health domain. UNICEF followed up the summit with individual national plans of action to reach the goals, and has published an annual *Progress of Nations* to monitor and report on progress.

Concurrent with the summit preparation, the movement to turn the Declaration of the Rights of the Child into the convention made headway. In 1990 the General Assembly adopted the convention, and thus far all member states of the UN have signed the convention, and all but the United States and Somalia have ratified the treaty. UNICEF's current programs are now firmly set in the context of rights. In recent years, UNICEF has not only successfully promoted the convention, but has also undertaken programs in the fields of child labor and the removal of land mines.

There have been impressive gains as a result of UNICEF's contribution to various public health programs. About 7 million young lives are now saved each year as a result of immunization and oral rehydration. Polio has been eliminated from the Americas. Guinea worm cases in Africa have been reduced by 97 percent. An estimated 90 million infants worldwide are protected from a significant loss of intelligence quotient and learning ability because their families use iodized salt that stops iodine deficiency. In spite of the gains, the review of the year 2000 goals scheduled to take place in September 2001 is likely to show that the majority of the targets have not been met. HIV/AIDS (human immunodeficiency virus/acquired immunodeficiency syndrome) has become a major killer of children in Africa. The gap between countries and within countries has continued to widen. Few countries have paid heed to the Summit For Children call for 20 percent of national development investment in the social sector and

20 percent of international development assistance in the social field.

With its role in the summit, however, UNICEF played a major role in setting the international public health agenda for the last decade of the twentieth century, and the General Assembly Special Session for Children in September 2001 is likely to influence public health activities in first decade or two of the new millennium.

UNICEF faces the twenty-first century invigorated by prospects in tackling problems that impact harshly on children in developing countries. With deepening poverty and a widening gap between the rich and poor, plus escalating violence as a result of armed conflict and civil disturbances, child health and women's health will remain major foci of UNICEF.

Malaria, immunization, and micronutrient disorders are among old problems receiving substantial new infusions of funds. HIV/AIDS programs and safe motherhood activities will also be expanded in the years to come. Given the activism of many nongovernmental organizations, including secular, professional, and service-based organizations, and the potential collaboration of the commercial sector, UNICEF's cooperation with the civil society is likely to increase in the years to come.

FUNDING SOURCES

Beginning in 1946 with a modest residue of funds from the defunct UN Relief and Rehabilitation Agency, UNICEF has grown to be a sizable development and humanitarian organization with an annual budget of around $1 billion. It operates entirely on voluntary contributions from both governmental and private sources. In addition to regular contributions, many governments also make special contributions for specific purposes, especially during emergencies. A network of thirty-seven national committees, registered as nonprofit entities in the industrialized countries, inform the public about the needs and rights of the child and raise funds to support UNICEF.

UNICEF has undertaken pioneering work with public personalities, including those in the performing arts or athletics, to generate public support for public health issues. A roster of goodwill ambassadors provides effective support in reaching specific audiences. Income from private sources includes the sale of greeting cards, the Halloween Trick for Treat for UNICEF campaign, television appeals, and special events such as concerts and sports activities. Substantial grants from private foundations, such as the ones created by Ted Turner and Bill Gates, are making private income an increasingly important resource for UNICEF.

As an operating agency of the United Nations, UNICEF is headed by an executive director, who is appointed by the Secretary General of the UN in consultation of its thirty-six-member executive board. Board members are in turn elected by the Economic and Social Council of the UN. There have only been four executive directors, all U.S. citizens, since its inception. Maurice Pate, a banker with experience in humanitarian relief, was the first. Pate steered the organization in its formative years and built its foundation. Henry R. Labouisse, a lawyer and the first foreign-aid chief for President John F. Kennedy, succeeded Pate. James P. Grant, another lawyer and president of the Overseas Development Council, followed Labouisse. Grant launched CSDR/GOBI and orchestrated the UN Summit for Children. Carol Bellamy, a lawyer and a former Director of the Peace Corps, succeeded Grant as executive director in 1995.

With a global staff of nearly 5,600, UNICEF operates from its headquarters at the United Nations in New York. There are eight regional offices—in Bangkok, Katmandu, Amman, Abidjan, Nairobi, Bogota, Tokyo, and Geneva—and 125 field offices serving 161 countries. UNICEF representatives at the country level have considerably more authority and resources than those of its sister UN agencies, but they generally serve under the leadership of the UN resident coordinator.

JACK CHIEH-SHENG LING

(SEE ALSO: *Alma-Ata Declaration; Child Health Services; Infant Mortality Rate; International Development of Public Health; International Health; International Nongovernmental Organizations*)

BIBLIOGRAPHY

Black, M. (1987). *The Children and the Nations*. Australia: Macmillan Co.

—— (1996). *Children First, The Story of UNICEF Past and Present*. New York: Oxford University Press.

Keeny, S. M. (1957). *Half the World's Children: A Diary of UNICEF at Work in Asia.* New York: Association Press.

Speigelman, J. (1986). *We Are the Children.* New York: Atlantic Monthly Press.

UNICEF (1980–2000). *State of the World's Children Reports.* New York: Author.

UNINSURANCE

"Uninsurance" is the lack of any health insurance coverage, either from private sources, such as an employment-based or privately purchased health plan, or from public programs such as Medicare, Medicaid, or the Children's Health Insurance Program (CHIP). While the problem of uninsurance is not unknown in other industrialized countries, the magnitude of the problem is greatest in the United States, where the social safety net is less extensive. In the United States, nearly all persons sixty-five years old and older are covered by at least Medicare. In 1999, an estimated 42.5 million Americans of all ages had no health insurance coverage. Among children up to age eighteen, 14 percent were uninsured in 1999. The proportion of the population without any coverage has been increasing steadily over the past two decades. In 1999, however, coverage increased among most population groups, although it is unclear whether this represents a new trend or simply a fluctuation.

Because more than 80 percent of persons under age sixty-five who have any health care coverage obtain it through employment, decreases and increases in employment-based health insurance coverage are the primary determinants of the number of uninsured people. Thus, the number of uninsured had been increasing, over the long run, primarily due to declining employment-based health insurance.

In the United States, the population groups with the highest uninsured rates are low-income persons (both in working and nonworking families); people of color (particularly Latinos); young adults; workers employed in small firms; and workers employed less than full-time throughout the year. Over 80 percent of all the uninsured are workers or are in a family headed by a working adult, and about half are in families headed by a person employed full-time.

Health insurance coverage is the second strongest predictor of use of health care services, after health status. The lack of health insurance is widely regarded as the primary barrier to accessing and using health care services, particularly for preventive care and for management of chronic conditions.

E. RICHARD BROWN

(SEE ALSO: *Access to Health Services; Ethnicity and Health; Health Care Financing; Medicaid; Medicare; National Health Insurance; National Health Systems; Poverty*)

UNITED NATIONS HIGH COMMISSIONER FOR REFUGEES

Persecution, political violence, natural disasters, armed conflict, and other catastrophic events are among the numerous reasons that, throughout history, millions of people have had to flee their homes as refugees and seek protection in other countries. Organized efforts to protect and assist refugees while finding lasting solutions to their problems can be traced back to 1919 and the founding of the League of Nations. Due to the large numbers of refugees that resulted from World War I, the Russian revolution, and the collapse of the Ottoman Empire, the League of Nations, in 1921, created the position of High Commissioner to deal with the problems of displaced persons.

Initially, the office of the High Commissioner addressed the needs of refugees from Europe, but later became more involved with displaced persons from other nations, including Syria. At that time, refugee assistance focused on defining the status of refugees, helping them with employment, and protecting them from further expulsion.

In 1945 The League of Nations was replaced by the United Nations (UN), and in 1947 the UN created a new agency called the International Refugee Organization (IRO) to deal with matters affecting displaced persons. However, this organization only addressed the needs of refugees from Europe. In 1951 the office of the United Nations High Commissioner for Refugees (UNHCR) was created to replace the IRO. In contrast to the former organization, the UNHCR was charged with addressing refugee problems around the world.

The main role of The United Nations High Commissioner for Refugees is to protect and assist refugees in finding durable solutions to their displacement, addressing their special needs, and promoting and monitoring states' adherence to the 1951 UN Refugee Convention in order to provide adequate protection to the refugees in their respective territories.

UNHCR activities changed significantly during its first half century of existence. For example, the scale of UNHCR operations was greatly increased, with offices in more than 120 nations around the world in 2001. In addition to permanent solutions to the long-term needs of refugees, the organization provides assistance with many more immediate concerns for survival. Initially, the UNHCR focused primarily on facilitating the flow of refugees. Now it also provides material support such as food, shelter, health care, education, and other related social services. It has also designed special programs to meet the specific needs of groups such as women, children, adolescents, the elderly, and those who are suffering from the effects of war trauma. Additionally, the UNHCR has developed programs that assist displaced people within their own countries, returnees, asylum seekers, and stateless people. Finally, the UNHCR works hand in hand with other United Nations agencies, peacekeepers, military forces, regional agencies, human rights organizations, and other international and local organizations and agencies.

Since its establishment in 1951, UNHCR has had as its primary mission the goal of meeting the needs of those forcibly displaced. However, the agency faces continuing challenges such as limited funding, difficult working environments, military threats, large numbers of displaced persons, and often overwhelmingly poor health conditions. Finding clear, lasting, and meaningful solutions to refugee problems around the world is extremely difficult due to complex political, economic, social, and related barriers. However, with more than 20 million refugees worldwide today—and another 24 million displaced persons—there is an obvious need for the UNHCR and other humanitarian organizations to work jointly to ensure peace and tranquility by mobilizing resources that support displaced persons.

MICHELE YEHIELI
CLEMENTINE MUKESHIMANA

(SEE ALSO: *Famine; Genocide; International Health; Natural Disasters; Refugee Communities; Terrorism; War; World Health Organization*)

BIBLIOGRAPHY

UNHCR (2000). *The State of the World's Refugees 2000. Fifty Years of Humanitarian Action.* Available at http://www.unhcr.ch/.

UNITED STATES AGENCY FOR INTERNATIONAL DEVELOPMENT (USAID)

The United States Agency for International Development (USAID) is an independent government agency that provides economic development and humanitarian assistance to advance U.S. economic and political interests overseas. This type of activity started in the United States in 1947 with the Marshall Plan, the forerunner of current development programs. President John F. Kennedy established the USAID in 1961 to promote development around the globe. The agency is currently based in Washington, with field missions abroad. USAID programs have provided aid in Africa, Asia and the Near East, Latin America and the Caribbean, Central and Eastern Europe, and the independent states of the former Soviet Union. The structure of the agency is shown in Figure 1.

To promote development, USAID partners with other U.S. government agencies, U.S. businesses, private voluntary organizations, indigenous groups, and universities. USAID contracts with more than 3,500 U.S. firms and over 300 U.S.-based private voluntary organization (PVOs).

The agency works in five principal areas crucial to achieving U.S. foreign policy objectives: promoting economic growth; advancing democracy; delivering humanitarian assistance to victims of famine and other population-wide emergencies; protecting the public's health and supporting family planning; and protecting the environment.

Figure 1

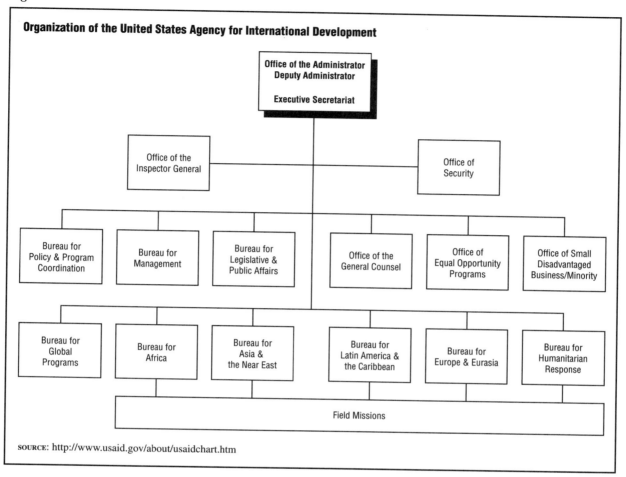

Organization of the United States Agency for International Development

SOURCE: http://www.usaid.gov/about/usaidchart.htm

When considering a nation for development assistance, USAID looks at a number of important factors, including strategic interests, a country's commitment to social and economic reform, and a willingness to foster democracy.

FOREIGN AID

What happens in the developing world has a dramatic impact on America's economic prosperity, environment, and public health. The fortunes of the United States are closely linked to those of other nations. Air pollution, the AIDS (acquired immunodeficiency syndrome) epidemic, rapid population growth, and deforestation are only a few examples of the many problems in the developing world that touch American lives. U.S. development programs reflect the nation's compassion

for the poorest of the poor and America's interest in a more prosperous and peaceful world.

Foreign assistance is seen as an investment in creating the markets of the future, preventing crises, and helping advance democracy and prosperity. Foreign aid creates U.S. jobs and advances American economic well-being.

Economic and humanitarian assistance is also an investment in the future of America's economy. Foreign assistance fosters an enabling environment for U.S. trade and investment in developing nations by establishing fair business codes, viable commercial banks, and reasonable tax and tariff standards. Foreign assistance helps create the stable and transparent business standards by which U.S. companies need to operate. Between 1990 and 1995, exports to developing and transition countries increased by nearly $99 billion. This growth supported nearly 2 million U.S. jobs. Foreign assistance has often resulted in a huge payoff in terms of creating export markets for U.S. goods and services. For example, the United States now exports more to South Korea in just one year than was given to that country in total foreign assistance during the 1960s and 1970s.

HUMANITARIAN RELIEF

The United States has a long and generous tradition of providing assistance to the victims of man-made and natural disasters. Humanitarian assistance has been viewed as both an act of national conscience and an investment in the future. USAID is the world leader in providing assistance to the victims of floods, famine, conflict, and other crises around the globe.

Each year the U.S. government provides food, shelter material, and relief assistance to millions of people around the world who are affected by disasters and conflict. For example, following the mass exodus from Rwanda to Zaire in 1994, tens of thousands of refugees lost their lives due to a cholera epidemic that swept through refugee camps. USAID Disaster Assistance Response Teams and U.S. military forces were sent to the region to assist in establishing a clean-water distribution system to combat the epidemic. These efforts, along with other donors, helped stem one of the largest humanitarian crises of the decade.

CHILD HEALTH PROGRAMS

Among the most important of USAID's public health programs have been its child health programs. USAID has supported child health programs since 1975, intensifying its efforts in 1985 with the Child Survival Initiative. The initiative, carried out in collaboration with host governments and international organizations, has resulted in a 10 percent decline in infant mortality in USAID-assisted countries. Today more than 4 million infant and child deaths are prevented annually due to health services provided by USAID and its partners. These programs include oral rehydration therapy (ORT); acute respiratory infections (ARI); immunizations; breastfeeding; vitamin A; health technologies; malaria; guinea worm;

river blindness (onchocerciasis); displaced children and orphans; and war victims.

Oral Rehydration Therapy (ORT). A simple, inexpensive, and easily administered sugar-salt solution for treatment of dehydration from diarrhea was developed through USAID-assisted programs in Bangladesh. It is estimated to save the lives of 1 million children annually, and is one of the most important medical advances of the century. USAID financed the basic research on ORT, and has led the global effort to ensure that ORT is widely available and correctly used. ORT has been successfully used in recent cholera epidemics in Latin America, Asia, and Africa as well as in treating epidemics in refugee camps in Rwanda and Zaire.

Acute Respiratory Infections (ARI). To combat ARI, now the leading cause of death among children under five years of age, USAID has supported the development of new means of diagnosis and treatment involving the training of health workers, counseling of mothers, and the development of effective communication messages. In 2000 USAID supported ARI programs in thirty-seven countries and funded research on vaccines to prevent ARI. USAID-supported research on behavioral change, drug resistance, and potential preventive technology for controlling ARI is also underway.

Immunization. In 1980 fewer than 5 percent of children in developing countries were immunized against measles, diphtheria, pertussis, polio, and tuberculosis. In 2000 more than 80 percent were protected against these diseases. Immunization programs prevent close to 3 million child deaths annually from measles, neonatal tetanus, and tuberculosis.

Poliomyelitis (a viral infection of the spinal cord) has historically caused lameness in young children. It can also cause paralysis of the respiratory control mechanism, require assisted breathing, or result in death. Polio has been successfully eradicated from the western hemisphere and the western Pacific, and efforts are underway to achieve global eradication by the year 2005. There was more than a 90 percent decline in the reported polio cases worldwide from 1988 to 2000. By mid-2000, 150 countries had reported zero cases of poliomyelitis.

Following the breakup of the Soviet Union, USAID carried out emergency immunization support programs in the Central Asian Republics. Millions of doses of vaccine and huge quantities of cold-chain equipment were provided while immunization systems were rebuilt.

Breastfeeding. USAID has established a model program to promote breastfeeding that is being used to train health professionals from developing countries. The program, in conjunction with UNICEF, is currently providing assistance to more than forty countries in establishing "baby-friendly" hospitals to encourage breastfeeding.

Vitamin A. USAID-supported research has shown that vitamin A supplementation can substantially reduce child mortality in vitamin A-deficient populations. Vitamin A programs are now underway in fifty countries. Indonesia, which reported in 1978 that thirteen of every thousand children under the age of five suffered from night blindness, is now free of nutritional blindness due to vitamin A deficiency. In Central America, because of a vitamin A sugar fortification program, childhood blindness has been prevented in more than half a million children.

Health Technologies. USAID has also invested in research on health technologies. A single use, automatic self-destruct syringe, which prevents the reuse of soiled syringes and needles, has the potential to interrupt the transmission of hepatitis B and C, HIV/AIDS (human immunodeficiency virus/ acquired immunodeficiency syndrome), Chagas' disease, and malaria. Vaccine vial monitors (indicators placed on vaccine vials that show if vaccines should be discarded due to heat exposure) are now being used by UNICEF for poliomyelitis vaccine. New technologies now also make it possible for traditional birth attendants and midwives to provide safe care and home delivery by using kits that include strips to detect protein in urine, low cost delivery kits, and color-coded scales that identify low birth weight infants.

Malaria. USAID has had success in malaria-related research and in programs to fight the increasing incidence of the disease in various countries, including El Salvador, Pakistan, Nepal, Thailand, India, and Sri Lanka. New antimalarials are now used as alternative treatments in the face of drug-resistant malaria. Insecticide-impregnated mosquito nets also provide protection against malaria infection. The development of an effective vaccine is underway through a joint domestic and international effort. Since 85 percent of the malaria occurs in Africa, USAID is focusing its efforts to reduce the burden in the region.

Guinea Worm. As a result of its partnerships, more than a 97 percent reduction in the incidence of guinea worm has been achieved. Eradication of the disease is expected.

River Blindness (Onchocerciasis). The Onchocerciasis Control Program (OCP), launched in 1974 by the World Bank, the World Health Organization, the United Nations Development Programme, the Food and Agriculture Organization of the United Nations (FAO), and other organizations to eliminate river blindness as a public health problem, has eliminated onchocerciasis transmission in seven African countries. This program has prevented an estimated 350,000 cases of river blindness and the infection of 10 million individuals, and it has made possible the reopening of 250,000 square kilometers of fertile agricultural land for settlement and economic development.

Maternal Health Programs. Over 600,000 women die annually of causes related to pregnancy and childbirth. The vast majority of women in the developing world prefer to give birth at home. The major immediate causes of maternal mortality—hemorrhage, obstructed labor, eclampsia, (a serious complication, which includes high blood pressure, seizures, and sometimes bleeding), and unsafe abortions—are preventable with known technologies. In addition, millions of women suffer direct complications of pregnancy and delivery, the consequences of which include decreased quality of life, compromised ability to care for children, and diminished productivity.

USAID, along with the World Bank and UNICEF, have made efforts to reduce maternal mortality and promote maternal health by supporting cost-effective approaches to improve pregnancy and reproductive-health services; the increased utilization of essential obstetric services; and improved quality of care through training and quality-assurance programs. Specifically, efforts have been directed toward promoting behavioral change in those instances where traditional practices are harmful (such as restricting nutrient rich foods during pregnancy or speeding labor with potentially harmful local herbs), and training birth attendants, nurses, and midwives in the use of clean and safe birthing techniques. Support has also been provided for tetanus toxoid immunization of mothers to prevent neonatal tetanus.

Family Planning. Further reductions in maternal illness and death requires making family planning services available to all who need them. Twenty-five percent of maternal deaths could be prevented through the provision of family planning services that allow women to prevent unwanted pregnancies and unsafe abortions, and to time their pregnancies for greater safety. More than 100 million couples in developing countries would like to space or limit births, but lack accurate information and access to quality family planning services.

Improving access to family planning is also essential to improving child survival. Babies born less than two years apart are twice as likely to die in the first year of life as those born after an interval of at least two years. If the mother of an infant becomes pregnant again too soon, she may discontinue breast-feeding, putting her infant at greater risk of illness and death. Adequate birth spacing can prevent one in four infant deaths in developing countries.

In addition, children born to women younger than twenty years old are more likely to die before their first birthday than those born to mothers between the ages of twenty and twenty-nine. Children born to mothers over forty, and born to mother who have already had three or more children, are also more likely to die. One hundred thousand women die each year from the consequences of unsafe abortions. Family planning enables couples to prevent unintended pregnancies, thereby protecting themselves from the risks of unsafe abortions.

Since 1965, family planning programs supported by USAID have helped prevent unintended pregnancies in over seventy countries. USAID supports efforts to strengthen the provision of family planning information and services, as well as research to expand the choice of contraceptive methods and improve the quality of care. Contraceptive use has increased dramatically in many countries, from less than 10 percent in 1965 to over 45 percent in 2000. More than 50 million couples worldwide use family planning as a direct result of USAID programs. As a result, the average number of children per family has dropped from more than six to just over four. Family planning programs are improving maternal health by contributing to declining abortion rates in Eastern Europe. Family planning has also helped prevent the spread of HIV/AIDS by encouraging condom use and other reproductive-health measures.

HIV/AIDS. In December 2000, the World Health Organization (WHO) reported that more than 47 million people had been infected with HIV. The vast majority of people infected with HIV remain asymptomatic for years, allowing the disease to spread unknowingly. As the epidemic of AIDS evolves, it creates new pressures for overburdened social, health, and economic infrastructures in countries where resources are already limited and competing demands are increasing.

USAID has initiated HIV/AIDS prevention programs in fifty countries in the developing world, providing prevention-education training, technical and financial support, and the sale or distribution of condoms in developing countries.

USAID has been involved in social-marketing programs, in the development of improved, cost-effective approaches for sexually transmitted disease diagnosis and treatment; in behavior change interventions; and in providing assistance with the incorporation of HIV/AIDS in national development planning.

Displaced Children and Orphans and War Victims. The USAID Displaced Children and Orphans Fund has assisted and reunified thousands of children separated from their families as a result of wars in Ethiopia, Liberia, Mozambique, the former Yugoslavia, Angola, and Rwanda. It has provided assistance to others displaced by the AIDS epidemic or for social, economic, or political reasons. More than twenty thousand civilian victims of war have received prostheses and rehabilitation assistance from the USAID Patrick J. Leahy War Victims Fund.

KENNETH J. BART

(SEE ALSO: *Canadian International Development Agency; Economics of Health; Global Burden of Disease; International Development of Public Health; International Health; International Nongovernmental Organizations; International Sanctions, Health Impact of; Nongovernmental Organizations, United States; Policy for Public Health; UNICEF; World Bank)*

BIBLIOGRAPHY

USAID (1998). *The Fiscal Year 1998 Accountability Report.* Washington, DC: Author.

—— (1998). *Child Survival: A 13th Report to Congress.* Washington, DC: Author.

—— (1999). *From Commitment to Action.* Washington, DC: Author.

—— (1999). *Status Report on the Year 2000.* Washington, DC: Author.

UNITED STATES CONSUMER PRODUCT SAFETY COMMISSION

The U.S. Consumer Product Safety Commission (CPSC) is an independent federal regulatory agency whose primary mission is to insure that consumer products are safe to use and will not cause injuries or death.

The CPSC was created in 1972 by Congress as part of the Consumer Product Safety Act (CPSA). Congress directed the CPSC to "protect the public against unreasonable risks of injuries and deaths associated with consumer products." The commission has jurisdiction over about 15,000 types of consumer products—from automatic-drip coffee makers to toys to lawn mowers. (Other federal agencies have jurisdiction over certain specific products, such as motor vehicles, foods, drugs, cosmetics, alcohol, tobacco, firearms, pesticides, aircraft, and boats.)

The CPSC enforces other laws in addition to the Consumer Product Safety Act. The Federal Hazardous Substances Act (FHSA) requires the labeling of hazardous household substances. A 1988 amendment to the FHSA, the Labeling of Hazardous Art Materials Act, requires special labeling of certain art materials. The 1994 Child Safety Protection Act pertains to toys, balls, and other possible choking hazards to children. Under that act, the CPSC also developed a bicycle helmet safety standard. The Poison Prevention Packaging Act requires child-resistant packaging for certain drugs and hazardous household substances. The CPSC also issues and enforces regulations under the Flammable Fabrics Act and the Refrigerator Safety Act.

The president of the United States nominates the CPSC commissioners, who must be confirmed by the Senate. One of these commissioners serves as chairman. While the CPSA provides for five commissioners, in recent years Congress has appropriated money only for three.

MECHANISMS OF CONSUMER SAFETY

To accomplish its mission to reduce the unreasonable risk of injuries and deaths associated with consumer products, the CPSC has certain tools at its disposal.

Recalls. The CPSC can initiate recalls of dangerous consumer products, resulting in their repair, replacement, or a refund of their purchase price. Every year, hundreds of products with safety, or potential safety, problems are recalled. The commission is especially vigilant about checking for potentially unsafe toys and children's products.

Mandatory Safety Standards. The CPSC issues and enforces mandatory safety standards. For example, to reduce deaths and injuries associated with children under age five who play with cigarette lighters, a mandatory safety standard was established requiring disposable and novelty lighters to be child-resistant. The CPSC can also ban consumer products if no feasible standard would adequately protect the public, and it can seek civil and criminal penalties against companies that break the law.

Voluntary Standards. The CPSC works with industry to develop many voluntary safety standards. This method was used to develop a voluntary safety standard on baby walkers, making them less likely to fall down stairs. In addition, the CPSC may ensure safer products by meeting with companies and getting them to agree to change their product. This happened in addressing the problem of young children strangling in the loops of window blind and curtain cords. The commission met with manufacturers and persuaded them to eliminate the loops in these cords. The industry later adopted a voluntary safety standard.

Research. The CPSC conducts research on potential product hazards. CPSC scientists and researchers look for new or emerging consumer product hazards and try to find solutions to existing product hazards. Since the 1970s, the CPSC has operated the National Electronic Injury Surveillance System (NEISS), which tracks injuries in U.S. hospital emergency departments and allows the commission to make national injury estimates. The NEISS often serves as an early-warning system about problems with specific consumer products.

Communication/Partnerships. The CPSC communicates with and educates the public by working with the media, state and local governments, and private organizations; and by responding to consumer inquiries. The commission also develops cooperative partnerships with businesses and other organizations to create public health campaigns on many issues. For example, in cooperation with a national baby products company, a grassroots program called Baby Safety Showers was implemented. This program, conducted in hundreds of cities across the country, teaches young parents how to keep their babies safe.

The CPSC is located in Bethesda, Maryland, a suburb of Washington, D.C., and has field offices throughout the country. To learn more about the commission and to obtain information about a wide variety of home safety issues, consumers can visit CPSC's web site at http://www.cpsc.gov, or call its toll-free hotline at 1-800-638-2772.

ANN BROWN

(SEE ALSO: *Childhood Injury*)

UNITED STATES DEPARTMENT OF AGRICULTURE (USDA)

The particular contribution of the United States Department of Agriculture (USDA) to public health rests, for the most part, in its spawning of the great U.S. regulatory agencies: the Animal and Plant Health Inspection Service (APHIS); the Environmental Protection Agency (EPA); the Food and Drug Administration (FDA); and the Food Safety and Inspection Service (FSIS). Of these, APHIS and FSIS remain within the USDA, while the EPA became an independent agency in 1971 and the FDA became an independent agency in 1941 and then later became part of the Department of Health Education and Welfare (now the Department of Health and Human Services).

APHIS regulates plant and animal diseases mainly in order to protect economic interests. Some of the animal diseases, however, are transmissible to humans, including brucellosis (undulant fever) and tuberculosis. APHIS also is charged with keeping exotic animal diseases such as foot and mouth disease and bovine spongiform encephalopathy (BSE or mad cow disease) out of the United States. Epidemics of both these diseases among animals in several European countries during 2000 and 2001 have caused considerable fear of meat products as well as economic damage from extensive killing of animals to control the epidemics. Thus far during these outbreaks, however, no cases of either disease have been reported in the United States. Success in this area has marked APHIS as one of the most effective agencies of its kind in the world.

FSIS is charged with the inspection of meat, poultry, and eggs. A particularly large agency of more than 9,000 employees, FSIS is required by law to continuously inspect food animals during slaughter. This requirement is somewhat dated and is based on the dubious presumption that visual inspection is effective.

In order to modernize meat and poultry inspection, FSIS published a regulation in 1996 which has enabled the agency to employ the Hazard Analysis and Critical Control Point System (HACCP) as an added and improved safeguard. HACCP is a systems approach to food control that emphasizes prevention. First developed for the space program, HACCP is generally recognized as the most advanced system for ensuring safe food. Integral to the system is the identification of hazards that could contaminate the food and a comprehensive set of verification steps and audits that ensure the system has been effective. First adapted to a regulatory framework by the U.S. government, HACCP is now the standard of food inspection throughout the world. The Centers for Disease Control (CDC) has evaluated HACCP and concluded that it is, in fact, reducing food-borne disease from meat and poultry sources.

Egg inspection primarily consists of publishing standards for storage and temperature coupled with delegated collaboration with state and local officials. Egg safety concerns have been heightened by the advent of *Salmonella enteritidis* in the early 1980s. This organism found a new niche in the oviduct of laying chickens. While causing no disease to the bird, by seeding itself in the egg yolk it became a leading cause of salmonellosis in humans. Control programs center on eliminating the disease from breeder and laying flocks, as well as with consumer education programs designed to encourage adequate cooking of eggs. These interdiction programs have materially reduced human infection associated with the organism.

FSIS also operates two so-called "zero tolerance" programs—for *Listeria monocytogenes* and for *Escherichia coli 0157:H7*. Zero tolerance means that the presence of the organism at any level in a sample of ready-to-eat food is grounds for recall of the food from the marketplace. The largest food recalls in American history have resulted from this policy over the past two years. The *L. monocytogenes* program was initiated in 1988; a 1994 evaluation by CDC credited the program with a 25 percent reduction in human Listeriosis. The hemorrhagic *E. coli* program was implemented in 1994; human enterohemorrhagic *E. coli* has not particularly declined, but it also has not increased since the inception of the program in the midst of an annually progressing incidence.

FSIS has overseen a dramatic reduction in chemical contaminants of the meat and poultry supply. In the late 1970s and early 1980s, 10 percent or more of these foods were contaminated with anabolic steroids, antibiotics, pesticides, or heavy metals. Today, the levels of violative residues are below 1 percent and, in most meat commodities, levels are approaching zero. Violative levels are hazardous concentrations in foods. These accomplishments are due to a risk-based sampling program followed by sanctions against violators, due in part to a productive synergy with FDA's Center for Veterinary Medicine (CVM). CVM has banned or severely restricted a number of persistent agricultural chemicals such as diethylstilbesterol, sulfamethazine, and dimetridazole. CVM has acted on information developed with FSIS to both educate and prosecute farmers and veterinarians who do not use animal drugs correctly.

LESTER M. CRAWFORD

BIBLIOGRAPHY

Brown, M., ed. (2000). *HACCP in the Meat Industry.* Cambridge, UK: Woodhead Publishing Ltd.

Crawford, L. M., and Franco, D. A. (1993). *Animal Drugs and Human Health.* Basel: Technomics Press.

UNITED STATES DEPARTMENT OF ENERGY (USDOE)

The United States Department of Energy (USDOE) has a broad national mission that includes oversight of energy production and distribution. It also has a major role in the production of nuclear weapons, the safe storage of nuclear wastes, and the remediation of sites that have been contaminated as a result of the nation's atom bomb production program. DOE has a strong scientific component located in the DOE National Laboratories, which support research ranging from basic biologic processes to risk assessment.

While not a frontline public health agency, DOE engages in many activities that impact human health and the environment. These include its role in the national choice of energy sources, such as the different fossil fuels that emit varying levels of sulfur oxides, particulates, and nitrogen oxide air pollutants; nuclear energy with its attendant risks; and hydroelectric power sources, which also have ecological consequences. DOE is also heavily involved in research to develop more efficient and less-polluting automobiles. Within the DOE, the Division of Environmental Management and the Division of Environment, Health, and Safety have combined annual budgets of over $6 billion, which is used to clean up the legacy of atom bomb production and to protect worker and community health.

The secrecy surrounding the atom bomb program and a series of poor decisions on the part of DOE leadership have, at times, engendered distrust of the agency by local communities, scientific groups, and by Congress. This has led to many of its nuclear regulatory functions being placed under the independent control of the Nuclear Regulatory Commission and its worker surveillance programs largely placed under the direction of the Centers for Disease Control. It has also led to the funding of credible university-based organizations to work with the various stakeholders, such as the Consortium for Risk Evaluation with Stakeholder Participation. Compounding the issue of distrust is the public perception of grave risks associated with nuclear materials and the millennia-long half-lives of many radioactive compounds. A central issue for DOE is to find ways to safely and credibly provide stewardship of radioactive wastes for future generations.

BERNARD D. GOLDSTEIN

(SEE ALSO: *Automotive Emissions; Centers for Disease Control and Prevention; Nuclear Power; Nuclear Waste; Sulfur-Containing Air Pollutants [Particulates]*)

UNITED STATES DEPARTMENT OF HEALTH AND HUMAN SERVICES (USDHHS)

The United States Department of Health and Human Services (USDHHS) was officially created by President Jimmy Carter in 1980, when the Department of Education was fashioned out of the education component of the Department of Health, Education, and Welfare. It traces its beginning to the establishment of the Federal Security Agency by President Franklin Roosevelt in 1939. The Federal Security Agency became the Department of Health, Education, and Welfare (DHEW) in 1953 and then DHHS in 1980. In the 1990s, three major changes affected the DHHS: (1) on March 31, 1995, the Social Security Administration, with its more than 55,000 employees and $400 billion expenditures (in 1995) was established as an independent agency, with the commissioner of social security reporting to the president; (2) in 1995, the eight agencies of the U.S. Public Health Service were designated as operating divisions of DHHS, reporting to the secretary instead of reporting to the Assistant Secretary for Health (which they had done since 1968); and (3) in 1996, Congress terminated the federal Aid to Families With Dependent

Children's Program (commonly called welfare) and replaced it with block grants to states that stressed work instead of a minimum guaranteed payment for poor mothers and their children, thus dramatically reducing the federal role in welfare policy. The result of these changes was to make DHHS a de facto department of health.

The USDHHS is led by the Secretary of Health and Human Services Staff Offices (e.g., general counsel, Assistant Secretaries for Health, for Legislation, for Planning and Evaluation, for Public Affairs, and for Management and Budget, Director of the Office of Civil Rights), an independent inspector general and twelve operating divisions: (1) Administration on Aging; (2) Administration for Children and Families; (3) Health Care Financing Administration (Medicare and Medicaid); (4) Program Support Center; and the eight divisions that together constitute the U.S. Public Health Service: (1) Agency for Health Care Quality and Research, (2) Agency for Toxic Substances and Disease Registry, (3) Centers for Disease Control and Prevention, (4) Food and Drug Administration, (5) Health Resources and Services Administration, (6) Indian Health Service, (7) National Institutes of Health, and (8) Substance Abuse and Mental Health Services Administration.

In the year 2001, the expenditures by DHHS will exceed $400 billion, second only to the Social Security Administration. The largest expenditures will be for Medicare ($260 billion) and Medicaid ($123 billion), followed by the NIH ($20 billion), the Administration for Children and Families ($17 billion), to the smallest grant-in-aid programs ($29 million) of the Agency for Healthcare Research and Quality. The DHHS employs more than 50,000 individuals, mainly in the Indian Health Service and NIH.

The DHHS administers over 300 grant-in-aid programs, primarily to state and local governments for a variety of public health and social service programs, to universities for research, and to a range of nonprofit organizations and institutions (e.g., hospitals and community health centers).

The secretary's responsibilities include overseeing the hundreds of public health and social service programs, as well as Medicare and Medicaid. The secretary also oversees the Food and Drug Administration (FDA), which is the federal government's primary public health regulatory agency. In addition, the secretary advises the president on a range of health and social services policies. When President Roosevelt initiated the Federal Security Act in 1939 it was his desire to unite all federal agencies "concerned with the promotion of social and economic security, educational opportunity and the health of the citizens of the nation." In the intervening years the DHEW included these functions and expanded rapidly in the 1960s, with the advent of President Johnson's great society programs. In the 1970s, environmental health programs were moved to the EPA; in the 1980s education and vocational rehabilitation programs moved to the newly created Department of Education; and in 1995 the Social Security Administration (the core of the Federal Security Agency) became an independent agency. Despite these changes, the DHHS remains the largest federal department and one of the most complex to lead and manage.

PHILIP R. LEE, ANNE M. PORZIG,
BRIAN PUSKAS, JO IVEY BOUFFORD

(SEE ALSO: *Administration for Children and Families; Agency for Healthcare Research and Quality; Centers for Disease Control and Prevention; Food and Drug Administration; Health Care Financing Administration; Health Resources and Services Administration; National Institutes of Health; United States Public Health Service [USPHS]*)

BIBLIOGRAPHY

Berkowitz, E. (1998). "Health and Human Services, Department of." In *A Historical Guide to the U.S. Government,* ed. G. T. Kurian. New York: Oxford University Press.

UNITED STATES PREVENTIVE SERVICES TASK FORCE (USPSTF)

The United States Preventive Services Task Force (USPSTF) is a group of nongovernmental experts convened by the U.S. Department of Health and Human Services to review published literature and develop recommendations for the use of clinical preventive services. The task force are experts chosen for their experience in the evaluation of clinical evidence and its application to the care of patients. The first task force patterned itself on a previous program in Canada. Its report, entitled *Guide to Clinical Preventive Services,* appeared in 1988. The second task force met between 1990 and 1995 and published a second edition of the guide in 1996. This second edition contained recommendations on 53 screening tests, 11 counseling interventions, 13 immunizations, and 6 medications to prevent illness. The third task force convened in 1998.

The concept of preventing disease probably began in the 1790s with Edward Jenner's cowpox vaccination against smallpox. The eradication of smallpox and the near-eradication of polio are among the triumphs of preventive medicine. "Disease prevention"—appropriate in the case of smallpox and polio—is a misnomer in most cases. "Risk reduction" is a more apt description of what preventive services actually do. Counseling about seatbelt use, immunization against influenza, and medications to prevent osteoporosis and fractures are examples of preventive services that reduce the risk of illness or injury. Other preventive services, exemplified by a screening test, detect disease before it can do harm. The goal of breast cancer screening is to detect cancer before it spreads beyond the breast. As with many diseases, especially cancers, early detection improves the chances for effective treatment.

A recommendation to provide a preventive service establishes a policy that will apply to everyone. Airbags are a good example. All cars have them, yet very few people will have an accident in which airbags will function to save their lives. This situation is typical of most preventive services: The target condition occurs infrequently in healthy people. Therefore, many people are exposed to the risks of airbags for each person who survives an accident because of airbags. This example shows that a recommendation for a preventive service should have solid evidence that its benefits exceed any harms. This fact is the principal justification for convening experts to evaluate and using a systematic approach to this task.

The current United States Preventive Services Task Force exemplifies a thorough approach to the evidence. Once the task force decides to make recommendations about a topic (e.g., screening for diabetes), a federally funded university-based group of scholars searches the published literature for evidence about the effect of the preventive service on health outcomes. The group evaluates the evidence, picks the best research, and summarizes it in tabular form and in an evidence report. The task force meets four times a year to decide on the quality of the evidence and to formulate a recommendation. These recommendations vary in their conviction depending on the strength of the evidence.

Before making a recommendation, the task force considers two features of the evidence. First, is the evidence valid? In other words, does the preventive service really do what the evidence seems to say? To form this judgment, the task force must be sure that the preventive service (e.g., lowering serum cholesterol) rather than other factors (such as a healthy lifestyle) is responsible for a reduction in the frequency of a disease such as coronary heart disease. Second, how large is the effect of the preventive service? If the evidence is strong and the preventive service has a large health effect, the task force will make a strongly favorable recommendation. Otherwise, the task force may recommend against doing the preventive service, or it may simply say that the evidence is too weak to make a recommendation for or against the preventive service.

The task force publishes supporting evidence to justify each of its recommendations. Each publication consists of a description of the burden of suffering from the target condition, the effect of the preventive service on the risk of the target condition, recommendations of other organizations, and a discussion of special aspects of the evidence. Each publication begins with a concise description of the recommendation and a summary rating of the strength of the evidence and ends with a description of the clinical intervention that physicians would provide.

HAROLD C. SOX

(SEE ALSO: *Clinical Preventive Services; Prevention; Prevention Research; Preventive Health Behavior; Preventive Medicine; Primary Prevention*)

BIBLIOGRAPHY

United States Preventive Services Task Force (1996). *Guide to Clinical Preventive Services*. Baltimore, MD: Williams and Wilkins. Also available at http://www.apchr.gov/clinic/cpsix.htm.

Woolf, S. H, and Sox, H. C. (1991). "The Expert Panel on Preventive Services: Continuing the Work of the U.S. Preventive Health Services Task Force." *American Journal of Preventive Services* 7:326–330.

UNITED STATES PUBLIC HEALTH SERVICE (USPHS)

The eight agencies of the United States Public Health Service (USPHS) are the major public health component of the U.S. Department of Health and Human Services (USDHHS). The central mission of the PHS is to protect the health of the country's population. The action plan for the PHS has been translated into the main goals of *Healthy People 2010*: (1) increase quality and years of healthy life, and (2) eliminate health disparities.

In order to achieve these broad goals, *Healthy People 2010* includes four broad categories of action: (1) promote healthy behaviors; (2) promote healthy and safe communities; (3) improve systems for personal and public health; and (4) prevent and reduce disease and disorders. Within these four broad categories are twenty-eight priority areas (e.g.. improve the health, fitness, and quality of life of all Americans through the adoption and maintenance of regular, daily physical activity), and within these twenty-eight priority areas are 467 specific objectives. For each of the priority areas, PHS agencies (operating divisions in the USDHHS) are designated to coordinate activities directed toward achieving the objectives. The PHS periodically reviews progress toward achieving the *Healthy People* objectives.

The PHS administers hundreds of grant-in-aid programs, ranging from grants to support basic laboratory research by investigators in university departments, to block grants to states for support of maternal and child health services. Many of these grant-in-aid programs have a very narrow focus, specifying in some detail the action that must be taken by grantees (e.g., a state agency), while other grants (e.g., the Prevention block grant) permit greater leeway by the grantees. In addition to its hundreds of grant-in-aid programs, the PHS conducts research in its own laboratories, regulates the food, drug, medical device, and cosmetic industries (through the Food and Drug Administration), and directly manages health care and public health programs for the Native American tribes living on reservations and in Alaskan villages.

While the PHS traces its origins to an act "for the relief of sick and disabled seaman" passed by Congress and signed into law by President John Adams in 1798, its modern structure dates to the Public Health Service Act of 1944, as well as to the organization of the Federal Security Agency (FSA) by President Roosevelt in 1939 (when the PHS was moved from the Treasury Department to the FSA), and to the creation of the Department of Health, Education and Welfare (DHEW) in 1953. Following a series of transfers of programs out of DHEW (environmental health in 1970, education in 1980, and social security in 1995), the modern home for the PHS was established. The name of the department was changed to Health and Human Services after the Office of Education was separated to create the Department of Education.

The PHS underwent a series of reorganizations beginning in 1966, which resulted in the assistant secretary for health becoming chief operations officer of the PHS in the early 1970s. During the next several decades there were organizational changes within the USPHS, but the leadership continues to rest with the assistant secretary for health.

The PHS was reorganized by the secretary of Health and Human Services in 1995 with the operating divisions (agencies) reporting to the secretary instead of the assistant secretary for health (who now heads the Staff Office of Public Health and Science). The eight PHS operating agencies are:

1. Agency for Toxic Substances and Disease (ATSDR)

2. Agency for Healthcare Research and Quality (AHRQ)

3. Centers for Disease Control and Prevention (CDC)

4. Food and Drug Administration (FDA)

5. Health Resources and Services Administration (HRSA)

6. Indian Health Service (IHS)

7. National Institutes of Health (NIH)

8. Substance Abuse and Mental Health Services (SAMHSA)

The assistant secretary for health heads the Office of Public Health and Science and is the senior advisor to the DHHS secretary on health and science. In that position, he or she leads cross cutting between initiatives as identified by the secretary who is now the head of the PHS and directs the activities of the major PHS agencies. The surgeon general reports to the assistant secretary for health and is considered the nation's spokesman on public health issues. Located in the Office of Public Health and Science are important program offices supporting the work of the assistant secretary of health and coordinating USDHHS programs such as the National AIDS Program Office, the Office of International Health, the Office of Emergency Preparedness, the Office of Women's Health, the Office of Minority Health, the Office of Disease Prevention and Health Promotion, the National Vaccine Program Office, and the President's Council on Physical Fitness and Sports. It should be noted that the Public Health Service has commissioned officers (physicians, dentists, nurses, engineers) assigned to all the PHS operating agencies. The functions of the PHS operating divisions are described below.

Agency for Toxic Substances and Disease Registry (ATSDR). The ATSDR performs specific public health functions concerning hazardous substances in the environment. This agency works to prevent exposure and to minimize adverse health effects associated with waste management emergencies and pollution by hazardous substances. The agency goals are to identify people at risk of exposure to hazardous substances, evaluate the degree of risk due to the presence of toxic agents in the environment, and prevent or mitigate adverse human health outcomes.

Agency for Healthcare Research and Quality (AHRQ). Established in 1999 by Congress from its predecessor agency, the Agency for Health Care Policy and Research, the AHQR focuses on quality of care and medical care outcomes, rather than the health system and health care policy. The agency is responsible for conducting and sponsoring research to enhance the quality, appropriateness, and effectiveness of health care services. In general, the primary aims of the AHRQ are to support research designed to improve the quality of health care, reduce its cost, and broaden access to essential services.

Centers for Disease Control and Prevention (CDC). The CDC acts as the lead PHS agency relating to the surveillance and identification of disease through epidemiological and laboratory investigations, and it is the primary agency administering grants to support public health programs, such as HIV/AIDS (human immunodeficiency virus/acquired immunodeficiency syndrome), sexually transmitted diseases (STDs), injury protection, immunization, and cancer screening, in DHHS. The CDC is composed of eleven major operating components. These include three program offices, Epidemiology, International Health, and Public Health Practice, and eight centers, Immunization, Chronic Disease Prevention and Health Promotion, Prevention of Infectious Diseases, Injury Prevention and Control, HIV and STD Prevention, Health Statistics, Environmental Health, and the National Institute for Occupational Safety and Health (NIOSH). With its headquarters in Atlanta, Georgia, it has personnel abroad and on local, state, and federal levels of public health to facilitate data collection, analysis and program implementation. In addition to controlling the introduction and spread of disease in the United States, the CDC provides assistance to other countries and international health organizations.

Food and Drug Administration (FDA). The FDA is charged with administering the Federal Food, Drug, and Cosmetic Act and several related public health laws. New medical devices, experimental drugs, biologics, cosmetics, food additives, and food labels are some of the everyday items under FDA scrutiny. The FDA, in cooperation with the United States Department of Agriculture, is the primary federal agency responsible for food safety. It must assure the safety of all imported goods (e.g., fruit and vegetables) as well as domestically produced foods, except meat and poultry. The FDA also protects the nation's food supply indirectly by monitoring the type of food given to livestock. The United States Department of Agriculture is responsible for meat and poultry safety.

Health Resources and Services Administration (HRSA). The HRSA is a large and complex agency with three major bureaus that administer numerous categorical grant-in-aid programs to the states. The HRSA attempts to improve access to medical care for the indigent, uninsured, rural residents, and other special-need populations. HRSA promotes quality health care to underserved populations with policies that range from training of minority primary-care physicians to the resources related to health care for federal prisoners. It is the agency responsible for providing health professions education programs to meet national needs. The National Health Service Corps Program is one such program sponsored by HRSA that aims to direct health care personnel to underserved areas. The HRSA supports community health centers and funds the Ryan White CARE (Comprehensive AIDS Resources Emergency) Act for people living with HIV/AIDS. Though it works to improve the resources for maternal and child health, and establishes policies in cooperation with the private sector, including policy for allocation of organ, bone, and tissue transplants.

Indian Health Service (IHS). Article I, Section 8 of the U.S. Constitution is the original legal basis for the federal government's responsibility to provide health services to American Indians and Alaskan Natives. The structure of the IHS has been shaped by numerous treaties, laws, Supreme Court decisions, and executive orders since the ratification of the Constitution. The goals of the IHS have been to ensure that comprehensive, culturally acceptable personal and public health services are available and accessible to all American Indian and Alaskan Native people. Because of limited resources, the hospitals, clinics, and public health programs of the IHS primarily serve Indian reservations and Eskimo villages. Currently more than half of all American Indians do not reside on reservations and are not eligible for these direct services provided by IHS. In recent years the IHS worked closely with tribes to transfer program management to the tribes. Limited funding by Congress has slowed this process. Currently, the IHS provides care for approximately 1.5 million Native Americans and Alaskan Natives in thirty-four different states. Depending on the resources available, the IHS attempts to provide a full range of preventive, primary medical care (hospital and ambulatory care), community health, alcohol programs, and rehabilitative services. The IHS contracts with non-HIS providers such as individual physicians, state and local public health agencies or tribunal health institutions when the agency's facilities, resources, or highly specialized medical services are not available.

National Institutes of Health (NIH). Headquartered in Bethesda, Maryland, the NIH is composed of twenty-seven separate institutes and centers, including the National Institute of Environmental Health Sciences, located in North Carolina. The mission of the NIH is to fund biomedical research in its own laboratories, and in universities, hospitals, private research institutions, and private industry, to develop new knowledge that can potentially improve the health of the population, the quality of medical care, and the understanding of disease processes. The research at NIH is focused primarily in basic biomedical and clinical research.

Substance Abuse and Mental Health Services Administration (SAMHSA). SAMHSA was created in 1995, when the Alcohol, Drug Abuse, and Mental Health Administration (ADAMHA), created in 1973, was broken up and its research function transferred to NIH in three categorical divisions: Drug Abuse (NIDA), Alcohol Abuse and Alcoholism (NIAAA), and Mental Health (NIMH). The services programs (grant-in-aid program) was transferred to the newly created SAMHSA. The mission of SAMHSA is to improve the quality and availability of prevention, treatment, and rehabilitation services for persons suffering from alcoholism, substance abuse, and mental illness. SAMHSA's Center for Mental Health Services, Center for Substance Abuse Prevention, and Center for Substance Abuse Treatment work together and with other government and private organizations to build the infrastructure that facilitate community prevention and treatment. The agency funds programs and conducts its own studies and studies in conjunction with the NIH and other agencies, to improve treatment methods. SAMHSA provides its services primarily through block grants and contracts with state health agencies, in order to help reduce illness, death, disability, and cost to society caused by substance abuse and mental illness.

Currently, specific challenges facing the PHS include the threat of bioterrorism, the global HIV/AIDS epidemic, and assuring safety of the blood and food supply. Major problems and challenges include:

1. Applying the growing body of knowledge of the multiple determinants of health of populations, including health behaviors, human biology, the physical environment, the socioeconomic environment, and health care, to federal and state health policies and programs.

2. Continuing to support advances in science and technology, including those in biomedical research, social and behavioral sciences, computer science and informatics, nanotechnology, and other areas.

3. Developing the potential of the National Health Information Infrastructure (NHII), based on the Internet and the World Wide Web, to foster connectivity among the parties invoked in achieving healthier communities, improving patient safety, improving quality of health care, and contributing more directly to the health of individuals.

4. Respondent to the changing nature of the health problems in the United States, including the increased burden of chronic illness; sociobehavioral health problems (e.g., substance abuse, violence); the aging of the population; the increasing diversity of the population; the growing disparities in health status related to race; ethnicity and socioeconomic status; and the threats posed by infectious diseases.

5. Addressing the problems created at the state and local level by the current proliferation of categorical public health programs designed to deal with specific diseases, specific services, specific populations, specific providers, specific locations, or other categories.

6. Responding to the increasing importance of global health issues as country boundaries become more permeable to disease and as global markets determine the safety of food and the availability, quality and cost of pharmaceuticals, blood and medical devices.

The performance and impact of the U.S. health system (including both medical care and public health) in this complex environment can be significantly improved if a comprehensive strategy to promote public health is developed with leadership by the U.S. Public Health Service, and if supported with the necessary investments.

PHILIP R. LEE
BRIAN PUSKAS
ANNE M. PORZIG
JO IVEY BOUFFORD

(SEE ALSO: *Agency for Healthcare Research and Quality; Block Grants for Public Health; Centers for Disease Control and Prevention; Food and Drug Administration; Health Resources and Services Administration; Healthy People 2010; National Institutes of Health; United States Department of Health and Human Services [USDHHS]*)

UNIVERSAL HEALTH CARE

See National Health Systems *and* Uninsurance

UNIVERSAL PRECAUTIONS

These are procedures to be followed by all staff who are caring for a patient believed to be harboring a highly contagious dangerous pathogen, such as AIDS (acquired immunodeficiency syndrome), that is transmitted in blood, blood products, and other body fluids. Universal precautions were described in directives and guidelines issued by the Centers for Disease Control and Prevention (CDC) in 1987, and in standards published by the Occupational Safety and Health Administration (OSHA) in 1991. Revisions are published from time to time in *Morbidity and Mortality Weekly Reports (MMWR)*. Universal precautions in care of patients are an enhanced form of barrier nursing, but they are used also in handling pathology specimens that are known or suspected to be infected with dangerous pathogens. All medical, nursing, and laboratory staff, including mortuary attendants, wear gloves, waterproof aprons, gowns, masks, and protective eye shields to prevent exposure to pathogens of potential portals of entry for infection (nose, mouth, mucous surfaces, conjunctival membranes, abrasions and lacerations on the skin, etc.). Specific precautions are set out for surgical,

obstetric, and invasive diagnostic procedures, renal dialysis, dentistry, and mouth-to-mouth resuscitation. Surgical gloves must be worn when performing simple procedures such as drawing blood from veins and conducting intra-oral examination or manipulation. OSHA standards include procedures for cleaning and disposing of used surgical equipment, needles, and laundry, and for disposal of contaminated waste. Universal precautions are intended to supplement, not replace routine infection-control procedures, such as handwashing and the use of surgical gloves, and do not eliminate the need for other categories of disease-specific isolation measures, such as isolation procedures that are used for open pulmonary tuberculosis and "enteric" procedures used for cases of infectious diarrhea. Some patient advocates at first regarded the use of universal precautions as actually or potentially stigmatizing—tending to label patients as "contaminated" and therefore "bad," but this attitude has been overcome by careful explanation and the use of educational material.

JOHN M. LAST

(SEE ALSO: *Barrier Nursing; Sterilization*)

URBAN HEALTH

The health of those who live in the more densely populated areas of the world is of interest and concern for two reasons: (1) the large numbers of persons involved, and (2) the fact that the population density of an urban area changes the potential for both public health problems and public health solutions. The potential for problems includes increased exposure to large a number of individuals who can spread infectious conditions, larger volumes of waste products at risk of poor handling, the presence of pollutants, an apparent increase in stress, and a concentration of more serious mental health problems. Solutions are influenced by economies of scale in providing services, a more varied array of resources, and the potential for closer proximity to others with similar interests and needs. Opportunities to work with others who share a concern increases the likelihood of identifying appropriate actions and generating political support for solutions.

Over time, the population of the world has become much more urban. In 1900, 39.6 percent of the United States population was defined as "urban" by the Bureau of the Census; by 1990 the proportion considered urban was 75.2 percent. The definition of urban as used, however, does not include solely the densely populated centers such as Chicago or New York City. The Census Bureau considers any area with over 2,500 population to be urban; this is a "population center" many people are more likely to call a village or hamlet than a city. The definition more consistent with the common concept of an urban area includes communities of 100,000 or more, with a nucleus of at least 50,000 and surrounding communities that share a high degree of social and economic integration. By this definition, only the 276 major metropolitan areas of the United States are considered urban.

Social cohesion and social breakdown are the two ends of a spectrum describing the relationship people in a given setting experience. The greater the cohesion, the more likely the group is to work together, to share common values, and to find positive solutions to problems in ways that are inclusive of all members of the group. Conversely, when social breakdown has occurred, individuals are left to struggle with the challenges of living alone, people turn on one another in ways that are damaging, and problems accumulate to a level incompatible with a healthy life. Urban areas of today have within them neighborhoods that could be described as fully cohesive, but far too many urban areas are at, or are closer to, the other end of the spectrum.

AREAS OF CONCERN

The issue of urbanization is not just one of larger numbers of persons gathered into urban geopolitical units. The geographic size of a city makes a difference as well. For example, in central New York City (Manhattan), there are 52,419 people per square mile; in Cook County, Illinois (Chicago), 5,398; in Los Angeles County, California, 2,183; and in Dade County, Florida (Miami), 996.1. In contrast, the overall United States population density is 70.3 people per square mile; and in 1790 the nation had a population density of 4.5 people per square mile. The less concentrated population of today's sprawling urban areas present challenges of a different kind, such as the difficulties of organizing public transportation. Lack of mass transportation may mean increased pollution from

individual use of internal combustion engines, and it may mean that individuals lacking a personal car may have difficulty reaching health services.

From an economic perspective, urban populations experience some of the extremes of income inequality, with large differences in income between the highest- and lowest-earning segments of the population. Income inequality has been increasing in the United States over the last twenty-five years, and, for the low-earning segment, can have a significant negative impact on health. Areas with high income inequality and a low average income have been reported as experiencing nearly 140 deaths per 100,000 people, compared with a rate of 64.7 per 100,000 in other areas. This impact is greater for infants and those between 15 and 64 years of age. A study of thirty large metropolitan areas revealed that when poverty is concentrated within a geographic area, mortality is significantly elevated. Conversely, a concentration of affluence is associated with lower mortality, at least in the elderly.

Urban populations in the United States include large ethnic and racial minority populations. The combination of segregation and discrimination felt by minority groups in urban areas can also have an impact on health, whether due to limitations in access to health services, education, and jobs; or the increase in stress due to the tensions of being a minority population. Urban areas have been cited often, for example, for the failure of their police forces to respond equitably to members of minority populations. This has included disproportionate targeting of minorities as potential offenders (racial profiling), a lower level of response to complaints or requests for assistance, or outright disrespect or brutality. While none of these issues is uniquely urban, the concentration of population and the media visibility in a metropolitan area make this an even greater issue of concern.

As already identified, placing a large number of people in a small area increases the risk of health and illness problems. The closer proximity and higher rate of face-to-face contact has a direct impact on the rates of transmissible diseases such as tuberculosis and other respiratory infections. It is no surprise that the resurgence of tuberculosis experienced in the United States in the late 1980s and early 1990s began in New York. The high population density, and the use of large, poorly ventilated spaces as overnight sleeping accommodations for the homeless provided an ideal environment for the transmission of the bacillus. The fact that the public health resources were being strained by the arrival of another condition, HIV/AIDS (human immunodeficiency virus/acquired immunodeficiency syndrome), compounded the problem and meant that drug-resistant organisms were being shared. Health concerns as much as concerns for recreation space have been involved in the development of at least limited open spaces such as parks within concentrated urban areas.

The interrelationships of central urban areas to their surrounding suburbs has been the focus of study and attention from several perspectives. The decreased population density of suburban housing may mitigate some problems that are encountered in older urban settings. For example, there may be more open spaces for recreation or sport, and access to more remote areas is simpler. On the other hand, suburbs mean more widely dispersed individual homes, each needing access to utilities and transportation, and constructed in such a way that neighborhood cohesion may be difficult or impossible to develop. The availability of individual automobile transport in the United States has undoubtedly contributed to suburban sprawl, as have issues of social discrimination. These areas have also grown because of what has been labeled "urban flight": the movement out of cities of the more affluent as new waves of immigrants, often from different ethnic or racial groups, moved in. The apparent cost of maintaining or advancing a standard of living within the urban core was seen as too great. This flight, however, leaves older housing stock to be occupied by those of lower income levels, with less generation of taxes to support services, and the beginning of a downward spiral. When combined with the movement of industry because of restrictions on pollution, search for a cheaper labor pool, or simple displacement due to competition from elsewhere, the result can be a severe, area-wide depression. The cities of the so-called Rust Belt of the northeastern United States provide many vivid examples of this cycle.

Some of the health concerns in urban areas are the result of a loss of individual control. When a person is dependent on either walking or using a private vehicle on a seldom-used two lane road, there is much less need to be concerned about the behavior of others than if the person uses public transportation or walks or drives in a busy urban environment. In addition to the difficulties related to the increased numbers of encounters, there is an increased level of stress, which is known to increase the risk of illness. The density of urban populations and the associated stresses have also been associated with increased rates of violence and, in the second half of the twentieth century, an increase in crime associated with an increase in the distribution, sale, and use of illegal drugs. Some of the crime directly involved the drug distribution networks, as they competed with one another for turf; other crimes were committed by those who became addicted as they attempted to find the resources to support their addictions. For example, one occupational risk that has been studied is the risk of violence to convenience store employees. Of 1,835 robberies of convenience stores in eastern metropolitan areas in 1992 and 1993, 63 percent involved the use of a firearm, and 12 percent were associated with an injury to at least one employee. All five reported fatalities were firearm-related.

A major news story of the late twentieth century was the dramatic success of many urban areas in reducing violent crime. While observers are consistent in saying that no single action can be credited with bringing this about, it may have been the result of a combination of much more sophisticated and targeted policing and a demographic shift that meant a smaller population of young adults, the group most likely to be involved in crime.

Finally, cities are a center of immigration, both from rural areas (as evidenced by the population shift of the last century) and from other countries. Port cities (which may not be coastal in this age of airport travel) experience a constant influx of people from other cultures and climates. This may add to the health challenge in a number of ways. For example, during the period following the end of the Vietnam War in which a large number of refugees from Southeast Asia were arriving in the United States, many health care providers had to learn about an entirely new range of parasitic diseases that were endemic in these people's countries of origin. Beyond specific diseases, immigrants bring different expectations of the health care system, and a different understanding of the range of interventions appropriate to various disease states. Some immigrant health practices have moved toward the mainstream, as in the increasing use of acupuncture, once seen as an odd practice of the Chinese immigrant community. And the increasingly popular herbal remedies are an echo of the role the *botanica* plays in Hispanic cultures.

HOUSING

Assurance of safe housing has long been an issue for urban areas, and the history of the city is one of many cycles of housing development and reform. Failure to plan for housing infrastructure (water and sewer systems, electricity) when the population is moving into an urban area can result in extensive, substandard housing for those at lower income levels. This can be found in the *barrios, favelas*, and other overnight city extensions found around many cities in the developing world. In the United States, few such areas are visible (though they are reported to be growing around cities along the Mexican border). Substandard urban housing more often takes the form of older buildings in central city neighborhoods that have not been maintained and are not well-served by public or private services of any kind. Health hazards in such settings include exposure to lead-based paint, cockroach feces (implicated in the increase in asthma), temperature extremes, or unsafe windows and stairs.

In addition to issues of inadequate housing, the combination of a limited supply of affordable housing and low-income levels leaves some individuals and families with no place to call home. The homeless concentrate in urban areas. This may be in part due to the cost of housing in some urban areas, forcing people out of safe housing and into the streets. For example, the economic boom of the 1990s in New York City led to a tightened housing market; those serving the homeless reported a marked increase in families with children finding themselves without a permanent place to live. This has important implications for health care, as homelessness may be associated with a lack of a way to pay for care, and the struggle for safe shelter may obscure early indications of need for care and thus more serious illness problems later on. Housing policy that does not offer

ready assistance may also consider a person as having a home as long as there is some extended family member with room on the sofa or living room floor. While such an arrangement may work for a short time under emergency circumstances, the loss of privacy and crowding that results adds another dimension of stress to the risks of mental and physical ill health.

The investment of public funds in housing has met with mixed success. In some cities, the housing provided was poorly matched to the preferences and needs of the people who would be living there, and then allowed to deteriorate to the point that destruction was the only viable option. The implosion of the Pruitt-Igoe Houses in St. Louis, Missouri, in the 1970s was the first widely publicized destruction; many others followed. Other substandard housing has been removed under the guise of urban renewal, but has not always been replaced with appropriately affordable housing. The process of improving housing stock has often led to increases in cost, attracting a more affluent group. This gentrification leaves those at the lower end of the income scale still at risk and without suitable housing. Current public policy in the United States, directed by the Department of Housing and Urban Development, is focused on developing tenants as managers of public housing projects, under the theory that this will increase the likelihood that the property will not be allowed to deteriorate and that those involved in the management process will be learning new skills and improving their place in the general job market.

Another approach to insuring that the entire urban population has safe housing is through subsidies (vouchers) that underwrite a portion of the rent in the general housing market. Landlords are encouraged to participate in the program through tax incentives. News reports have often made much of this program, and of the fact that it may be associated with the integration of racial or ethnic groups that do not typically share neighborhoods. Some neighborhoods have been reported to be extremely resistant and even hostile to this approach; others have been welcoming and found it an enriching experience.

As would be true in rural as well as urban areas, control of indoor temperature is a significant issue. Experiences during periods of extreme heat during the 1990s have led to an increasing awareness of the risks, especially for the elderly or infirm in urban areas, when the temperature remains over 95 or 100 degrees Fahrenheit for several days. Windows may be locked shut for fear of intruders and fans or air conditioning may be seen as an expensive luxury. Neighborhoods attentive to the needs of the housebound during a severe winter (are they frozen in without adequate food? have we made adjustments in the cost of heating so that freezing is unlikely?) have not understood that there were perils at the other end of the thermometer. In areas in which housing is multilevel, and especially where it is high-rise, the isolation of individuals may mean that neighbors do not know who is alone and unable to make appropriate adjustments to either hot or cool weather, and excess media attention to crime and violence may distort views of personal safety and mitigate against cooperation.

FOOD AND WATER

Urban areas offer inhabitants little opportunity to obtain food other than through purchase. The larger the urbanized area, the further foods have to travel to reach stores and eventually households. This also makes "fresh" a relative term: the produce delivered straight from the field to the store is going to be much fresher when the journey is one hour than when it is one day. On the other hand, large concentrations of people make it economically reasonable to regularly import food from all over the globe, making formerly seasonal fruits and vegetables available year-round.

The issue of food availability in urban areas differentiates by income level, as does every other aspect of urban life and health. The cost of space in urban areas makes it less likely that large, modern supermarkets with volume pricing will be available; instead, food is purchased from small neighborhood shops, usually at higher prices. Further, in areas in which many live in smaller spaces (apartments and multiple occupancy buildings of all kinds) there may be less space to store less expensive bulk items. The combined impact of these factors is that the quality and quantity of food available to lower income families in urban areas means they will suffer nutritionally.

Some urban areas have made vacant space available for neighborhood gardens in which both produce and decorative plants may be grown.

During periods of population decline or urban renewal, the destruction of buildings makes lots available, and it may be good policy to encourage neighborhood use of the space for gardening. The return of economic development, however, may also abruptly make the land far more valuable as a space for building, leaving the gardeners bereft of land. The issue is not just that of the food produced, which represents only a small proportion of need, but the benefits of open space and positive activities.

Delivery of fresh water to residents was often one of the first public health activities taken up by municipal authorities in the eighteenth century. Using simple surface impoundment, wooden piping, and gravity, water that was not contaminated by urban sewerage and waste products could be made available to central pumps and to individual residences. Over time, the systems have become more elaborate, and contamination concerns have expanded to include not only the infectious diseases of the past and present, but a wide range of potentially damaging chemical agents associated with modern industrial life. The Environmental Protection Agency devotes a substantial proportion of its budget and energy to both the protection of water in its natural state (through the provisions of the Clean Water Act of 1977) and the assurance that drinking water is safe. The capacity of modern laboratories to measure the presence of material in water at a level of very few parts per billion has led to extensive debates about the level of purity that is achievable and reasonable. Whatever the outcome of these differences, it is very clear from mortality and morbidity figures that waterborne diseases in the United States are significantly fewer now than they were a century ago. Water systems need regular maintenance, however, and main pipes installed decades ago remain a regular rupture hazard in older urban areas.

For urban areas, concern about water is not only related to use for human consumption, it is a significant part of safety, given the role that water plays in control of fire. The concentration of housing and industry in urban areas has made fire safety an urban concern since the colonial era. Benjamin Franklin is cited as the father of the modern fire insurance and fire fighting systems in the United States. Urban areas devote an extensive portion of zoning and construction regulation to assuring that heating, cooking, and industrial fires, and electrical transmission systems, are such that the probability of fire is minimized. For example, every building over six stories high in New York City must be equipped with a rooftop water storage tank, assuring a volume and pressure of water adequate for fire suppression, should one occur. Municipalities have also led the way in the development of professional fire departments, with increasingly sophisticated training and equipment. In some communities, fire department personnel are involved not only in fire safety education as a community service, but they are active in health promotion (e.g., blood pressure awareness campaigns) and in a full range of injury prevention and emergency response. Studies done in New York City have also traced the origins of conditions conducive to drug abuse and the spread of HIV infection to decisions made during a time of fiscal crisis to close firehouses. As neighborhoods deteriorated, with fires destroying more buildings before they could be extinguished, boarded-up buildings became shelters for drug dealers and drug users, and the sharing of needles facilitated the rapid spread of the infection.

WASTE DISPOSAL

The concentration of populations in urban areas also means an increased accumulation of waste products. Removal of human waste and garbage is a major commitment in any city, whether the mechanism chosen is completely public or funded by a mixture of public and private resources. The treatment of human waste is costly, and new requirements that protect both people and the environment from contaminants has meant a steady investment in upgrading treatment facilities and building new ones. Treatment plants running at or near capacity in systems in which storm runoff drains into the common sewers may overflow or be bypassed during rainy seasons, causing downstream problems.

Trash and garbage that accumulate in urban areas must be disposed of safely. The old-fashioned garbage incinerator is no longer feasible, due to both volume of material and the air pollution caused by burning. Landfill disposal requires moving the material outside the urban boundary, and safety requirements for landfills have become increasingly stringent. While many areas do not want any waste disposal nearby, the acceptance

and processing of urban waste has been welcomed by some economically suffering rural areas. Trash from East Coast urban areas may be moved long distances by land or sea for final disposal. The volume of waste is directly related to the degree of attention paid to recycling of materials. Paper, glass, metal, and plastics all can be returned to use with proper treatment, but efforts to fully recycle met with varying degrees of success. Some urban areas have come very late to full recycling efforts, but most now offer curbside or individual pickup of separated recyclable materials.

At the same time as communities search for more ways to dispose of waste, attention to the siting of waste disposal has increased due to the awareness that racial and ethnic minorities have found themselves disproportionately exposed to these sites. Whether this is because landfills are deliberately located in minority communities, or their proximity is the indirect result of lower income levels and lower property values adjacent to environmental hazards, the practice has fueled both rage and concern, and government action has been taken to address the problem. This issue of environmental justice could be easily expanded to other land-use issues in urban areas, since neighborhoods with lower income levels and greater concentrations of minority populations generally have less open space for parks and playing fields, and the ones they have are often in poor condition. Lack of safe park space leaves low-income urban children playing in the street or other unsafe areas, increasing chances of injury.

Both air and noise pollution are of great concern in urban areas. In the United States, the Clean Air Act (1970) authorized the Environmental Protection Agency to take a number of steps to reduce pollutants, and there were notable improvements in the last part of the twentieth century. These changes have affected both industry (and may have driven manufacturing away from population centers) and private lives (in transportation changes). The need to move large volumes of materials into urban areas, and to move large numbers of people around within urban areas, means that the search to devise more environmentally sound and quiet means of locomotion and transportation will continue. The attachment to motor vehicles that has come over the last century poses a substantial barrier to needed change, however. As with the changing attention to drinking water, people must be concerned not only with visible particulate matter (smoke and ash from fireplaces) but with a wide range of chemicals associated with the increase of chronic disease.

HEALTH AND HEALTH SERVICES

Urban hospital systems have provided a critical link in access to health care. Many have a long history of service that dates to the waves of immigration and the epidemics of communicable diseases during the nineteenth and early twentieth centuries. Those that are publicly owned have been particularly important because of their continuity of presence, visibility, and obligation to serve all within the jurisdiction. One example of the continuing evolution of such systems is the shift from a combination of inpatient care, specialty clinics, and emergency rooms to community partnerships featuring community-oriented primary care. Shifts in payment approaches by public insurances such as Medicaid's use of prepaid group coverage requires adaptation to global and capitation payment methods, and has drawn some traditional patients (and their money) away from these public hospitals, leaving them strapped financially but still serving an essential function in urban areas.

While there are many negatives to health and health services in urban areas with large uninsured populations and antiquated care systems, there are also positives associated with urban health. The concentration of people means that specialized services are economically viable. It is medical services in urban centers that have pioneered many of the interventions now taken for granted and that are now being transferred to less populated areas. The person with a relatively unusual condition who lives in an urban area is more likely to find the needed care within close proximity than a similar individual in a rural location.

Urban areas have been leaders in developing services for the homeless and services targeted to individual racial and ethnic groups. For example, the United States Indian Health Service has supported the development of urban clinics to provide health services for the large numbers of Native Americans living in urban areas who are cut off

from culturally appropriate services that would be available on reservations. In neighborhoods without an adequate supply of health services, funding from the Health and Human Services Administration and the Substance Abuse and Mental Health Services Administration have allowed the creation of community-oriented ambulatory care programs. Services supported with these funds must have boards that include representatives of the community being served, and they have been marked by a high degree of acceptance.

In addition to services set up for the diagnosis and treatment of individual patients, urban health services also have a population-wide focus, provided by each jurisdiction's public health agency. These services are intended to prevent epidemics, protect against environmental hazards, prevent injury, promote and encourage healthy behavior, respond to disasters, and assure the quality and accessibility of health services. They date to the late nineteenth and early twentieth centuries, and had their beginnings as a response to epidemics such as typhoid and cholera. They continue to play an important role, though the diseases of interest have expanded. Today an urban health department (which may be several agencies, depending on local preference) monitors HIV infection, tuberculosis, asthma, diabetes, violence, child safety, tobacco control, suicide prevention, family planning, nutrition, and immunizations. The line between the services offered by a health department and those available from other publicly supported health services is an arbitrary one. In order to prevent disease and promote health, individuals must have access to personal care, and when it is not available elsewhere, the public health agency may provide it, at least in urgent circumstances. But where there are other resources for care, the public health agency can focus on system-level actions that will limit exposure of the population to risk factors and support health for all. This is best done in collaboration with citizen groups and other public health entities in an organized way. The Healthy Cities/Healthy Communities movement of the 1990s is one example of resources available to those interested in improving health.

Urban health is a complex web of both threats to health and supports to health. It cannot be understood apart from an appreciation for the size and density of the populations involved, and it continues to evolve as economics shift, technology advances, and public expectations develop. But the likelihood that urban areas will continue to concentrate people, problems, and opportunities makes its health concerns unique and important.

KRISTINE GEBBIE

(SEE ALSO: *Boards of Health; Clean Air Act; Clean Water Act; Community Health; Drinking Water; Environmental Determinants of Health; Environmental Justice; Ethnicity and Health; Healthy Communities; Inequalities in Health; Social Determinants; Substance Abuse; Urban Social Disparities; Urban Sprawl; Urban Transport; Violence; Wastewater Treatment*)

BIBLIOGRAPHY

Amandus, H. E.; Hendricks, S. A.; Zahm, D.; Friedmann, R.; Block, C.; Wellford, D.; Brensilver, D.; et al. (1997). "Convenience Store Robberies in Selected Metropolitan Areas." *Journal of Occupational and Environmental Medicine* 39(5):442–447.

Amick, B. C.; Levine, S.; Tarlov, A. R.; and Walsh, D. C. (1995). *Society and Health.* New York: Oxford University Press.

Anderson, R. J. (1997). "The CJ Shannaberger Lecture: Pitfalls in the Corporatization of Health Care." *Prehospital Emergency Care* 1(4):227–285.

Der-McLeod, D. (1997). "On Lok: Community-Based Long Term Care." *Continuum* 17(4):10–13.

Drum, M. A.; Chen, D. W.; and Duffy, R. E. (1998). "Filling the Gap: Equity and Access to Oral Health Services for Minorities and the Underserved." *Family Medicine* 30(3):206–209.

Hewett, N. C. (1999). "How to Provide for the Primary Health Care Needs of Homeless People: What Do Homeless People in Leicester Think?" *British Journal of General Practice* 49(447):819.

International Healthy Cities Foundation (2000). "What Is the Healthy Cities Movement?" Available at http://www.healthycities.org/.

Lynch, J. W.; Kaplan, G. A.; Pamuk, E. R.; Cohen, R. D.; Heck, K. E.; Balfour, J. L.; and Yen, I. H. (1998). "Income Inequality and Mortality in Metropolitan Areas of the United States." *American Journal of Public Health* 88(7):1074–1080.

Opdycke, S. (1999). *No One Was Turned Away.* New York: Oxford University Press.

Sachs-Ericsson, N.; Wise, E.; Debrody, C. P.; and Paniucki, H. B. (1999). "Health Problems and Service Utilization in the Homeless." *Journal of Health Care Poor and Underserved* 10(4):443–452.

Witzman, N. J., and Smith, K. R. (1998). "Separate But Lethal: The Effects of Economic Segregation on Mortality in Metropolitan America." *Milbank Quarterly* 76(3):341–373.

URBAN SOCIAL DISPARITIES

It is a truism of epidemiology that disease is not uniformly distributed across society—that some social groups or geographical areas experience higher disease rates, while other social groups or areas experience lower disease rates. Thus, some epidemiologists have investigated the relationship between social class or socioeconomic position and health or disease. These studies show that disease and mortality rates are higher in those urban areas or social classes where the incumbents are the least educated, and where household income is lowest, jobs are insecure, and where there is little wealth or political power. Similarly, disease and mortality rates are lower in those areas and social classes where the incumbents are the most educated, and where household income is highest, jobs are secure, and where wealth and political power are concentrated.

SOCIAL CLASS DEFINED

Richard Scase (following the trail blazed by Karl Marx) writes that social classes in the industrial era are inherent to capitalism—that differential control over the means of production (factories, restaurants, computers, software systems) produces different social classes. Thus the concept of "class" is important for understanding urban (or rural) social disparities in health and disease in capitalist societies. Dennis Gilbert (following both Karl Marx and Max Weber) defines a social class as a large group of families or households that are "approximately equal in rank to each other but clearly differentiated from other families" along the dimensions of occupational autonomy and security, education, income, wealth, and political power.

Gilbert in 1998 maintained that six classes adequately describe the American class structure:

a capitalist class (1% of households), an upper middle class (14%), a middle class (30%), a working (or lower middle) class (30%), the working poor (13%), and an underclass (12%).

- Capitalist households are composed of investors, heirs, and executives; their incomes average around $1.5 million per year (in 1995); and their main source of income is property, stocks, or other investments. Capitalists-to-be usually graduate from selective universities.

- Upper-middle-class households are composed of upper managers, professionals, and medium-sized business owners; their incomes average $80,000 per year, and their main source of income is from one (or two) salaries. Upper-middle-class professionals often have postgraduate credentials.

- Middle-class households are composed of lower managers, semi-professionals, and nonretail sales workers; their incomes average $45,000 per year; and some middle-class incumbents may not be college graduates.

- Lower-middle-class households are composed of operatives, low-paid craftsmen, clerical workers, and retail sales workers; their incomes average $30,000 per year; and they are typically high school graduates.

- Working poor households are composed of service workers, laborers, low-paid operatives, and clerical workers; incomes average $20,000; and many incumbents are not high school graduates.

- Underclass households are composed of unemployed or part-time workers; many incumbents depend on government assistance; their incomes average $10,000 per year; and many are not high school graduates.

Because wealth, job autonomy and security, and political power are hard to measure, epidemiologists have generally relied upon occupation, income, or education to characterize the class position of the people in their studies. However, relying on education or occupation as the only measure of social class may underestimate the true relationship between social class and disease. Social epidemiologists also argue that more attention should be paid to measuring the socioeconomic characteristics of neighborhoods and communities where people live. The reasoning behind this assertion is the hypothesis that the social environment (absence of safe parks for walking or exercise, for example) may have additional impacts on health that would be missed if the focus of measurement were household characteristics exclusively.

HOW SOCIAL CLASS AFFECTS HEALTH

The social class distribution in a community or urban area appears to affect both the general level of health as well as specific disease rates through a variety of mechanisms. One hypothesis is that the general susceptibility to disease is higher in the disadvantaged classes because of chronic exposure to stressful life events. The presumed biological mechanisms involve several aspects of the neuroendocrine system that adversely impact host resistance. Another hypothesis is that social class affects life chances from birth through old age—that is, disadvantaged circumstances early in life can set the stage for late onset chronic disease. Starting tobacco smoking and engaging in sedentary behaviors as a teenager from a disadvantaged lower-middle-class household, followed by the development of ischemic heart disease in middle age, would be an example of this life course phenomenon. Another mechanism through which social class can affect health is via differential access to high quality primary and specialty medical care.

EVERETT E. LOGUE

(SEE ALSO: *Social Class; Social Determinants; Urban Health; Urban Sprawl*)

BIBLIOGRAPHY

Berkman, L. F., and Kawachi, I. (2000). "A Historical Framework for Social Epidemiology." In *Social Epidemiology,* eds. L. F. Berkman and I. Kawachi. New York: Oxford University Press.

Gilbert, D. (1998). *The American Class Structure in an Age of Growing Inequality.* Belmont, CA: Wadsworth.

Lynch, J., and Kaplan, G. (2000). "Socioeconomic Position." In *Social Epidemiology*, eds. L. F. Berkman and I. Kawachi. New York: Oxford University Press.

Scase, R. (1992). *Class*. Minneapolis: University of Minnesota Press.

URBAN SPRAWL

Land use choices strongly affect public health. More or less direct effects on air and water pollution are well recognized, but other less direct but important impacts have only recently begun to reach public attention. "Urban sprawl" may be defined as development of low-population-density settlements around high-density cities, either by emigration from the core cities or by influx of new residents from elsewhere.

Sprawl results from thousands of personal decisions and from policies and subsidies that are outcomes of the electoral process. Special interests such as the highway and automobile lobbies spend vast sums to exert pressure; developers often state sincerely that they will build whatever the market demands. The fact that sprawl is in part subsidized by government policies—for example, building roads and sewers and supporting low gas prices partly at the expense of non-users, in effect providing greater subsidies for suburban than for low-income core-city housing—further emphasizing that the "choice" of living in sprawl development is not a simple free-market or quality of life option. In addition, in choosing sprawl over core city redevelopment, we are in effect incurring public health burdens.

RELATIVELY DIRECT EFFECTS OF SPRAWL ON PUBLIC HEALTH

Air Pollution. Life in sprawl developments demands up to three times as much driving as in high-density urban areas. Since high levels of the monitored pollutants can trigger loss of federal highway funds, affected metropolitan regions such as Atlanta are changing their development policies. Light rail and other forms of mass transit can reduce auto pollution in suitable situations but, in the absence of special planning, may not decrease sprawl.

Water Pollution. In 1998 the Environmental Protection Administration (EPA) reported that 35 percent of the nation's rivers and 45 percent of its lakes were polluted and not clean enough for swimming or fishing. Although some of the pollutants were from agricultural and industrial sources and landfills, many resulted indirectly from sprawl. For instance, increased bacteria come from overextended and overloaded sewer systems, overflows of "combined sewers," and leaking home septic systems. Road "runoff" of automobile oils and battery metals and road salt also contribute to water pollution and may affect public health.

Other Impacts of Increased Auto Usage. With increased mileage, higher speeds, and fewer sidewalks, pedestrian accidents have increased, especially among children and elderly, comprising some 13 percent of traffic accident fatalities in 1997 and 1998. Remarkably, 59 percent of pedestrian deaths occurred where there was no access to crosswalks, that is, in typical sprawl roadways. A related factor was the higher speeds prevalent in suburban (vs. urban) roads, since speed and fatality are highly correlated. If states were willing to spend highway funds on pedestrian safety, there are many short-term measures (e.g., "traffic calming," more crosswalks) that could be taken, but at some point, slowing of traffic will encounter public resistance. Another impact in typical sprawl development is the loss of easy access of the elderly to medical care, social services, and shopping once they stop driving; since mass transit is not generally available. This problem is bound to become more severe as the elderly begin to comprise some 20 to 25 percent of our population by 2050.

INDIRECT EFFECTS OF SPRAWL ON PUBLIC HEALTH

A few examples illustrate that there are also some indirect impacts of urban sprawl on public health.

Duplication of Medical Infrastructure. As hospitals expand to meet the needs of the more affluent and growing population, they often cannot afford to maintain medical centers both in a population-depleted or relatively poor inner city and in the suburbs.

Quality of Life and Health. The stress of commuting and congestion decreases time and energy for quality parenting and relaxation. The conversion of open space to roads and developments creates an environment without ready access to parks and nature. Abandonment of traditional neighborhoods results in a loss of sense of community, which in turn may lead to less community-based caring for children, the elderly, the ill, and the disabled. Finally, abandonment of and disinvestment in urban core cities leads to concentration of poverty and both racial and economic resegregation.

There are strong and often compelling social reasons or perceptions why many Americans prefer low-density suburban to urban living, beyond the known or hidden subsidies that promote this population shift. However, to the greatest extent possible, the public health impacts need to be consciously factored into the public costs of sprawl so that provisions are made to minimize these costs to those (especially inner-city residents) who are negatively affected and to offer everyone more balanced choices of places to live and work. The so-called "Smart Growth" movement offers a variety of land use choices that minimize the negative public health impacts discussed here.

NORMAN ROBBINS

BIBLIOGRAPHY

Jacobs, J. (1993). *The Death and Life of Great American Cities*. New York: Vintage Books.

Surface Transportation Policy Project (2000). *Mean Streets 2000: Pedestrian, Health, and Federal Transportation Spending*. Washington, DC: Author.

U.S. Congress, Office of Technology Assessment (1995). *The Technological Reshaping of Metropolitan America* (OTAH ETIH 643). Washington, DC: U.S. Government Printing Office.

URBAN TRANSPORT

One of the consequences of urbanization has been the need to transport people and goods to, from, and within cities. Urban transport for people has come to be dominated by the car in the twentieth century, and trucks have increasingly displaced trains for the movement of goods, while public transport, biking, and walking are less frequently used alternatives, especially in North America. The 1990 census in Canada found that 73 percent of working Canadians drove their own vehicle to work while 10 percent used public transport, 7 percent walked, and 1 percent bicycled. On average, North Americans now spend 5 percent of their time in motor vehicles.

Urban sprawl has made the ownership and use of at least one car almost essential for suburban residents. Such low density urban sprawl makes public transport uneconomical and results in high vehicle miles, high fossil fuel consumption, and high levels of air pollution and emissions of carbon dioxide, the main greenhouse gas (see Figure 1, which shows energy use compared to urban density for many world cities). One study in Ottawa, Canada, found that suburban residents walk or cycle one-third as much as people living in the central parts of the city, but they drive twice as far, consume twice as much energy, and produce twice as much pollution.

Unfortunately, these trends are being followed in the developing world; 52 percent of the increase in the world's motor vehicle fleet between 1996 and 2020 will occur in Asia and in Central and South America. On a global scale, transportation accounts for 60 percent of total oil consumption, and this consumption is expected to increase about 50 percent between 1993 and 2010, but twice as fast in the developing world and three times as fast in South Asia.

In addition to outdoor air pollution, the health consequences of urban transportation include in-vehicle air pollution, motor vehicle accidents (MVAs), noise, and a variety of mental and social affects, as well as the contribution transportation makes to global warming and fossil fuel depletion.

CONSEQUENCES OF URBAN TRANSPORT

Urban Air Pollution. Motor vehicles are a major source of nitrogen oxides (NO_x) and volatile organic compounds (VOCs)—which interact to form ground level ozone—and of microscopic particulate matter (PM_{10}). These are the key components of urban air pollution. Globally, outdoor air pollution results in 200,000 to 570,000 deaths annually, with 1.4 billion people exposed to urban air pollution above World Health Organization (WHO)

Figure 1

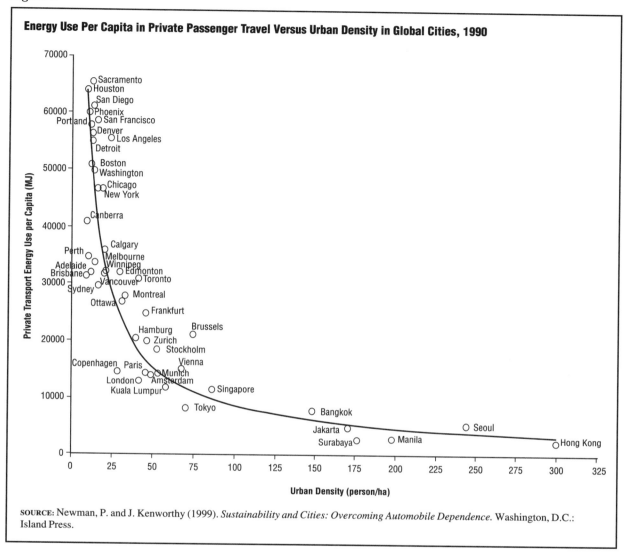

Energy Use Per Capita in Private Passenger Travel Versus Urban Density in Global Cities, 1990

SOURCE: Newman, P. and J. Kenworthy (1999). *Sustainability and Cities: Overcoming Automobile Dependence.* Washington, D.C.: Island Press.

guidelines. But deaths are only a small part of the problem. Far more serious are the huge numbers of people who become ill. The "health effects pyramid" for PM_{10}, for example, shows that for every death caused by this pollutant there will be 34 emergency admissions, 407 asthma days, 6,085 reduced activity days, and 18,864 acute respiratory symptom days.

In-Vehicle Pollution. A generally neglected aspect of urban transportation is the air quality inside motor vehicles—a place where North Americans spend as much time now as they do outdoors. Levels of benzene (a human carcinogen), carbon

monoxide, and nitrogen dioxide may be much higher inside the vehicle, especially in poorly maintained vehicles and in congested, slow moving traffic conditions such as those found in urban settings.

Motor Vehicle Accidents (MVAs). In 1996, MVAs in the United States accounted for 41,907 deaths, 3.5 million nonfatal injuries, and total societal costs in excess of $150 billion. In Canada in 1996, 3,082 deaths resulted from MVAs and there were 249,198 injuries. It is estimated that globally by 2030 there will be over 2 million MVA deaths and 50 million injuries annually, with 5.7

million people permanently handicapped. Accident rates are much higher in the developing world, up to 75 times more per licensed vehicle. These figures represent a huge human, social, and economic cost, with the economic cost estimated to be 1 to 2 percent of a country's gross domestic product (GDP). Although some of these accidents occur outside urban areas, transportation of people and goods to and from cities is a significant factor in this carnage.

Noise. Traffic is the principal source of noise pollution in the urban environment. The health effects include hearing loss, disturbance of sleep patterns, interference with communication, and degradation in the quality of life, according to WHO.

Mental and Social Effects. In Canada in 1992, only 8 percent of employed Canadians did not commute to work. Average commuting time was forty-eight minutes each day, but sixty minutes in the larger cities; 10 percent of commuters spent more than ninety minutes a day commuting. This contributes to stress (sometimes expressed as "road rage"), increased social isolation, and loss of time available for family and community life.

Global Warming. In 1994 in Canada, transportation was responsible for 31.4 percent of emissions of carbon dioxide. Per capita transportation-related CO_2 emissions in Canada and the United States are roughly three times that of other Western industrialized countries. The health impacts of global warming are likely to be significant, and mostly negative.

Other Effects. A 1994 Statistics Canada report refers to a number of other adverse environmental and health consequences of transportation, including increased urban runoff and thus water pollution, solid waste production, habitat destruction, and the partition or even destruction of neighborhoods. In addition, the private car is expensive to own and operate, which can be a real burden for people on low incomes, while urban congestion costs the local economy in terms of wasted fuel, lost time, and health effects. The Organization for Economic Cooperation and Development estimates the external costs of such unsustainable transportation systems to be 5 percent of the GDP.

ALTERNATIVE APPROACHES

This litany of adverse health and environmental impacts of transportation has resulted in a growing interest in alternative approaches, including more walking and biking, reduced goods transportation, and improved public transit. The health benefits of a good urban transit system are both direct and indirect. Direct health benefits include lower rates of respiratory and heart disease resulting from reduced pollution; lower accident rates because transit is a safer form of travel; and fitter and healthier people resulting from the more active lifestyle as people walk and bicycle more. Indirect health benefits may include less congestion, reduced commuting time, less noise, less stress, less cost, higher discretionary incomes (especially for low-income families), less social isolation, increased access for disadvantaged groups, the conservation of energy and resources, and reduced global warming.

Ultimately, a healthier urban transportation policy will require a significant change in urban development and land use practices and in the North American way of life. To improve public health in urban areas, it will be necessary to encourage more European-style urban developments with higher densities, mixed land use, strong support for public transport, the creation of pedestrian and bike routes, and policies to restrict the use of private vehicles.

TREVOR HANCOCK

(SEE ALSO: *Ambient Air Quality [Air Pollution]; Built Environment; Climate Change and Human Health; Ecological Footprint; Healthy Communities*)

BIBLIOGRAPHY

Elmson, D. (1996). *Smog Alert: Managing Urban Air Quality*. London: Earthrscan.

Fletcher, T., and McMichael, A. J., eds. (1997). *Health at the Crossroads: Transport Policy and Urban Health*. Chichester: John Wiley.

Newman, P., and Kenworthy, J. (1999). *Sustainability and Cities: Overcoming Automobile Dependence*. Washington, DC: Island Press.

Schwela, D., and Zali, O., eds. (1999). *Urban Traffic Pollution*. London: E. and F. N. Spon.

Statistics Canada (1994). *Human Activity and the Environment*. Ottawa: Author.

U.S. Department of Health and Human Services (1998). *Healthy People 2010 Draft Objectives*. Washington, DC: U.S. Public Health Services.

Whitelegg, J. (1997). *Critical Mass: Transport, Environment and Society in the 21st Century*. London: Pluto/World Wide Fund for Nature.

World Resource Institute (1998–1999). *World Resources*. New York: Basic Books.

URINALYSIS

Urinalysis is an important test used in diagnosing diseases of the genitourinary tract. Urine is examined for pH and specific gravity by chemical and direct microscopic methods. The presence and concentration of various chemicals such as proteins, ketones, bilirubin, glucose, and nitrite are measured. Chemical metabolites also may be screened through urinalysis. In urinalysis, microscopic examination is performed to quantify the cellular urinary components, including red and white blood cells, fungi, and bacteria. The presence and concentration of cellular components, combined with the results of chemical analyses, give important clues for diagnosis of genitourinary diseases.

BIJAN SHEKARRIZ
MARSHALL L. STOLLER

(SEE ALSO: *Genitourinary Disease; Urine Cytology; Urine Dipstick*)

URINE CYTOLOGY

Urine typically contains epithelial cells shed from the urinary tract. Urine cytology evaluates this urinary sediment for the presence of cancerous cells from the lining of the urinary tract, and it is a convenient noninvasive technique for follow-up analysis of patients treated for urinary tract cancers. For this process, urine must be collected in a reliable fashion, and if urine samples are inadequate, the urinary tract can be assessed via instrumentation. In urine cytology, collected urine is

examined microscopically. One limitation, however, is the inability to definitively identify low-grade cancer cells and urine cytology is used mostly to identify high-grade tumors.

BIJAN SHEKARRIZ
MARSHALL L. STOLLER

(SEE ALSO: *Genitourinary Disease; Urinalysis*)

URINE DIPSTICK

A urine dipstick is a colorimetric chemical assay that can be used to determine the pH, specific gravity, protein, glucose, ketone, bilirubin, urobilinogen, blood, leukocyte, and nitrite levels of an individual's urine. It consists of a reagent stick-pad, which is immersed in a fresh urine specimen and then withdrawn. After predetermined times the colors of the reagent pad are compared to standardized reference charts.

The urine dipstick offers an inexpensive and fast method to perform screening urinalyses, which help in identifying the presence of various diseases or health problems. This test should be interpreted with caution, however, due to numerous limitations, including inaccurate results due to medications and collection techniques. Abnormal values need to be confirmed with more precise quantitative measurements.

BIJAN SHEKARRIZ
MARSHALL L. STOLLER

(SEE ALSO: *Genitourinary Disease; Urinalysis*)

UTERINE CANCER

Endometrial adenocarcinoma, or uterine cancer, is the most common genital cancer in women over forty-five years of age in the United States. Approximately 36,000 new cases are diagnosed each year, and 6,300 women ultimately die of the disease. The lifetime incidence is approximately 22 per 100,000. In over 90 percent of the cases, the earliest symptom is abnormal or postmenopausal bleeding. Almost 70 percent of uterine cancers are diagnosed early (while being confined to the uterus), and therefore are more apt to be cured. Uterine cancer is associated with hypertension, diabetes, and obesity. Hyperestrogenic states, pelvic radiation, and tamoxifen increase the risk of developing endometrial cancer.

THOMAS J. RUTHERFORD

(SEE ALSO: *Cancer; Cervical Cancer*)

BIBLIOGRAPHY

American College of Obstetrics and Gynecologists (1991). *Carcinoma of the Endometrium.* ACOG technical bulletin, no. 162. Washington, DC: Author.

Boronow, R. C.; Morrow, C. P. et al. (1984). "Surgical Staging in Endometrial Cancer: Clinicopathologic Findings of a Prospective Study." *Obstetrics and Gynecology* 63:825.

V

VACCINE-PREVENTABLE DISEASES

See Immunizations

VACCINES

See Immunizations

VALUES

See Benefits, Ethics, and Risks *and* Ethics of Public Health

VALUES IN HEALTH EDUCATION

The delivery and acceptance of health-education and health-promotion programs are influenced by personal, religious, environmental, cultural, political, and economic factors, all of which help create and are affected by individual and societal values. Values are an integral part of people's everyday lives, even though individuals do not often consciously determine how their values influence their ideas or behavior. One common definition of values is that they are notions or ideas upon which we place worth. Values are influenced by cultural background, gender, religious affiliation, and membership in social groups. Values therefore become internalized and affect motivation, thoughts, and behavior. In other words, they become standards that guide one's behavior and they are part of one's identity. Undergoing a values clarification process helps individuals to not only recognize their own values, but understand how their values can assist in making future choices.

A "value system" is the organization of beliefs that guide individual behavior. This system is composed of instrumental and terminal values. Instrumental values are those that involve modes of behavior such as honesty, cheerfulness, independence, and obedience. These values lead to terminal values, or endstates, which include happiness, pleasure, social recognition, and wisdom. Both levels of values affect behavior, and conflicts between opposing values need resolution. Consider the conflict adolescents experience when they are told by their parents not to smoke but are encouraged to do so by their peers. In this instance, there is a conflict between obedience, an instrumental value, and social recognition, a terminal value. Resolving such a conflict becomes an individual decision based upon prioritized values. If an adolescent determines that obedience is more important than social recognition, acting on this choice and making related decisions will follow.

Two pairs of contrasting values are significant for this discussion: contentment versus attainment, and pleasure versus self-fulfillment and growth. Contentment can be accomplished by a reduction of desires. The satisfaction received from one desire will lead to more desires, which can lead to discontent if the desires are not attained. On the other hand, attainment of specific objects or goals may lead to a better or healthier life. Focusing on achieving pleasure, such as physical or emotional pleasure, is often given precedent over achieving self-fulfillment and growth, which relies more on internal, self-evaluation processes. However, when the latter occurs, new goals, or the restructuring of previously developed goals, results. When health is considered in light of the above information, the following observations can be made: (1) attaining a life that is rich in variety and activities may be considered healthy; and (2) one's experiences of poor health, either having poor health oneself, or being exposed to other's experiences of poor health, can be the stimulus to evaluate how one attains self-fulfillment through the creation of more appropriate goals.

Values that affect health also affect health education and health promotion on two levels—the individual level and the societal level. At the individual level, values determine whether certain health behaviors are acceptable, whether the individual will engage in them, and whether health-education and health-promotion programs are acceptable. As already stated, once values are established, they need to be acted upon through decisions that are made by the individual. Returning to the example of the adolescent conflicted over smoking, while prioritizing values may lead an individual to choose not to smoke, exposure to a variety of health messages through the media or through the school environment may also influence this decision. The adolescent may have come to value having a physically fit and healthy body and decided to engage in healthful behaviors. In doing so this individual will have undergone self-evaluation and created goals for specific health behaviors.

When health-education and health-promotion programs are being developed, the audience's values need to be considered. This will affect, among other things, what topics are included, the way in which the topics are presented, and whether both genders or certain age groups will be included in the planning and delivery phases. Consider a health-education project that was conducted with a Hutterite colony. This religious sect lives a communal agrarian lifestyle, separate from mainstream society. An assessment of health issues within the colony generated information about their values and how these influenced their lifestyle and behaviors. Based upon this information, health-education sessions were planned

and implemented regarding the handling of life-threatening emergencies. Because Hutterites value self-sustaining behaviors such as farming over academic learning, the colony members do not complete high school. Therefore, when the sessions were planned, handouts were prepared in easily understood terms with numerous diagrams to illustrate the points. The colony is governed through an internal system that includes several men within key positions. These individuals were consulted when planning the health-education sessions to ensure their acceptance. Research that focuses on health assessments can be conducted in a manner that links the findings to the individual's values, thereby ensuring that new or refined health-education and health-promotion resources are appropriately determined.

At the societal level, values make a significant contribution to public health. Two basic values in public health are cooperation and collaboration. Health care systems in most countries, regardless of whether or not they are based upon the principles of universal accessibility or affordability, focus upon an illness-care system. Illness-care is only directed at those experiencing ill health, either acute or chronic. This is an expensive system to maintain, forcing the numerous caregiving agencies in countries with a large private sector to compete for clients for financial reimbursement rather than collaborate with other agencies in providing care. Even in countries with a publicly funded health system, there is competition for adequate resources to maintain both an illness-care and a wellness-care system. Wellness-care is focused on healthy individuals to assist them in maintaining or improving their health. Not surprisingly, regardless of what system is available, illness-care is given the priority. Hence, although health-education and health-promotion programs exist, they are not always given a high priority within health agencies. The public at large also has difficulty in creating a societal value which emphasizes wellness-care for several reasons. First, illness-care is more visible through the presence of acute health facilities and the media attention given to medical breakthroughs. Second, the lack of extensive and prolonged exposure to a variety of health-education and health-promotion programs lessens the overall benefits and the integration of such programs into the public's everyday lives. Despite these limitations, such programs have the potential to influence and alter individual and societal values and subsequent behaviors, if they are appropriately delivered. One example is the public acceptance of the use of seat belts, a practice which has become commonplace due to the implementation of various health-education programs and strategies as well as the public's prioritization of values related to health and safety.

More recent discussions of values and their impact on health have called into question the manner in which health education and health promotion is being delivered. In an issue of *Social Science Medicine*, in 1998, Olav Forde discussed at length the emphasis on achieving a lifestyle that is free of risk. Forde wrote that life has become medicalized due in part to an increase in health and risk awareness, which stems from the media concentration on diseases that capture the public's attention and concern. Such attention is enhanced by health professionals who encourage the continual flow of health information to the public while continuing to base their interventions on people's fear of disease and obsession with health. Thus, engaging in a healthy lifestyle, and in certain behaviors, becomes parallel to avoiding risk. The more crucial concern is the link between the unnecessary emphasis on the prevention of risk and the inappropriate change in societal values in relation to health. Consequently, *healthism* is becoming the principal life value. Values such as tolerance and nonconformity are questioned when there is such emphasis on avoiding risk because there is an expectation that everyone will act in a manner that will lower individual risk and, ultimately, the public's risk. A shift such as this can lead individuals to experience guilt, blame, and intolerance if they do not adhere to such values and behaviors. Diversity of thoughts and action is less acceptable because conformity becomes the expectation. Health-education and health-promotion workers, unconsciously or not, incorporate these attitudes in their work with individuals and communities, further contributing to this shift in values.

Values are constantly being altered according to the changing context within which they are located. It has been suggested that values for the twenty-first century will be empowering, caring, and cooperating. Such changes will likely be debated and examined to ensure that the relationships between values and health education and health promotion are sound ones and that they can lead to health behaviors that will result in an optimal level of health for the public.

JUDITH C. KULIG

(SEE ALSO: *Anthropology in Public Health; Cultural Anthropology; Cultural Appropriateness; Cultural Identity; Cultural Norms; Customs*)

BIBLIOGRAPHY

Brunt, H. (1998). "Canadian Hutterites." In *Canadian Transcultural Nursing*, eds. R. E. Davidhizar and J. N. Giger. St. Louis, MO: Mosby.

Farthing, M. (1997). "Health Education Needs of a Hutterite Colony." *The Canadian Nurse* 8:20–26.

Forde, O. H. (1998). "Is Imposing Risk Awareness Cultural Imperialism?" *Social Science Medicine* 47(9): 1155–1159.

Gutt, C. A. (1996). "Health and Wellness in the Community." In *Nursing Care in the Community*, ed. J. M. Cookfair. St. Louis, MO: Mosby.

Hyland, M. E. (1997). "Health and Values: The Values Underlying Health Measurement and Health Resource." *Psychology of Health* 12:389–403.

Liaschenko, J. (1999). "Can Justice Coexist with the Supremacy of Personal Values in Nursing Practice?" *Western Journal of Nursing Research* 21(1):35–50.

Ray, D. W., and Flynn, B. C. (1980). "Competition vs. Cooperation in Community Health Nursing." *Nursing Outlook* 10:626–630.

Rokeach, M. (1973). *The Nature of Human Values.* New York: Free Press.

Spradley, B. W., and Allender, J. A. (1996). "Health Care Economics." In *Community Health Nursing*, eds. B. W. Spradley and J. A. Allender. Philadelphia, PA: Lippincott.

—— (1996). "Values and Ethical Decision Making in Community Health." In *Community Health Nursing*, eds. B. W. Spradley and J. A. Allender. Philadelphia, PA: Lippincott.

VARICELLA

See Chicken Pox and Shingles

VDRL TEST

In connection with syphilis control, the standard test for measuring nontreponemal antibodies is the Venereal Disease Research Laboratory (VDRL) test. In this test, heated serum or unheated cerebrospinal fluid is mixed with reagin (a purified mixture of lipids such as cardiolipin, lecithin, and cholesterol) on a glass slide, and flocculation, or clumping, of the mixture is read microscopically as "reactive" (if clumping occurs) or "nonreactive" (if there is no clumping). Like the rapid plasma reagin (RPR) test, the VDRL test can be quantitated by examining serial dilutions of serum and can be used to follow the course of illness, including the response to therapy. The VDRL usually becomes reactive within the first few weeks after infection, peaks during the first year, and then slowly declines, so that low titers (levels) are seen in late syphilis. It can revert to negative in the absence of treatment in about 25 percent of cases. Although regarded as the gold standard for the diagnosis of neurosyphilis, the VDRL test may be negative in 40 to 73 percent of patients. Recent immunization, other bacterial and viral infections, and certain chronic conditions (e.g., liver disease, malignancy) can result in false positive test results, though titers are usually low (less than 1:8 dilution) under these circumstances.

JUDITH E. WOLF

(SEE ALSO: *Antibody, Antigen; Fluorescent Treponemal Antibody Absorption; RPR Test; Syphilis*)

BIBLIOGRAPHY

Hook, E., and Marra, C. (1992). "Acquired Syphilis in Adults." *New England Journal of Medicine* 326:1060–1069.

Wolf, J. (1997). "Syphilis." In *Current Diagnosis*, 7th edition, eds. R. Conn, W. Borer, and J. Snyder. Philadelphia, PA: W. B. Saunders.

VECTOR-BORNE DISEASES

From the perspective of infectious diseases, vectors are the transmitters of disease-causing organisms that carry the pathogens from one host to another. By common usage, vectors are considered to be invertebrate animals, usually arthropods. Technically, however, vertebrates can also act as vectors, including foxes, raccoons, and skunks,

which can all transmit the rabies virus to humans via a bite. Arthropods account for over 85 percent of all known animal species, and they are the most important disease vectors. Arthropods may affect human health either directly by bites, stings, or infestation of tissues, or indirectly through disease transmission. Several genera of arthropods play a role in human disease, but mosquitoes and ticks are the most notable disease vectors. The most significant mode of vector-borne disease transmission is by biological transmission by blood-feeding arthropods. The pathogen multiplies within the arthropod vector, and the pathogen is transmitted when the arthropod takes a blood meal. Mechanical transmission of disease agents may also occur when arthropods physically carry pathogens from one place or host to another, usually on body parts.

The transmission of vector-borne diseases to humans depends on three different factors: the pathologic agent; the arthropod vector; and the human host (see Figure 1).

The majority of vector-borne diseases survive in nature by utilizing animals as their vertebrate hosts, and are therefore zoonoses. For a small number of zoonoses, such as malaria and dengue, humans are the major host, with no significant animal reservoirs. Intermediary animal hosts often serve as a reservoir for the pathogens until susceptible human populations are exposed. The vector receives the pathogen from an infected host and transmits it either to an intermediary host or directly to the human host. The different stages of the pathogen's life cycle occur during this process and are intimately dependent upon the availability of suitable vectors and hosts. Key components that determine the occurrence of vector-borne diseases include: (1) the abundance of vectors and intermediate and reservoir hosts; (2) the prevalence of disease-causing pathogens suitably adapted to the vectors and the human or animal host; (3) the local environmental conditions, especially temperature and humidity; and (4) the resilience behavior and immune status of the human population.

Vector-borne diseases are prevalent in the tropics and subtropics and are relatively rare in temperate zones, although climate change could create conditions suitable for outbreaks of diseases such as Lyme disease, Rocky Mountain spotted fever, malaria, dengue fever, and viral encephalitis in temperate regions. There are different patterns of vector-borne disease occurrence. Parasitic and bacterial diseases, such as malaria and Lyme disease, tend to produce a high disease incidence but do not cause major epidemics. An exception to this rule is plague, a bacterial disease that does cause outbreaks. In contrast, many vector viral diseases, such as Yellow fever, dengue, and Japanese encephalitis, commonly cause major epidemics.

There has been a worldwide resurgence of vector-borne diseases since the 1970s including malaria, dengue, Yellow fever, louse-borne typhus, plague, leishmaniasis, sleeping sickness, West Nile encephalitis, Lyme disease, Japanese encephalitis, Rift Valley fever, and Crimean-Congo hemorrhagic fever. Reasons for the emergence or resurgence of vector-borne diseases include the development of insecticide and drug resistance; decreased resources for surveillance, prevention and control of vector-borne diseases; deterioration of the public health infrastructure required to deal with these diseases; unprecedented population growth; uncontrolled urbanization; changes in agricultural practices; deforestation; and increased travel. Changes have been documented in the distribution of important arthropod disease vectors. The yellow fever mosquito, *Aedes aegypti* has reestablished in parts of the Americas where it had been presumed to have been eradicated; the Asian tiger mosquito, *Aedes albopictus*, was introduced into the Americas in the 1980s and has spread to Central and South America; and the blacklegged tick, *Ixodes scapularis*, an important transmitter of Lyme disease and other pathogens, has gradually expanded its range in parts of eastern and central North America.

Control measures for vector-borne diseases are important because most are zoonoses that are maintained in nature in cycles involving wild animals and are not amenable to eradication. Therefore, control methods generally focus on targeting the arthropod vector. These include undertaking personal protective measures by establishing physical barriers such as house screens and bed nets; wearing appropriate clothing (boots, apparel that overlap the upper garments, head nets, etc.); and using insect repellents. Environmental modification to eliminate specific breeding areas, or chemical biological control measures to kill arthropod larvae or adults may also be undertaken. Areas such as ports and airports should be rigidly monitored, with control measures utilized to prevent

Figure 1

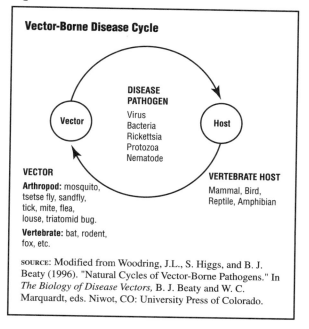

Vector-Borne Disease Cycle

Vector → DISEASE PATHOGEN (Virus, Bacteria, Rickettsia, Protozoa, Nematode) → Host

VECTOR
Arthropod: mosquito, tsetse fly, sandfly, tick, mite, flea, louse, triatomid bug.
Vertebrate: bat, rodent, fox, etc.

VERTEBRATE HOST
Mammal, Bird, Reptile, Amphibian

SOURCE: Modified from Woodring, J.L., S. Higgs, and B. J. Beaty (1996). "Natural Cycles of Vector-Borne Pathogens." In *The Biology of Disease Vectors*, B. J. Beaty and W. C. Marquardt, eds. Niwot, CO: University Press of Colorado.

important arthropod disease vectors from entering the country. Some efforts to control vector-borne diseases focus on the pathogen. For example, there are vaccines available for diseases such as Yellow fever, tick-borne encephalitis, Japanese encephalitis, tularemia, and plague. The vertebrate host and/or reservoir may also be the target for control measures. For example, vaccination of fox against rabies in Europe and Canada is an effective means to reduce the threat of rabies. In addition, reduction of host reservoirs, such as rodents and birds, from areas of human habitation may lessen the risk for contracting certain vector-borne diseases such as plague and St. Louis encephalitis.

It is clear that people will always have to live with vector-borne diseases, but maintenance of a strong public health infrastructure and undertaking research activities directed at improved means of control—possibly utilizing biological and genetic-based strategies, combined with the development of new or improved vaccines for diseases such as malaria, dengue and Lyme disease—should lessen the threat to human health.

HARVEY ARTSOB

(SEE ALSO: *Arboviral Encephalitides; Communicable Disease Control; Malaria; Plague; Zoonoses*)

BIBLIOGRAPHY

Beaty, B. J., and Marquardt, W. C. (1996). *The Biology of Disease Vectors*. Niwot, CO: University Press of Colorado.

Goddard, J. (2000). *Infectious Diseases and Arthropods*. Totowa, NJ: Humana Press.

Gubler, D. J. (1997). "Resurgent Vector-Borne Diseases as a Global Health Problem." *Emerging Infectious Diseases* 4(3):442–450.

VETERINARY PUBLIC HEALTH

In 1999, a study group on veterinary public health (VPH), convened jointly by the World Health Organization (WHO), the Food and Agriculture Organization of the United Nations (FAO), and the Office International des Epizooties (OIE), and including twenty-eight experts from eighteen countries, defined veterinary public health as "The contribution to the complete physical, mental, and social well-being of humans through an understanding and application of veterinary medical science."

The contribution of veterinary science to human health has been fundamental and sustained over millennia. It is not generally appreciated that this contribution pertains not only to livestock and food production, animal power, and transportation, which have laid the basis for most urban societies around the world. The study and management of animal diseases have also laid the basis for much of what is known about the dynamics and management of infectious human diseases, and has aided in the promotion of environmental quality.

Calvin Schwabe, one of the most important figures in veterinary public health in the twentieth century, has traced and documented the roots of the healing professions to healer-priests in the Nile Valley. Because cattle and horses were so important for sustainable food supplies, transport, and the military cohesion of ancient empires, these animals were very carefully observed and husbanded. In addition, the integrative view of healers in Egyptian and Greek cultures allowed lessons of comparative anatomy and diseases learned from the slaughter, hunting, and sacrifice of animals to be applied readily to the healing of primates. Even today, both human and veterinary medical practice draw upon the same pool of comparative, multispecies biomedical research.

RELATIONSHIPS TO PUBLIC HEALTH

If we narrow the focus of veterinary public health to those aspects that are directly pertinent to the practice of public health, rather than to human health in general, three broad areas of involvement become clear. Although these are sometimes characterized in historical terms, or in terms of "rich country-poor country" divisions, these different facets of veterinary public health are in fact ongoing, in complementary and often synergistic fashion, in most parts of the world.

Veterinary public health, in the first place, grows from its relationship to food production, usually by investigating and controlling animal diseases that threaten either food supplies or animal transportation and labor, which are essential elements in food production throughout much of the world. A second facet of veterinary public health relates to control of the transmission of zoonotic diseases, either directly or through foods. This is reflected in a wide array of activities, including research and control of infectious agents in meat and milk, rabies vaccination campaigns (both of wildlife and domestic animals), monitoring arboviruses and Lyme borreliosis in populations in wildlife, and hydatid disease control programs.

These first two facets are widely recognized as veterinary public health activities. The third facet, however, is less widely known. In many parts of the world, veterinarians, because of their knowledge of animal diseases, as well as the ecological, economic, and human cultural contexts of these diseases, have been instrumental in developing and implementing new methods of promoting sustainable public health that are ecosystemically grounded, culturally feasible, and economically realistic.

Many veterinary public health activities are reflected in the nature of veterinary involvement in public health institutions in North America and Europe. Veterinary activities involving disease control and health management in animal populations, and their integration of clinical, pathological, and epidemiological practices, often preceded similar activities in human medicine by decades, or, in some cases, centuries. It was in the area of food hygiene, however, that veterinary contributions to public health were first formally institutionalized. In Europe, particularly in Germany, veterinarians in the nineteenth and twentieth centuries were integral to the development of food hygiene laws and meat inspection systems, initially to curb large outbreaks of trichinosis.

In the aftermath of World War II, the U.S. Public Health Service's Communicable Disease Center, later named the Centers for Disease Control and Prevention (CDC) established a veterinary public health unit. James Steele, the first chief public health veterinarian in the CDC, was also active in promoting the veterinary public health unit in the World Health Organization. Martin Kaplan, another American veterinarian, became the first director of this unit. Both men expanded the traditional European emphasis on veterinary-directed food-safety programs to include investigations into the epidemiology and control of zoonoses. The 1960s and 1970s saw a reduced interest in veterinary public health, particularly in North America, because major infectious diseases were thought to be under control, and public health epidemiologists focused their efforts largely on chronic diseases such as heart disease and cancer. Although veterinarians were deeply involved in improving the understanding of these conditions by studying them in animal populations, many scientists and laypeople still had an image of veterinary public health practitioners as meat inspectors in a slaughterhouse. In 1975, the veterinary public health unit within the CDC was officially disbanded. Even during this time, however, several veterinarians were making strong contributions to public health through the CDC. Joe Held, a graduate of the Epidemic Intelligence Service of CDC, went on to become director of the National Institutes of Health Division of Research Services, Assistant Surgeon General, and director of the Pan American Zoonoses Center in Argentina.

Some within the CDC have argued that veterinary skills have been put to much broader use since the disbanding of the veterinary public health unit. In 1997, Peter Schantz, a veterinary parasitologist at CDC, documented that there were fifty-nine veterinarians at CDC assigned to eleven different centers, institutes, or program offices. Besides programs carrying out research and control of zoonotic diseases, veterinarians worked as epidemiologists and research scientists on other infectious diseases—including HIV/AIDS (human immunodeficiency virus/acquired immunodeficiency syndrome)—and on the national immunization program, environmental health, occupational health, and international health.

It was really only when infectious diseases began to reemerge as a global problem in the 1980s and 1990s that veterinary public health came back into prominence. This is largely because veterinary education, traditionally oriented to farm livestock, has been at the forefront of understanding the epidemiological features of infectious diseases in populations. It is no accident, for instance, that the protective effects for a population of vaccinating part of that population is termed a "herd effect." Furthermore, the wide scope of veterinary education lends itself well to studying and controlling zoonotic and food-borne illnesses, which became important areas of interest at the beginning of the twenty-first century.

Animal diseases may threaten human health in two ways: (1) they may threaten the animal populations that serve as food, transportation, or traction power in the fields; and (2) through zoonotic diseases, that are transmissable to humans.

NONZOONOTIC ANIMAL DISEASES OF PUBLIC HEALTH IMPORTANCE

Cattle plague, or rinderpest, which affects all cloven-hoofed animals, may serve as an example of how an epidemic disease in animals may have catastrophic effects on public health through a variety of indirect ways. The virus which causes rinderpest, related to canine distemper and human measles, was once endemic in Central Asia and made periodic forays into Europe, where it killed off tens of millions of cattle in the eighteenth century, despite strong quarantine measures, stimulating the creation of Europe's first veterinary schools. Rinderpest arrived in the lower Nile Valley with the British campaigns into the Sudan in 1884 through 1885. The prosperous cattle cultures further south, however, were initially protected by the Sahara Desert. Then, in 1889, the Italian army invading Eritrea brought cattle with them for provisioning. The disease then spread south in great devastating waves, killing millions of cattle and destroying the wealthy, cattle-based sub-Saharan civilizations. A third of the Ethiopian human population is estimated to have died as a result of this cattle plague. In what is today Tanzania, fewer than 5 percent of 4.5 million cattle survived. Villages disappeared, pastoral people were forced to become sedentary, and sedentary people lost their beasts of burden. About two-thirds of the Masai people starved to death. The way was opened up for European settlers and Bantu agriculturalists, who, of course, viewed their conquests as signs of superiority rather than as an exercise in carpet-bagging. One white South African source is quoted as saying that "the ravages of rinderpest, although reducing the native to poverty, has not been without beneficial results, and the native has now learnt humility to those to whom he is subordinate." Many wildlife species, especially large ungulates like buffalo, eland, giraffe, and kudu were decimated, and carnivores, deprived of their normal food, took to open attacks on people and other nonsusceptible species.

The disease also destroyed, initially, the natural hosts for tsetse flies, which spread blood-borne trypanosome parasites that cause sleeping sickness in people; the disease thus disappeared from wide areas of its historic habitat. Both wildlife and the scrub woodlands that support tsetse flies rebounded more quickly than the cattle and their associated grasslands. This created misconceptions among Europeans about the nature of African civilizations, the ecology of Africa in general, and about the zoonotic nature of sleeping sickness. Many sub-Saharan African ecosystems have, at different points in history, self-organized around wildlife-woodland species and cattle-grassland species. Current conservation efforts have been directed to conserve the wildlife-woodland system, which is also more hospitable to tsetse flies and endemic sleeping sickness. This is one of many examples where the veterinary activities, if allowed to take their appropriate place alongside ecologists and human health practitioners, can make profound contributions to our understanding of sustainable public health.

More recently, the public health effects of major epidemics of such nonzoonotic animal diseases as foot-and-mouth disease and both classical and African swine fever have been buffered and softened by social and economic safety nets, as well as rapid veterinary, public health, and economic responses.

ZOONOSES

The second way in which animal diseases may be of importance for public health is when the agents that cause them can be transmitted to people. The World Health Organization (WHO) defines zoonoses as "those diseases and infections, [the agents of] which are naturally transmitted between [other] vertebrate animals and [people]." This is a good, clear definition, and includes most of the diseases, such as rabies, brucellosis, tuberculosis, Q Fever, Lyme disease, salmonellosis, hydatid disease and sleeping sickness, which are conventionally viewed as being zoonoses. However, this definition is often stretched to include many infections that people share with other animals, either directly or indirectly. In some cases (such as histoplasmosis and blastomycosis), animals create conditions which allow the disease organisms to proliferate more easily. This broader net also includes other animal-associated illnesses—such as allergies—as well as the beneficial effects of animal ownership, ranging from lowered blood pressure and survival after heart attacks to serving as substitute social networks in time of crisis for elderly people.

Most often, humans are accidental hosts of zoonotic agents. The exceptions are some tapeworms, such as *Taenia solium*, *Taenia saginata*, and *Diphyllobothrium latum*, for which humans are the definitive host. In these cases, the agent is recycled back to people when they ingest meat from pigs, cattle, and fish, respectively, which have had the misfortune of ingesting infested human feces. These diseases are clearly tied to public hygiene measures as well as animal feeding practices.

Zoonoses may be classified according to their maintenance cycles. Direct zoonoses, such as leptospirosis, hantaviruses, and anthrax, may be perpetuated in nature by a single vertebrate species. Cyclozoonoses have maintenance cycles that require more than one vertebrate species, but no invertebrates. *Echinococcus multilocularis*, a tapeworm of canids that goes through intermediate stages in ruminants or omnivores, is an example. Metazoonoses require both vertebrates and invertebrates, such as ticks or mosquitoes, to complete their life cycle. American trypanosomiasis (Chagas disease, spread by triatomid "kissing bugs"), Lyme Disease (spread by deer ticks), plague (spread by rat fleas), and leishmaniasis (Kala-Azar, spread by sand flies) are metazoonotic diseases.

Saprozoonoses depend on inanimate reservoirs or development sites, such as soil, water, or plants, as well as vertebrate hosts. Toxoplasmosis, a single-celled intestinal parasite of cats which requires days to weeks in the environment to develop into an infective larval stage, and which infects people either through environmental contamination or through undercooked meat, is one example. *Toxocara canis* and *T. catis*, which exist as roundworm infections in dogs and cats, require an external environment to become infective for people. Children pick these larvae up in contaminated playgrounds and develop visceral larva migrans (VLM) or ocular larva migrans (OLM) when the larval forms move through the human body. Finally, mycotic infections such as blastomycosis, which can spend their entire life cycles externally, are also examples of saprozoonoses.

FOOD-BORNE ZOONOSES

After a half century of seeming to be under control, food-borne diseases reemerged in the 1980s as a major class of human infections. Most of the agents associated with the current worldwide increases in cases of food-borne diseases—*Salmonella* DT104; *Salmonella enteritidis*; *Escherichia coli* 0157:H7; *Campylobacter jejuni*; *Listeria monocytogenes*; and the prions associated with bovine spongiform encephalopathy (mad cow disease) and its human form, new variant Creuzfeldt-Jakob disease (nvCJD)—have their reservoirs in animal populations. In most cases, they cannot be controlled without a full, multispecies understanding of the food chain, from "stable to table." Veterinary public health has therefore become a much more active field of inquiry and activity than it was in the mid–twentieth century.

The reasons for the global increases in food-borne diseases are complex, and have revealed weaknesses in how modern agriculture is organized. Industrialized agriculture tends to encourage economies of scale to keep prices down, and large groups of animals are often gathered into one place. Poultry and swine are often kept in large groups throughout their lives. Cattle may be kept in a dispersed manner when young, but are then gathered into large feedlots for fattening. Since the conditions which promote epidemics are a function of the size of the susceptible population and the probability of adequate contact (itself a function of the agents and the methods of spread), these large populations of animals are vulnerable to epidemic diseases. In an attempt to control this vulnerability, veterinarians have worked closely with various livestock industries to set up "herd health" or "flock health" programs. When these have broken down—as all programs eventually do, especially those requiring high labor, energy, or educational inputs—there have been catastrophic epidemics of diseases such as hog cholera, salmonella, or foot-and-mouth disease. But these economies of scale have also created epidemic conditions for agents which may not only affect the livestock themselves.

No matter how they are kept, most livestock, or livestock products such as milk, are processed in centralized facilities. At some point in the modern food system, the bacteria and viruses from a wide variety of sources are brought together in one place. This allows not only for cross-contamination, but for wide dispersal of the agents so gathered, since these centralized processing industries must, in order to remain economically viable, serve large populations.

The biological effects of these economies of scale have been exacerbated by the economic pressure to become more efficient; hence animal "wastes" (organs and parts of animals not considered fit for human consumption) have been reprocessed (rendered) into protein supplements (meat and bone meal, or MBM) through various heat and chemical processes. These allow animals to grow faster or produce more milk. Economically, this seems to make sense. Ecologically, however, this has created ideal conditions for the spread and enhancement of food-borne illnesses. Well before the epidemic of BSE in Britain in the 1980s and 1990s, salmonellosis was known to increase and be magnified throughout the food system through the synergistic effects associated with scale and efficiency.

The epidemic of BSE in the United Kingdom had several contributory factors. Not the least of these was a large ratio of sheep (40 million, compared with 8 million in the United States) to cattle (12 million, compared to 104 million in the United States). Furthermore, there was a high prevalence of scrapie-infected sheep in the United Kingdom (scrapie is a well-known but little understood transmissible spongiform encephalopathy of sheep). Thus, in the United Kingdom, rendered animal protein was 14 percent sheep-derived, compared to 0.6 percent in the United States, and much of the sheep-derived MBM came from scrapie-infected sheep. Then, in the late 1970s, changes in the economic value of tallow and fats and deregulation of the rendering industry affected the proportion of MBM processed with hydrocarbon fat solvents, which fell from about 70 percent in the mid-1970s to about 10 percent in the early 1980s. It is hypothesized that this helped create conditions which allowed infective prions to slip through the system.

The BSE epidemic not only clarified some of the weaknesses in how post–Word War II agriculture was organized. It also uncovered some structural problems in the relationships between veterinary and human public health. The first cases of BSE in cattle were reported in 1986. Within two years, it became clear that there was a serious epidemic of a new disease in cattle underway, and a series of well-designed veterinary epidemiological studies were done. As the epidemic unfolded, the emphasis shifted between concerns for BSE as an animal disease, to BSE as a public health, economic, and sociopolitical problem. Although the epidemic was brought rapidly under control through various draconian measures, the lack of formal structures to link these various concerns in a systemic manner has been costly not only in terms of lives lost to nvCJD, but also through the broad, preventable, public health impacts mediated through economic and agricultural restructuring. Public health workers have tended to view transmissible spongiform encephalopathies (TSEs) such as CJD as rare, geographically widespread, and species-specific. However, those who worked with animal TSEs such as scrapie saw them as endemic in many countries, with evidence that they were capable of crossing species barriers. An integrated veterinary public health system might have made much earlier use of this information.

As indicated earlier, *Salmonella* epidemics in poultry had identified the recycling of animal proteins back into animal feeds for reasons of efficiency as problematic even before the BSE epidemic. Similarly, the use of antimicrobials in animal feeds—again for reasons of efficiency and

cost—had underlined the fact that there could be serious public health consequences to such practices. There was evidence in the 1970s that feeding of antimicrobials to animals for growth promotion or as prophylaxis could promote the spread of resistant bacteria. What also became apparent was how easily bacteria can share genetic coding for resistance, and the degree to which resistance to various drugs might be linked. An understanding of the ecology of microbial populations in the food chain has improved, even as new strains of multidrug resistant bacteria, such as *Salmonella* DT104, have emerged as serious human pathogens in North America and Europe. The links between microbial ecology, veterinary practices, and public health have made this an increasing area of concern for veterinary public health practitioners.

OTHER ZOONOSES

If agricultural activities have created epidemic conditions for food-borne diseases and problems with antibiotic resistance, they have also contributed—along with land use and climatic and cultural changes—to creating ecological conditions suitable for a range of other zoonoses. Among these, arboviruses—small, simple RNA viruses carried by arthropods (insects, spiders, crustaceans)—are particularly sensitive to changes in habitat and climate. Arboviruses multiply in the arthropods, which transmit them between vertebrate hosts. Thus, the incidence and spread of infection is sensitive to increases in standing water (mosquito breeding sites), which can be caused by irrigation systems as well as increased rainfall and temperature due to global climate changes. Hence, they often appear in seasonal epidemics. The feeding habits of the mosquitoes (whether they favor one host, or switch according to availability) are also important. For many of these viruses, small mammals and birds act as important reservoirs because they provide a steady supply of new, susceptible hosts.

Of the 535 arboviruses catalogued, some 100 are known to cause human illness, ranging from general fevers and muscle and joint pain to hemorrhagic symptoms and encephalitis. Many of these also cause similar illnesses in domestic animals. Large, long-lived vertebrates may actually serve to slow an epidemic since they develop strong immunity and, because they tend to develop low-level viremias, are not considered an important source of reinfection for other animals. These include various equine encephalitis viruses, which have been well studied for decades, such as those associated with Western, Eastern, and St. Louis Encephalitis; as well as others, like West Nile virus, that emerged as major concerns (at least in Europe and North America) at the turn of the millennium. They also include the agents of Rift Valley fever, yellow fever, and Japanese encephalitis. Even dengue fever, which is transmitted by the yellow fever mosquito *Aedes aegypti*, may have its origins in a treetop jungle cycle between wild primates and sylvatic mosquitoes.

The relationships between emerging infectious diseases and global environmental change have been stimulated not just by arboviral infections. At least two direct zoonoses—hantavirus pulmonary syndrome and leptospirosis—are sensitive to these changes. A few years ago, few people outside of military circles had ever heard of hantaviruses. Military people knew about them because they caused epidemic hemorrhagic fevers and kidney problems for troops in South Korea. Over three thousand United Nations personnel were infected. Indeed, this version of the disease has been reported around the world for many decades. Only in 1993, when a new version of the disease seemed to emerge in the American southwest, did something approaching panic spread through the medical community. This illustrates a global rule of disease emergence: diseases are important if politically or economically powerful people deem them to be so.

Being associated with drought, floods, and plagues of rodents, the story of hantavirus pulmonary syndrome has strong biblical resonances. In the spring of 1992, six years of drought in the Four Corners region of the southwestern United States ended in torrential rains. In the wake of the floods came piñon nuts and grasshoppers, and then a plague of deer mice. In one year, the deer mouse population increased tenfold, bringing the little creatures into much closer contact with farmers and other rural residents. By the time the mouse population started declining in 1993, forty-two people had succumbed to an illness that started with fever, nausea, and vomiting and ended, for twenty-six of the forty-two, with fluid in the lungs, and then death. This emergence of hantavirus pulmonary syndrome demonstrated that the disruption of ecosystems, whatever the cause, was not merely an "environmental" issue.

In many ways, hantavirus infection is similar to leptospirosis. Both are associated with spiral-shaped bacteria that prosper in warm moist places like kidneys and bladders. Neither of these diseases require a flea or other invertebrate to help complete their life cycle. The difference between hantaviruses and leptospires is that the leptospiral bacteria can survive longer in the environment, and thus are more likely to be directly affected by changes in temperature and rainfall patterns as a result of global environmental changes. Leptospirosis is believed to be the mystery killer disease which appeared in Nicaragua in 1996 after extensive flooding. Both leptospires and hantaviruses, however, are spread through rat urine and its aerosolized forms and both are closely associated with agricultural and military occupations that demand intensive meddling in restructured natural environments where rats make their homes. Hantaviruses may have started as pathogens of poor housing conditions and poverty, but the North American middle-class infatuation with visiting, or living in, "natural landscapes" has spread these agents to all socioeconomic levels.

Concern with food-borne and other emerging infectious diseases, many of which are zoonotic, has certainly broken down many barriers between veterinary and "mainstream" public health. The presence of veterinary epidemiologists at international public health conferences is no longer considered an aberration. Veterinarians are active in most public health departments in industrialized countries. ProMED, the important international electronic list-serve for reporting emerging infectious diseases, brings plant, animal, and human reports into one forum. Veterinary epidemiologists and pathologists, together with human health researchers and ecologists, have characterized many of the environmentally and agriculturally related public health problems of importance in the twenty-first century. All of these trends point to a return to the roots of "one medicine" as practiced by the great poly-mathic biologists of the nineteenth century. But these new activities take comparative medicine one step further, as they consider the ecological and cultural contexts in which diseases occur.

ECOSYSTEM-BASED VETERINARY PUBLIC HEALTH

Arboviruses and other wildlife and environmentally related zoonoses have renewed interest among veterinary public health practitioners in ecology and medical geography, and in techniques of investigation, analysis, and presentation involving spatial statistics and geographic information systems. These, combined with new environmental management techniques, have resulted in several innovative initiatives to promote public health through ecosystem-based approaches. The Network for Ecosystem Sustainability and Health, an international network of researchers from a variety of disciplines and communities, has had strong veterinary involvement from the beginning, as has the International Society for Ecosystem Health. The Center for Conservation Medicine links the veterinary college at Tufts University with Harvard Medical School and the Wildlife Preservation Trust. A nationally coordinated professional veterinary elective in ecosystem health was developed in 1993 and delivered jointly by the four Canadian veterinary colleges. From the point of view of understanding and promoting public health in a sustainable fashion, these integrative initiatives were long overdue.

Veterinary public health, growing from an orientation toward animal populations, and chastened by economic limits, has always drawn strongly on epidemiological methods of investigation and control. Before the twentieth century, many of these methods were based on various ecological observations, as well as military and agricultural necessity. As early as the fourth century, Marcus Terrentius Varro, observing diseases of livestock in Rome, noted that "there are bred [in swamps] certain minute creatures which cannot be seen by the eyes, which float in the air and enter the body through the mouth and nose and cause serious disease." Based on this kind of understanding, population-health management, quarantine, mass treatments, and mass vaccinations were a well-developed method of controlling animal diseases well before they became standard public health practices.

The International Society for Veterinary Epidemiology and Economics (ISVEE) symposium brings together every three years researchers and frontline workers from around the world who deal with the ecological and cultural dynamics of zoonotic and animal diseases that affect public health. As the global public health movement matures, one can only hope that veterinary and nonveterinary public health practitioners can be more openly integrated into new organizational frameworks that take advantage of their complementary and synergistic understanding of what it means to create healthy and sustainable human communities on earth.

DAVID WALTNER-TOEWS

(SEE ALSO: *Bovine Spongiform Encephalopathy; Centers for Disease Control and Prevention; Climate Change and Human Health; Ecosystems; Emerging Infectious Diseases; Epidemics; Epidemiology; Food-Borne Diseases; International Health; Prions; Salmonellosis; Vector-Borne Diseases; Zoonoses*)

BIBLIOGRAPHY

Palmer, S. R.; Soulsby, L.; and Simpson, D. I. H. (1998). *Zoonoses: Biology, Clinical Practice, and Public Health Control.* Oxford, UK: Oxford University Press.

Schwabe, C. W. (1978). *Cattle, Priests, and Progress in Medicine.* Minneapolis: University of Minnesota Press.

—— (1994). *Veterinary Medicine and Human Health,* 3rd edition. Baltimore, MD: Williams & Wilkins.

VanLeeuwen, N. N. O., and Waltner-Toews, D. (1998). "Ecosystem Health: An Essential Field for Veterinary Medicine." *Journal of the American Veterinary Medical Association* 212:53–57.

Waltner-Toews, D. (2001). "An Ecosystem Approach to Health and its Applications to Tropical and Emerging Diseases." *Cadernas de Saúde Publical Reports on Public Health* 17(Supp.):7–22.

See also the journal *Emerging Infectious Diseases* at http://www.cdc.gov/ncidod/eid/ and the World Health Organization at http://www.who.int, where veterinary public health activities are integrated into various parts of the site.

VIDEO DISPLAY TERMINALS

See Ergonomics *and* Information Technology

VIOLENCE

The public health approach to the study and prevention of interpersonal violence was given formal recognition in 1984 when Surgeon General C. Everett Koop stated: "Violence is every bit as much a public health issue for me and my successors in this century as smallpox, tuberculosis, and syphilis were for my predecessors in the last century." As the injury and death toll from violent behavior have become increasingly evident, multidisciplinary scholarship in the study of violence has emerged and expanded at an unprecedented pace.

The most widely accepted definition of violence—sometimes termed "intentional inter-personal injury"—is: "behavior by persons against persons that intentionally threatens, attempts, or actually inflicts physical harm" (Reiss and Roth, 1993). The closely related terms "aggression" and "antisocial behavior" are generally applied to lesser forms of violence and include, but are not limited to, behaviors that are intended to inflict psychological harm as well as physical harm.

The public health approach to the study and prevention of violence entails a four-step process: (1) data collection of violence-related problems, assets, and resources; (2) assessment of the possible causes of violence through risk-factor identification; (3) the establishment and evaluation of violence prevention strategies; and (4) the dissemination and implementation of effective strategies. Public health, then, is inherently a research-driven and prevention-oriented science. This approach complements and overlaps with the narrower focus of criminology, which is primarily concerned with forms of violence that constitute crimes and with policies and practices that deter and punish perpetrators.

VIOLENT VICTIMIZATION

Epidemiological data on violence are derived from three primary sources: (1) hospital, emergency medical service, and medical examiner records; (2) police reports and arrest records (and other agency records, such as child protective services for reports of child abuse); and (3) self-report surveys and interviews. In addition, specialized studies that address the particular dynamics and contexts of violence have proven to be important to the understanding and prevention of violence.

The most complete and accurate violence-related datasets are those on homicide victims. In the United States, the overall homicide victimization rate has fluctuated during the twentieth century from fewer than two homicides per 100,000 in 1900 to a high of nearly eleven homicides per 100,000 in 1980. In 1998, 17,893 individuals were murdered in the United States, which translates into an average daily death toll of forty-nine people. The worldwide 1998 homicide rate was 12.5 per 100,000, significantly higher than the U.S. homicide rate of 6.2 per 100,000. Nevertheless, data from the 1980s reveal that among the forty-one most developed countries, the United States has the third highest homicide rate.

Because violence is not evenly distributed throughout the population, these overall homicide rates provide only a partial picture of homicide's toll. Most notably, homicide victimization in the United States is most prevalent among youth. In 1998, homicide was the second leading cause of death among fifteen- to twenty-four-year-olds. Racial disparities in homicide rates are also disturbingly high. During the second half of the twentieth century, African Americans were murdered at five to eleven times the rate of their white counterparts. Gender differences are equally as dramatic, with males murdered at approximately ten times the rate of females. Finally, the risk of homicide is higher in urban than nonurban areas as well as within neighborhoods characterized by concentrated poverty. Neighborhood social disorganization also increases the probability of violence victimization as well as perpetration.

In comparative studies conducted in the 1990s, the homicide victimization rates in the United States, particularly among children and adolescents, were shown to be several times higher than those in any other industrialized country. In fact, the homicide rate for children under sixteen years old in the United States was five times higher than the corresponding homicide rate for the next twenty-five richest countries combined. The reasons for these elevated homicide rates in the United States are not fully understood; however, probable causes include easier access to firearms, more common and severe patterns of income disparities, and higher levels of racial and ethnic diversity in conjunction with racist and xenophobic attitudes and behaviors.

The question of mechanism, or the means by which people are murdered or injured, is another critical piece of information with respect to our understanding and prevention of violence. The examination of mechanism was particularly helpful in understanding the tremendous increase in homicide victimization rates of adolescents in the United States from 1987 to 1993, and the subsequent downturn through 1998. When the data are disaggregated by mechanism, a clear picture emerges: These trends over time can be accounted for by changes in the number and proportion of youth murdered with a firearm (see Figure 1). The changes in gun use during this period are generally attributed to three major factors: the crack epidemic—which had the effect of destabilizing local drug trafficking markets, rendering them more volatile and violent—and the subsequent petering out of this epidemic; changes in economic opportunity; and changes in policing policy for gun violations.

Most assaultive behavior, however, does not result in death. In 1997 more than 1.75 million people in the United States were treated for assaultive injuries in emergency departments, and more than 10 million individuals aged twelve and over reported that they had been victims of violent crimes. These and other data reveal that young people, African Americans, and males are disproportionately victimized by nonlethal forms of violence, though these disparities are less pronounced than for homicide victimization.

VIOLENCE PERPETRATION AND ASSOCIATED RISK FACTORS

The number and characteristics of individuals who commit murder cannot be precisely determined because of limitations in law-enforcement reporting systems and because identifying information about perpetrators are only available for cases in which an arrest is made or the perpetrator is otherwise identified. Still, some reasonably sound information about adolescents who murder is available: About nine in ten are male, more than half are African American, approximately half act alone, most kill individuals who are close in age and of the same ethnic background, and most use a firearm. The peak or modal age among homicide perpetrators occurs in the late teens and early twenties.

Since the rampage shooting at Columbine High School in the spring of 1999, much concern

about violence at schools has been aired, and fears that such events could happen anywhere have emerged. Contrary to these perceptions, however, the number and rate of youth-initiated school violence—both lethal and nonlethal—generally decreased, or at worst remained relatively stable, during the 1990s. Like the homicide victimization rates, the overall juvenile homicide perpetration rate, as well as the aggregate juvenile offending rate for serious forms of violence, rose precipitously in the late 1980s, peaked during the early to mid-1990s, and then decreased through the beginning of the twenty-first century. School-based homicides constitute only 1 percent or fewer of all homicides committed by young people, and schools remain one of the safest environments for children and adolescents.

Equally important to estimating the scope of violence perpetration among youth are efforts to identify risk factors—the characteristics that when present increase the probability that a young person will subsequently engage in violent acts. There are five important aspects of risk factors. First, risk factors tend to be additive—the more risk factors that are present, the more elevated the risk of violence. A single risk factor generally has low predictive power. Even among those children and adolescents with multiple risk factors, few will become violent. Second, risk factors occur, and need to be addressed, at multiple levels, including individual, family, peer group, school, and neighborhood or community levels. Third, different risk factors pertain to different points in the lifespan, with family-level factors playing a greater role for younger children, and peer group and neighborhood factors playing a greater role for older children. Fourth, some risk factors are specific to certain types of violent behavior (e.g., risk factors for sexual violence may be quite different than those for robbery). And fifth, the severity of risk-factor exposure is likely to increase or decrease risk proportionately (e.g., extreme and chronic child abuse is likely to have a more profound effect than lesser forms of child maltreatment).

Several literature reviews have been undertaken on risk factors that increase the probability that children and young teens will subsequently engage in violent behavior. These reviews have sorted out risk factors into two categories: risk factors during the childhood years and risk factors

Figure 1

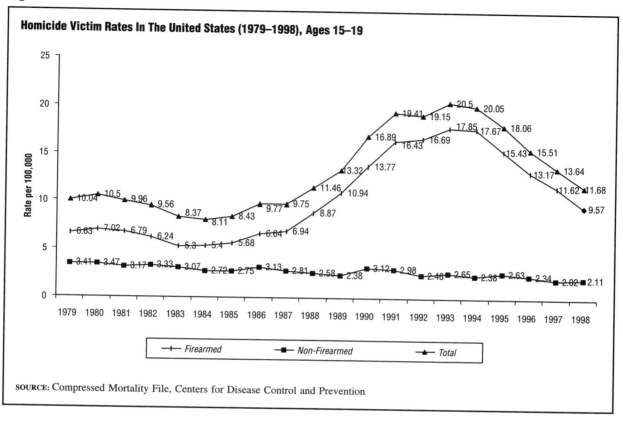

Homicide Victim Rates In The United States (1979–1998), Ages 15–19

SOURCE: Compressed Mortality File, Centers for Disease Control and Prevention

during the early adolescent years. Risk factors during infancy, and even perinatally, have also been identified, (e.g., child abuse and neglect). This entire body of research, however, is relatively new and far from exhaustive. Therefore, some factors that may in reality increase subsequent risk for violence perpetration may not have been identified in the extant literature because they have been inadequately researched or because of their complexity—the potency of a risk factor may be significantly affected by specific contextualized circumstances (e.g., bystander support), neighborhood norms, and personal history. Similarly, one factor may only become a risk factor, or may become a more potent risk factor, when it occurs in tandem with another factor.

During childhood, the two most powerful predictors of subsequent violence perpetration are substance use and delinquency. Additional, less potent risk factors include aggressive behavior; family violence; inconsistent, overly lax, and harsh disciplinary practices; association with antisocial

peers; and poor attitudes toward schooling. Media violence has been shown to increase aggression in the short term, but such exposure has not been linked directly to violent adolescent behavior. Conversely, attempts to reduce violence through media advocacy (e.g., the "Squash It" campaign) have not been shown to reduce rates of violence significantly.

During the early adolescent years, three major and interrelated risk factors have been identified: weak associational ties with nondelinquent peers; strong associational ties with antisocial and delinquent peers; and gang membership. Gang membership, in particular, appears to fulfill important psychological needs with regard to peer acceptance and belonging, as well as the need for enhanced social status, particularly for unpopular youth and for those youth who feel socially powerless. Because gangs serve these fundamental needs, efforts to dissuade young people from joining youth gangs is a more efficient strategy than trying to entice them out of the gang after they have joined, particularly since gangs typically promise to provide valued incentives such as money, power and status, excitement, and, for males, promises of sexual "favors." On the other hand, to ignore current gang members, or rely exclusively on punitive law enforcement efforts, is an inefficient and ineffective violence reduction strategy. Community-based outreach efforts in association with community policing operations are required. Such efforts need to address the psychological, interpersonal, and economic needs of gang members; they should be based upon multiple sources of information about local gang activity; and they should include collaborative efforts involving the police, schools, social service agencies, former gang members, and grassroots organizations.

Additional risk factors during the early adolescent years include antisocial behavior, attending a school in which gangs are prevalent, having been a victim of a violent crime, and residing in a high-crime neighborhood and/or in neighborhoods that have high levels of social disorganization.

While quantitative risk factor analyses are important, qualitative studies based on in-depth interviews, focus groups, and intensive field studies of particular groups of youth provide insights into the dynamics underlying risk-factor analyses and point to additional factors, or combinations of factors, that may be fruitful to study. These studies are important given the generally weak overall predictive power yielded from risk-factor analyses. Examples of such studies include James Garbarino's 1999 study of children and adolescents who have committed violent crimes, Elijah Anderson's 1999 study of the impact of street and cultural norms in an impoverished African-American section of Philadelphia, John Devine's extensive 1996 field studies of school violence in New York City, and Felix Padilla's in-depth 1992 study of the dynamics and culture of a Latino gang in Chicago. These richly textured studies, and others like them, capture the complex and tragic nature of acts of violence. They also provide insights about the psychological logic and developmental history of those who commit violent acts, reminding us that even the most vicious forms of violence can ultimately be understood, though not justified, as uniquely human responses to a volatile mix of difficult circumstances and experiences combined with specific personality and character dynamics.

PREVENTION STRATEGIES

Four major interrelated approaches to the prevention of violence have been articulated: (1) the inculcation or enhancement of protective factors (factors that reduce the probability of violence perpetration among individuals exposed to known risk factors) and/or a corresponding reduction in the number or severity of risk factors, (2) the adoption of self-contained violence prevention programs, (3) the specification of generic strategies (e.g., social skills training) derived by grouping effective and promising programs according to the approach they adopt and the specific program characteristics they utilize, and (4) the elucidation of framing principles that guide the establishment and implementation of programs.

The use of mechanical and electronic surveillance devices (e.g., metal detectors), and the establishment of laws, law enforcement policies, judicial processing, and incarcerative practices remain primarily in the domain of criminology and need to be better integrated with public health approaches. One successful example of this kind of comprehensive and integrated approach was established in Boston. This strategy involved several agencies and programs working together to reduce gun and gang-related violence. The police, probation officers, and courts addressed surveillance, interdiction, and enforcement; legislators passed tougher penalties for gun-related violence; researchers conducted analyses of gun violations; and social workers and religious leaders counseled at-risk youth in the use of nonviolent conflict resolution techniques and offered employment opportunities and program activities. Other approaches to violence prevention, such as changes in public policies, (e.g., foster care policies, school reform, and employment and housing strategies), have received only passing attention within the public health field, with the notable exception of the significant attention paid to firearm policies.

The study of protective factors has been spurred by the long-standing observation that some children who are exposed to several known risk factors do not become violent or otherwise seriously impaired. The task, then, is to identify common characteristics or circumstances that buffer these resilient children from the ill effects of exposure to known risk factors. The scientific study of protective factors, however, is in its infancy and the evidence from this small body of literature is suggestive rather than conclusive.

The most well-documented protective factor is maintaining conventional values, including the rejection of aggressive or violent behavior as an appropriate means to resolve conflict. This characteristic is associated with the peer-level protective factor of associating with peers who hold prosocial values. At the family level, a warm and supportive relationship with one's parents or guardians and engagement in familial bonding activities have been associated with reduced levels of aggression.

As children move into the more high-risk adolescent years, family factors alone do not continue to exert a powerful protective effect. The innoculative effects of protective factors appear to require developmentally appropriate exposures at each stage of development. At the school level, commitment to school has been identified as a protective factor. Finally, because neighborhood and societal change are so difficult to study in controlled studies, and also so challenging to address, protective factors at these levels have not been identified.

The development and implementation of self-contained violence prevention programs has a long-standing history. The introduction of scientific methods to assess the effectiveness of such programs, however, only commenced in the 1980s, with the number and rigor of such evaluations accelerating rapidly during the 1990s. Still, scientific evaluations are very costly and only a small proportion of programs now in use at schools and in communities have been rigorously evaluated.

The programs that have been evaluated are generally highly structured, implemented by professionals, and developed at academic institutions. While this body of research has revealed that some programs do indeed reduce rates of aggression and violence (and that some programs clearly do not work), it is inaccurate to assume that programs that have not been evaluated do not work, or conversely, that they are effective.

It is also inaccurate to conclude that programs that have been shown to be effective will work equally well in all settings and contexts. Very little is known about whether, or how, programs need to be adapted from one setting to another. Some programs may not work equally well for males and

females, some may work well in urban but not rural settings, and some programs may work in one cultural context but not another. Some programs are appropriate for all children or youth within a designated age range (universal, or primary, prevention), some are appropriate for children and youth exhibiting or possessing known risk factors (selective, or secondary, prevention), and some programs are appropriate for youth who have already engaged in violence or serious delinquent behavior (indicated, or tertiary, prevention).

In the late 1990s and early 2000s, several compendia of effective, promising, and ineffective violence prevention programs were issued. These include reports by the Surgeon General, the Centers for Disease Control and Prevention, the Center for the Study and Prevention of Violence, the Office of Justice Programs, the National Research Council, the Violence Institute of New Jersey, M. W. Lipsey and D. B. Wilson (1998), and M. B. Greene (1998). The major strategies that have been shown to be effective, along with brief descriptions of illustrative programs, are summarized below; however, readers interested in a full explication of such strategies, along with detailed descriptions of effective and promising programs, are urged to consult sources listed in the bibliography.

The most widely adopted violence prevention strategy emphasizes social skills training to resolve conflict without resorting to aggressive or violent tactics. Social skills training programs generally utilize structured and interactive curricula (e.g., role playing) and are usually classroom based. One example of an effective social skills training programs is Promoting Alternative Thinking Strategies, or PATHS. This program is designed for children from kindergarten through fifth grade and focuses on five specific skills: emotional literacy, self-control, social competence, positive peer relations, and interpersonal problem solving. School-based sessions are taught for approximately thirty minutes each, and the program developers recommend that these lessons should be taught three times per week.

A second overall strategy focuses on parent training and family dynamics. This approach is both educational and therapeutic and based on the theory that a caring, supportive, and stable family life will provide the initial grounding to deter children from subsequently engaging in aggressive, delinquent, or violent behavior. Most commonly, programs are designed to work with parents of young children and are focused on parental decision making, communication, monitoring and sanctioning strategies, and on educating parents about child development. Several family-based strategies have been shown to be highly effective in reducing aggressive and/or violent behavior.

Home visitation, in which therapeutic guidance is provided to parents in their residence, has gained much recognition in recent years. One of the most effective home visitation programs is the Nurse Home Visitation Program, in which a trained nurse visits the home setting during the latter stages of pregnancy through the point at which the child reaches age two. Long-term follow-up studies indicate that the adolescent children of program participants had significantly fewer arrests than control-group adolescents. In addition, two family-oriented programs for adolescents who have exhibited violent and delinquent behavior have also been shown to be effective: Functional Family Therapy and Multisystemic Therapy. Both programs provide intensive family and individual therapy, as well as guidance to parents in addressing practical and everyday problems, and both have effected significant reductions in subsequent delinquent and violent behavior.

A defining feature of a third approach to violence prevention is the central role played by young people in the program's operation and implementation. Four principles underlie such programs: (1) young people understand their own peer culture and what kinds of program components are feasible; (2) young people provide a typically untapped human resource; (3) program norms are more readily diffused through the network of involved youth; and (4) the involvement by young people in implementing such programs provides an alternative for antisocial, violent, and delinquent behavior. The most popular of this class of programs is school-based peer mediation, in which a trained student mediates a dispute between two other students with the goal of establishing a mutually agreed-upon peaceful solution. Other types of programs engage young people in community organizing or advocacy activities. While the small number of peer-operated programs that have been rigorously evaluated has not shown significant reductions in violent or delinquent behavior, the theoretical promise of these programs, the fact that many types of youth-led programs have not been evaluated, and the inherent complexity in evaluating such programs suggest that a decision to forgo or eliminate such programs is premature. Nevertheless, sound policy also suggests that programs should be discontinued if they continuously fail to demonstrate their effectiveness.

Another class of programs utilizes psychoeducational strategies to reduce the likelihood of engagement in violent behavior. The most well-known type of program within this class of programs is mentoring. While not all mentoring programs are effective, the Big Brothers Big Sisters program model has been rigorously evaluated and shown to be an effective violence prevention strategy. Stand-alone individual counseling, however, is considered an ineffective violence prevention strategy.

Another type of program involves counseling and supportive services for youth who have been exposed to violence, either as victims or as witnesses—both of which are risk factors for subsequent perpetration. In one such program, the Child Development Community Policing Project, police officers receive training in child development and the dynamics of psychological trauma and work together with mental health clinicians—who receive training in police practices and culture—in identifying and responding to children who have been exposed to violence. This program illustrates the potential value of integrating clinical and law enforcement approaches.

Finally, some programs are hybrids, either combining two or more of the approaches outlined above or not fitting neatly into any of the four approaches. One "hybrid" is Olweus's Bullying Prevention Program. This program has several key features, including skills-based classroom training, parent involvement, policy development, "hot spot" analysis, and counseling. Evaluations of this program suggest that it is effective in reducing levels of bullying and harassment. Indeed, multicomponent programs are generally viewed as preferable, particularly for high-risk youth.

Public health efforts to address gun-related violence also do not fit neatly into any of the approaches outlined above. Strategies to reduce gun violence include the promotion of laws and policies that reduce access to guns (some evidence of effectiveness); the adoption of mechanical and electronic means to make guns safer, such as trigger locks and personalized guns (the consistency and quality of such devises are variable and none has been adequately evaluated); educating children in safe gun practices (ineffective); gun buybacks (ineffective); and public information campaigns (no evaluations have been conducted).

As indicated above, an alternative way to approach violence prevention programming is by establishing a set of framing principles that inform their development. While this cannot be done without examining what is known from evaluation studies and from risk and protective factor analyses, it is too early in the evolution of such studies to simply extract these principles from the programs that have been subject to rigorous evaluation and proven to be effective or promising. Some of the principles listed below, therefore, owe more to findings in other areas of public health than they do to the violence prevention field per se. Some principles have been described in earlier parts of this article (e.g., that no single program or approach works equally in all settings and circumstances). What follows is a brief though not exhaustive list of such principles.

The first principle, known as local ownership, suggests that programs will be most successfully operated if the residents in the targeted neighborhood and the specific group of individuals for whom the program is designed to help are centrally involved in the planning, operation, and administration of the program. A second principle multidisciplinarianism, suggests that insights, methods, and approaches from multiple disciplines are needed in developing and implementing violence prevention programs. A third principle, collaboration, suggests that no single agency or group can successfully operate a program in isolation: Violence prevention programs are inherently neighborhood-based and require the engagement of multiple stakeholders.

A fourth principle suggests that a strength-based focus should be emphasized—focusing exclusively on deficits without drawing upon the strengths and interests of the individuals the program is designed to help and the resources available in the community will reduce the probability of success. A fifth principle suggests that committed leadership is necessary for the successful planning and implementation of violence prevention programs. Similarly, staff development is also critical: An untrained, unsupported, and unsupervised staff simply will not succeed in program implementation. Staff also need to be temperamentally suited to the populations with which they work.

Program accessibility is also critically important: If a program is sited in an undesirable location (turf issues are very important for young people), is sited in a difficult-to-get-to location, or is physically unwelcoming or uninviting, then the program will simply not attract participants. Specificity is also important: Programs need to set specific and measurable objectives, otherwise they tend to flounder and evaluation is rendered unfeasible. A final principle is local fit; A program's design and objectives should be derived from a thorough and multipronged assessment of the nature and extent of the violence-related problems in the neighborhood in which the program will be implemented. Additionally, new programs need to fit well into the context of existing programs and strategies.

Perhaps it is fitting to end with a quote from Surgeon General David Satcher, taken from his preface to the Surgeon General's report on youth violence: "As a Nation, we possess knowledge and have translated that knowledge into programs that are unequivocally effective in preventing much serious youth violence."

MICHAEL B. GREENE

(SEE ALSO: *Abuse; Adolescent Violence; Antisocial Behavior; Crime; Domestic Violence; Gun Control; Homicide; Prevention; Reckless Driving; Safety; Street Violence; Suicide; Terrorism; War*)

BIBLIOGRAPHY

Alexander, J. F. (1998). *Functional Family Therapy*. Boulder, CO: Institute for Behavioral Science.

Anderson, E. (1999). *Code of the Street: Decency, Violence, and the Moral Life of the Inner City*. New York: Norton.

Arredondo, S.; Aultman-Bettridge, T.; Johnson, T.; Williams, K.; and Ninneman, L. (1998). *A Study of Youth*

Handgun Violence. Boulder, CO: Center for the Study and Prevention of Violence.

Berkowitz, L. (1993). *Aggression: Its Causes, Consequences and Control.* New York: McGraw-Hill.

Blum, R. W.; Beuhring, T.; and Rinehart, P. M. (2000). *Protecting Teens: Beyond Race, Income and Family Structure.* Minneapolis, MN: Center for Adolescent Health, University of Minnesota.

Blumstein, A., and Wallman, J., eds. (2000). *The Crime Drop in America.* New York: Cambridge University Press.

Centers for Disease Control and Prevention (1997). "Rates of Homicide, Suicide, and Firearm-Related Death among Children—26 Industrialized Countries." *Morbidity and Mortality Weekly Report* 46(5):101–105.

Devine, J. (1996). *Maximum Security: The Culture of Violence in Inner-City Schools.* Chicago: University of Chicago Press.

Elliott, D. S., ed. (2001). *Youth Violence: A Report of the Surgeon General.* Atlanta, GA: Office of the Surgeon General.

Elliot, D. S., and Tolan, P. H. (1999). "Youth Violence, Prevention, Intervention, and Social Policy." In *Youth Violence: Prevention, Intervention, and Social Policy,* eds. D. J. Flannery and C. R. Huff. Washington, DC: American Psychiatric Press.

Fagan, J., and Wilkinson, D. L. (1998). "Social Contexts and Functions of Adolescent Violence." In *Violence in American Schools,* eds. D. S. Elliot, B. A. Hamburg, and K. R. Williams. New York: Cambridge University Press.

Federal Bureau of Investigation (1993). *Age-Specific Arrest Rates and Race-Specific Arrest Rates for Selected Offenses: 1965–1992.* Washington, DC: Author.

Garbarino, J. (1999). *Lost Boys: Why Our Sons Turn Violent and How We Can Save Them.* New York: Free Press.

Gilligan, J. (1996). *Violence: Reflections on a National Epidemic.* New York: Random House.

Greene, M. B. (1996). "Youth and Violence: Trends, Principles and Programmatic Intervention." In *Minefields in Their Hearts: A Mental Health Handbook for Children in War and Communal Violence,* eds. R. J. Apfel and B. Simon. New Haven: Yale University Press.

—— (1998). "Youth Violence in the City: The Role of Educational Interventions." *Health Education and Behavior* 25(2):175–193.

Henggeler, S. W. (1997). *Treating Serious Antisocial Behavior in Youth: The MST Approach.* Washington, DC: U.S. Department of Justice.

Herrenkohl, T. I.; Magiun, E.; Hill, K. G.; Hawkins, J. D.; Abbott, R. D.; and Catalano, R. F. (2000). "Developmental Risk Factors for Youth Violence." *Journal of Adolescent Health* 26:176–186.

Howell, J. C. (2000). *Youth Gang Programs and Strategies.* Washington, DC: Department of Justice.

Krug, E. (1999). *Injury: A Leading Cause of the Global Burden of Disease.* Geneva: World Health Organization.

Lipsey, M. W., and Derson, J. H. (1998). "Predictors of Violent or Serious Delinquency in Adolescence and Early Adulthood: A Synthesis of Longitudinal Research." In *Serious & Violent Juvenile Offenders,* eds. R. Loeber and D. P. Farrington. Thousand Oaks, CA: Sage Publications.

Lipsey, M. W., and Wilson, D. B. (1998). "Effective Intervention for Serious Juvenile Offenders: A Synthesis of Research." In *Serious and Violent Juvenile Offenders,* eds. R. Loeber and D. P. Farrington. Thousand Oaks, CA: Sage Publications.

Marans, S., and Berkman, M. (1997). *Child Development–Community Policing: Partnership in a Climate of Violence.* Washington, DC: Office of Juvenile Justice and Delinquency Prevention.

McCord, J.; Widom, C. S.; and Crowell, N. A., eds. (2001). *Juvenile Crime, Juvenile Justice.* Washington, DC: National Academy Press.

Mercy, J. A.; Rosenberg, M. L.; Powell, K. E.; Broome, C. V.; and Roper, W. L. (1993). "Public Health Policy for Preventing Violence." *Health Affairs* 12(4):7–25.

Milne, J. S., and Hargarten, S. W. (1999). "Handgun Safety Features: A Review for Physicians." *Journal of Trauma Injury* 47(1):145–150.

Murphy, S. L. (2000). *Deaths: Final Data for 1998.* Atlanta, GA: Centers for Disease Control and Prevention.

Nourjah, P. (1999). *National Hospital Ambulatory Medical Care Survey: 1997 Emergency Department Summary.* Atlanta, GA: Centers for Disease Control and Prevention.

Office of Juvenile Justice and Violence Prevention (1999). *Promising Strategies to Reduce Gun Violence.* Washington, DC: Author.

Olds, D. (1998). *Prenatal and Infancy Home Visitation by Nurses.* Boulder, CO: Institute for Behavioral Science.

Olweus, D. (1993). *Bullying at School.* Malden, MA: Blackwell Publishers.

Padilla, F. (1992). *The Gang as an American Enterprise.* New Brunswick, NJ: Rutgers University Press.

Petersilla, J. (1990). "Conditions that Permit Intensive Supervision Programs to Survive." *Crime and Delinquency* 36:126–145.

Rand, M. (1998). *Criminal Victimization 1997.* Washington, DC: Bureau of Justice Statistics.

Reiss, A. J., and Roth, J. A., eds. (1993). *Understanding and Preventing Violence.* Washington, DC: National Academy Press.

Rennison, C. M. (2000). *Criminal Victimization 1999: Changes 1998–99 with Trends 1993–99.* Washington, DC: U.S. Department of Justice.

Sampson, R.; Raudenbush, S. W.; and Earls, F. (1997). "Neighborhoods and Violent Crime: A Multilevel Study of Collective Efficacy." *Science* 277:918–924.

Sherman, L. W.; Gottfredson, D.; MacKenzie, D.; Eck, J.; Reuter, P.; and Bushway, S. (1997). *Preventing Crime: What Works, What Doesn't, What's Promising.* Washington, DC: Office of Justice Programs.

Snyder, H. N., and Sickmund, M. (1999). *Juvenile Offenders and Victims: 1999 National Report.* Pittsburgh, PA: National Center for Juvenile Justice.

Steinberg, L. (2000). "Youth Violence: Do Parents and Families Make a Difference?" *National Institute of Justice Journal* 243:30–38.

Thorton, T. N.; Craft, C. A.; Dahlberg, L. L.; Lynch, B. S.; and Baer, K. (2000). *Best Practices of Youth Violence: A Sourcebook for Community Action.* Atlanta, GA: Centers for Disease Control and Prevention, National Center for Injury Prevention and Control.

Tierney, J. P.; Grossman, J. B.; and Resch, N. L. (1995). *Making a Difference: An Impact Study of Big Brothers Big Sisters.* Philadelphia, PA: Public/Private Ventures.

U.S. Department of Education (1999). *1999 Annual Report on School Safety.* Washington, DC: Author.

Violence Institute of New Jersey (2001). *SourceBook of Drug and Violence Prevention Programs for Children and Adolescents.*

Wintemute, G. J. (1999). "The Future of Firearm Violence Prevention." *Journal of the American Medical Association* 282(5):475–478.

VIRAL INFECTIONS

See Communicable Disease Control

VIRCHOW, RUDOLPH

Rudolph Virchow (1821–1902) was one of the towering figures of nineteenth-century medicine, pathology, and social reform. He studied medicine in Berlin and taught there for a great part of his life, with interludes in Silesia and Würzburg. His primary field was pathology, to which he made prolific contributions, including the founding in 1847 of *Archiv für pathologische Anatomie und Physiologie* (known as "Virchow's Archives"), which still survives as a leading journal of pathology. In 1848 he served on a commission to investigate an epidemic of typhus, for which he wrote a penetrating report criticizing the social conditions that fostered the spread of the disease. He had already established a reputation as a crusading social reformer, and this report consolidated that reputation. He has since been identified as much with what came to be called "social medicine" as with his primary specialty of pathology.

Virchow's writings and speeches are full of observations and recommendations about ways to improve people's health by improving their economic and social conditions. He helped to shape the health care reforms introduced in Germany under Otto von Bismarck. He entered politics, serving in the German Reichstag (1880–1893), while also directing the Pathological Institute in Berlin. His prolific writings, while mainly on topics in pathology, included many essays and addresses on social medicine and public health. These writings remain relevant over one hundred years after they were first written. Virchow also contributed substantially to anthropology, paleontology, and archeology.

JOHN M. LAST

(SEE ALSO: *History of Public Health; Social Medicine; Typhus, Epidemic*)

BIBLIOGRAPHY

Virchow, R. (1985). *Collected Essays on Public Health and Epidemiology,* ed. and trans. L. J. Rather. Canton, MA: Science History Publications.

VIRUSES

See Pathogenic Organisms

VISION DISORDERS

Human vision is dependent on the successful interaction of optical structures in the eye. When these structures malfunction, vision disorders occur. The key to treatment and resolution of these disorders is early detection through regular eye exams and prompt consultation with an ophthalmologist when problems occur.

The best way to describe how vision works is to use the analogy of a camera. The pupil manages the incoming light rays, opening and closing—like a camera shutter—according to the amount of light available. These light rays are progressively refracted and focused by three structures: the cornea, a transparent, convex cover over the iris and pupil in front of the eye; the lens, a spherical body behind the cornea, and the vitreous humor, a gelatinous substance that fills the back of the eyeball. It is important that the rays be in sharp focus when they reach the retina, a sensory membrane that lines the back of the eye and acts like film in a camera. The retina converts the light rays into electrical signals that are sent to the brain by way of the optic nerve. The brain then translates these electrical signals into what we know as sight.

Refractive Errors. The most common vision disorders are refractive errors—specifically nearsightedness, farsightedness, and astigmatism. In each case, the eye does not refract the incoming light properly, so the image is blurred. While they are not diseases, refractive errors affect every age range and comprise the largest treatment effort of ophthalmologists. Refractive errors can be successfully corrected with eyeglasses, contact lenses, and laser refractive surgery.

Cataract. A cataract results when the normally transparent lens of the eye clouds, blurring vision. Most cataracts are age-related, advancing slowly and progressively until functional blindness occurs. Cataract cannot be prevented or cured with medication or optical devices, but it can be successfully treated through a surgical procedure that removes the damaged, natural eye lens and replaces it with a permanent, intraocular lens implant. The procedure has over a 90 percent success rate. After refractive errors, cataract is the most common vision disorder.

Macular Degeneration. Located in the retina, the macula is responsible for central vision. When people have macular degeneration, they can no longer bring the center of the picture they see into focus. The most common type of the disease is age-related, and there are two forms: "wet" and "dry." Whereas the wet form comprises only about 10 percent of cases, it causes the greatest vision loss,

striking quickly and without warning as a result of erupting blood vessels. The dry form is characterized by a slow, progressive loss of vision from the thinning and tearing of the macula. Although both forms are being extensively researched, definitive causes and treatments have not yet been identified. Age-related macular degeneration is the leading cause of blindness in most developed countries.

Glaucoma. Glaucoma is a disease of the optic nerve. If the aqueous humor (the clear fluid that fills the front of the eye) does not drain properly, intraocular pressure builds, damaging the optic nerve and causing blind spots to develop. When the entire nerve is destroyed, blindness results. If glaucoma is detected and treated in the early stages, loss of vision can be averted. However, the disease is chronic and cannot be cured or reversed. Unfortunately, the early stages are symptomless. Once symptoms occur, usually manifested by loss of peripheral or side vision, irreversible vision loss has already taken place. Treatment consists of medication and/or surgery, depending on the type of glaucoma, the patient's medical history, and the stage of the disease. Glaucoma is the leading cause of blindness worldwide and the second-leading cause in developed countries.

Diabetic Retinopathy. Retinopathy is a side effect of diabetes and occurs as a result of fluctuations in the body's blood sugar, a daily problem for diabetics. When blood sugar fluctuates over time, it affects the blood vessels in various parts of the body, including the retina of the eye, where the blood vessels can break and bleed, causing blurred vision. The longer a person has diabetes, the higher the risk of retinopathy; good diabetic control can forestall the disease, however. Signs of retinopathy often occur before symptoms appear. Treatment includes the use of laser photocoagulation to seal leaking blood vessels. Often undetected and untreated, diabetic retinopathy is the leading cause of visual disability among working-age people.

Retinal Degenerations. Retinal degeneration is an umbrella term for a number of hereditary and degenerative disorders that range from mild to profound vision loss and blindness. Retinitis pigmentosa is the most common type of retinal degeneration, affecting one in three thousand people. Its many forms have widely varied symptoms, and onset and progress of the disease can be slow or rapid. In general, symptoms occur in childhood or young adulthood. Patients complain of night blindness followed by loss of visual field. There is no treatment, though researchers are hopeful that genetic therapies may be possible in the future.

Strabismus. Unlike most other vision disorders, strabismus is a physical defect. One or both of the eyes are misaligned and point in different directions. One eye may look ahead while the other eye points up, down, in, or out. Strabismus is more common in children than in adults. In adults it can be a side effect of head trauma or brain disorder. Treatment may involve eyeglasses, an eye patch (in some cases), or surgery on the eye muscles.

BARBARA L. PAWLEY

(SEE ALSO: *Diabetes Mellitus*)

BIBLIOGRAPHY

O'Toole, M. (1997). *Miller-Keane Encyclopedia & Dictionary of Medicine, Nursing, & Allied Health,* 6th edition. Philadelphia, PA: W.B. Saunders.

VITAL STATISTICS

Vital statistics are perhaps the most widely used national, state, and local data for identifying and addressing major public health issues. In the United States, legal authority for the registration of vital events (births, deaths, marriages, divorces, fetal deaths, and induced terminations of pregnancy [abortions]) resides with the states, and individually with New York City, the District of Columbia, and the U.S. territories. The states are the legal proprietors of these data and are responsible for maintaining registries and issuing copies of the records.

The existence of a national data system of registration-based vital statistics depends on a cooperative relationship between the states and the federal government. This relationship has evolved over many decades, with its initial beginnings in the early development of the public health movement and the creation of the American federal vital statistics system.

THE HISTORY OF VITAL STATISTICS

The registration of births, marriages, and deaths has a long history in the United States, beginning with registration laws enacted by the Grand Assembly of Virginia in 1632 and the General Court of the Massachusetts Bay Colony in 1639. In enacting this legislation, the early settlers, who were predominantly English, were following English customs. Thus, Virginia law required the clergy to keep a record of all christenings, marriages, and burials in their parishes. The Massachusetts law differed from Virginia's in two important respects: it called for the recording of vital events (births, deaths, and marriages) rather than church-related ceremonies; and it placed responsibility for registration of vital events on government officials rather than the clergy. Little or no statistical use was made of such records, however—along with wills and property inventories, they were regarded primarily as statements of fact essential to the protection of individual rights, especially those relating to the ownership and distribution of property.

The impetus for the use of vital records as the basis of a public health data system came from the realization that records of births and deaths, particularly records of deaths by cause of death, could provide information needed for the control of epidemics and the conservation of human life through sanitary reform. The origin of vital statistics in the modern sense can be traced to an analysis of the English bills of mortality published by John Graunt in 1662. Similarly, the clergyman Cotton Mather noted, in 1721, during a severe smallpox epidemic in Boston, that more than one in six of the natural cases died, but only one in sixty of the inoculated cases died.

In the nineteenth century, the industrial revolution resulted in rapid urbanization, overcrowding of cities, and a deterioration of social and living conditions for large sectors of the population. Public health reformers became acutely conscious of the need for general sanitary reform as a means of controlling epidemics of disease, particularly cholera. These early sanitarians used the crude death statistics of the time to arouse public awareness of the need for improved sanitation, and in the process they pressed for more precise statistics through effective registration practices and laws.

The work of Edwin Chadwick (1800–1890) and Dr. William Farr (1807–1883) in England and of Lemuel Shattuck (1793–1859) in Massachusetts was instrumental in the development of public health organization and practice, including the recording of vital statistics. Thus, the history of public health is largely the history of vital registration and statistics.

The United States Constitution provided for a decennial census but not a national vital registration system. To obtain national data on births, marriages, and deaths, the decennial censuses in the latter half of the nineteenth century included questions about vital events, such as: "Born within the year," "Married within the year," and "Disease, if died within the year." These census items were soon recognized as inefficient and the results as deficient. Therefore, when the Bureau of the Census was made a permanent agency of the federal government in 1902, the enabling legislation authorized the bureau to obtain annually copies of records filed in the vital statistics offices of those states and cities having adequate death registration systems and to publish data from these records. This marked the birth of the National Vital Statistics System. Ten states and cities provided death records to the Census Bureau in 1902. In 1915, birth registration was added to the system, and by 1933 all states were registering live births and deaths and providing the required data.

In 1946 responsibility for collecting and publishing national vital statistics was transferred from the Census Bureau to the U.S. Public Health Service, first in the National Office of Vital Statistics and later (1960) in the National Center for Health Statistics (NCHS). In 1987 NCHS became part of the Centers for Disease Control and Prevention of the U.S. Department of Health and Human Services.

In the early part of the twentieth century, the Bureau of the Census received unit record data from the states in hard copy or microfilm. States were reimbursed for copying efforts at four cents per record. Data were transcribed (later key entered) at both the national and state levels, as both states and federal government produced statistics. In 1971 NCHS began an experiment with the state of Florida to receive data on computer tape. This effort expanded and evolved over time, and by 2000, electronic processing and transmission was

the norm. NCHS provides partial funding support for state vital statistics efforts and also works with states to implement standards for data elements, editing and coding specifications, quality control procedures, and data transmission schedules.

VITAL STATISTICS DATA FILES

The National Vital Statistics System includes several major electronic data files, each containing the demographic and health information recorded on all events that occur in the United States. Birth data are recorded in the "natality file," which includes characteristics of mother's age, race, Hispanic origin, education, residence, marital status, month of pregnancy, month prenatal care began, tobacco use, and weight gain during pregnancy. Characteristics of the birth include birth weight, length of gestation, sex, plurality, method of delivery, and congenital anomalies.

The "mortality file" variables include residence, place of occurrence, month of death, age, race, Hispanic origin, birthplace, sex, education, marital status, and underlying and multiple causes of death. The "fetal death file" includes data on all fetal deaths of twenty weeks or more gestation. The characteristics of the mother and the delivery are similar to those for natality, but also include the fetal or maternal conditions causing death.

The "linked birth/infant death data system" includes three separate files: a numerator file with linked birth-infant death records for infants who died during the period; a denominator file of data for all births; and a file of the relatively few infant death records that were not linked to birth certificates.

Unlike the natality and mortality systems, detailed data for marriages and divorces have never covered the entire United States. With data year 1996, NCHS ceased collecting detailed marriage and divorce data from the states that had been providing unit records. Monthly counts of the number of marriages and divorces continue to be obtained from each state.

Data and reports from these files are available at the NCHS web site http://www.cdc.gov/nchs/nvss.htm.

VITAL STATISTICS MEASURES

The vital statistics system provides counts of the number of times specified vital events have occurred. These counts are useful in themselves. For example, the numbers of births and deaths are used in the estimation of population size. For most purposes, however, other statistical measures are needed. For example, comparisons of births in one place with those in another requires information on the population size of each area. The simplest and cleanest method of making such comparisons is to compute rates that relate the events to the population exposed to the risk of the event (e.g., the number of births to the number of women of child-bearing age).

Many types of relative numbers are used in the analysis of vital statistics. Those used most frequently in the United States are listed below. The reader can find additional information about the definition and computation of these statistics in the works of Weeks (1996), Shryock and Siegel (1976), or Pollard et al. (1991).

Crude rates. The number of events in a given time period divided by the population at risk produces crude rates. The result is multiplied by a constant (typically 1,000 or 100,000) for ease of presentation. Common crude rates include birth, death, marriage, and divorce.

Specific rates. Crude rates may be limited to a specific group, such as deaths from a specified cause or in a specific age group, or births to unmarried women.

Age-adjusted rates. Age-adjustment is a technique used to eliminate the effect of the age distribution of the population on mortality rates. Since the frequency of death varies with age, a measure free of the influences of population composition is needed to make comparisons between areas or over time.

Infant mortality rates. Infant mortality rates reflect the risk of deaths to infants under the age of one year. For infant deaths, the most commonly used estimate of the population at risk (denominator) is the number of live births during the period.

Life tables and life expectancy. A life table is used to measure the effect of mortality on longevity. It shows the mortality experience of a hypothetical group of infants born at the same time and subject to the mortality rates of a specific population group. A life table provides numerous statistics; perhaps the most widely used is life expectancy at birth.

INTERNATIONAL CLASSIFICATION OF DISEASES

Causes of death are classified for purposes of statistical tabulation according to the *International Classification of Diseases* (ICD), which is published by the World Health Organization. Traditionally, a single cause of death is selected for statistical tabulations. When the certifying physician indicates that more than one cause contributed to death, a procedure is required for selecting the single cause to be tabulated. The ICD provides the basic ground rules used to code and classify causes of death, to identify the underlying cause of death, and to compensate for inconsistencies in the reported cause-of-death statement. It also includes definitions of terms such as "underlying cause of death," "live birth," "maternal death," as well as tabulation lists which define the cause-of-death groupings to be used for international comparisons. The ICD delineates the format of the medical certification of death and specific regulations regarding the compilation and publication of statistics on diseases and causes of death.

VITAL STATISTICS AND THE PRACTICE OF PUBLIC HEALTH

Over several centuries of development, the vital registration system in the United States has evolved into the primary source of fundamental public health information. Data on deaths, especially causes of death, have been critical for identifying, tracking, and eventually understanding and controlling epidemics of communicable diseases. Today, mortality data are used to study trends and differentials in all kinds of causes of death, both chronic and communicable, as well as those due to homicide, suicide, and unintentional injuries. Infant mortality has traditionally served as a key indicator of general health conditions in a given population. The availability of mortality statistics for small geographic units, such as counties, has contributed uniquely to the value of these data for epidemiologic investigations and surveillance.

Statistics obtained from birth certificates, fetal death reports, and the linked birth/infant death file provide a wealth of information about infant health. Statistics on birth weight, length of gestation, smoking during pregnancy, access to prenatal care, complications of labor and/or delivery, and obstetric procedures are monitored by health care providers and epidemiologists specializing in infant and child health.

In the arena of public policy, vital statistics also provide fundamental information. For example, teen pregnancy and nonmarital childbearing are topics of continuing interest in national welfare policy. Similarly, national health policy is very much concerned with the problem of health disparities among various race and ethnic groups. In these and many other important policy issues the vital statistics system constitutes a frontline source of information that leads to action programs, yields indicators of effectiveness, and generally guides the practice of public health.

Vital statistics are one of the few data systems that are generally available throughout the world. The United Nations and the World Health Organization have led efforts to standardize registration practices, definitions, and statistical measurement. Most countries have at least a rudimentary vital statistics system, and while there are inter-country variations, countries generally adhere to similar registration principles and statistical measures. These data are widely used to make international comparisons of life expectancy, cause-specific mortality, infant deaths, and other important measures. Vital statistics are also used for monitoring population growth, through measures such as total fertility rates. The United Nations publishes many international vital statistics comparisons in its *Demographic Yearbook*.

MARY ANNE FREEDMAN
JAMES A. WEED

(SEE ALSO: *Abortion; Bills of Mortality; Biostatistics; Birth Certificates; Birthrate; Census; Certification of Causes of Death; Chadwick, Edwin; Farr, William; Graunt, John; Infant Mortality Rate; International Classification of Diseases; Life Expectancy and Life Tables; Mortality Rates; National Center for Health Statistics; Rates; Rates: Adjusted; Rates: Age-Adjusted; Shattuck, Lemuel; Statistics for Public Health*)

BIBLIOGRAPHY

Hetzel, A. M. (1997). *History and Organization of the Vital Statistics System.* Hyattsville, MD: National Center for Health Statistics.

Pollard, A. H.; Farhat, Y.; and Pollard, G. N. (1991). *Demographic Techniques,* 3rd edition. Elmsford, NY: Pergamon Press.

Shryock, H. S.; Siegel, J. S.; and Associates. (1976). *The Methods and Materials of Demography,* condensed by E. G. Stockwell. New York: Academic Press.

Smith, D. P. (1992). *Formal Demography.* New York: Plenum Press.

United Nations Department of Economic and Social Affairs (1999). *1997 Demographic Yearbook.* New York: United Nations.

Weeks, J. R. (1996). *Population, An Introduction to Concepts and Issues,* 6th edition. Belmont, CA: Wadsworth.

World Health Organization (1992). *International Statistical Classification of Diseases and Related Health Problems,* 10th revision. Geneva: Author.

VLDL CHOLESTEROL

VLDL cholesterol is a minor lipid component of very low-density lipoprotein (VLDL) particles of VLDL particles. Triglycerides, which are present in five times the amount of cholesterol, are the more important lipid component of VLDL particles. VLDL cholesterol is only important in that it is calculated in a lipid profile in order to calculate the more important LDL cholesterol. Originally, LDL cholesterol was determined by a lengthy, laborious process called ultracentrifugation of serum. A much more rapid test became available based on the following Friedwald equation: Total cholesterol = LDL cholesterol + HDL cholesterol + VLDL cholesterol (VLDL cholesterol = triglycerides/5). One can rapidly and easily do a lipid profile by enzymatically measuring the important lipids—total cholesterol, HDL cholesterol, and triglycerides. Dividing triglycerides by five gives the relatively unimportant, but hard to measure, VLDL cholesterol, which is useful in then calculating the very important LDL cholesterol.

DONALD A. SMITH

(SEE ALSO: *Atherosclerosis; Blood Lipids; Cholesterol Test; HDL Cholesterol; Hyperlipidemia; LDL Cholesterol; Triglycerides*)

VO2 MAX

VO2 max, or maximum oxygen consumption, is an index of physical fitness and a measure of the maximum amount of oxygen that the body can utilize during exercise. Generating the energy needed in the muscles during exercise requires oxygen. Transporting oxygen from the outside air to the muscles involves the integrated function of several parts of the body, including the lungs, heart, blood, blood vessels, and the muscles which are the engines that produce the energy to do the physical work. Regular physical activity increases the body's ability to transport and utilize oxygen. This results in improved exercise tolerance and VO2 max, reflecting better fitness and aerobic capacity.

ANDREW L. RIES

(SEE ALSO: *Physical Activity; Pulmonary Function*)

BIBLIOGRAPHY

American College of Sports Medicine (2000). *ACSM's Guidelines for Exercise Testing and Prescription,* 6th edition. Philadelphia, PA: Lippincott Williams & Wilkins.

VOLUNTARY HEALTH ORGANIZATIONS

See Nongovernmental Organizations, United States

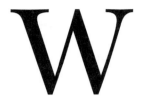

WAR

War is perhaps the most serious of all public health problems. Public health has been defined by the Institute of Medicine as "what we, as a society, do collectively to assure the conditions in which people can be healthy." Using this definition, war is clearly antithetical to public health. It not only causes death and disability among military personnel and civilians, but it also destroys the social, economic, and political infrastructure necessary for well-being and health. War violates basic human rights. As a violent method of settling conflicts, it promotes other forms of violence in the community and the home. War causes immediate and long-term damage to the environment. And war and preparation for war sap human and economic resources that might be used for social good.

DIRECT IMPACT ON HUMANS AND THE ENVIRONMENT

Worldwide, there were over 45 million deaths among military personnel during the twentieth century—a mean annual military death rate of 183 deaths per 1 million population. This rate was more than sixteen times greater than the reported rate for the nineteenth century, despite enormous progress in surgical treatment of war injuries and in the prevention and treatment of infectious diseases. In addition, since an increasing percentage of wars are civil wars or are indiscriminate in the use of weapons, civilians are increasingly caught in the crossfire. Civilian deaths as a percentage of all war-related deaths rose from 14 percent during

World War I to 90 percent during some wars of the 1990s. Moreover, during civil wars civilians may find it difficult to receive medical care and may be unable to obtain adequate and safe food and water, shelter, medicinal care, and public health services. The physical, mental, and social impacts of war on civilians are especially severe for vulnerable populations, including women, children, the elderly, the ill, and the disabled. Further, war is responsible for many million refugees and internally displaced persons.

INDIRECT IMPACTS ON HUMANS AND THE ENVIRONMENT

War also has a severe, indirect impact on humans and the environment through the diversion of human and economic resources. The governments of many developing countries spend five to twenty-five times more on military than on health expenditures. From this culture of violence people learn at an early age that violence is the way to try to resolve conflicts. War and preparation for war use huge amounts of nonrenewable resources, such as fossil fuels, as well as toxic and radioactive substances that cause pollution of the air, water, and land.

INDISCRIMINATE HARM TO NONCOMBATANTS

Of particular concern to public health is the indiscriminate harm done to noncombatants. This includes not only the use of so-called weapons of mass destruction, such as nuclear, chemical, and biological weapons, but also some uses of conventional weapons. Examples of the latter include the carpet bombing of Warsaw, Rotterdam, Coventry, Dresden, Hamburg, Tokyo, and other cities during World War II; and collateral damage caused by bombs and missiles in recent conflicts in Iraq, Serbia, and Kosovo. Anti-personnel land mines also cause indiscriminate injury and death and, like biological and chemical weapons, have been banned by international convention.

Chemical and biological weapons have been used since antiquity. Chemical weapons, which are used to produce toxic effects rather than explosions or fire, include vesicant agents such as mustard gas; agents producing pulmonary edema such as chlorine and phosgene; agents affecting oxidizing enzymes such as cyanide; and anticholinesterase inhibitors known as nerve agents. Chemical weapons were used extensively in World War I, leading to the negotiation of the Geneva Protocol of 1925, which banned the use of chemical and bacteriologic weapons. During World War II, chemical weapons were stockpiled by several nations, but were little used. The Chemical Weapons Convention (CWC), which was opened for signature in 1993 and entered into force in 1997, bans the development, production, transfer, and use of chemical weapons. The Organization for the Prohibition of Chemical Weapons (OPCW), headquartered in The Hague, has broad enforcement powers under the CWC. The United States and Russia are proceeding with destruction of stockpiles of chemical weapons, but there remains controversy about the health consequences of the methods being used. In 1995, the Aum Shinrikyo sect in Japan released nerve agent gas in the Tokyo subway, resulting in a number of deaths and many injuries. This incident heightened the concern about future use of chemical weapons.

Biological weapons, which are used to cause disease in living organisms, were developed and stockpiled by the United States, Great Britain, and other nations during World War II, but saw only very limited use by Japan in China. In 1969 the United States unilaterally renounced the use of biological weapons and announced the destruction of its stockpiles. The Biologic Weapons Convention (BWC), which was opened for signature in 1972 and entered into force in 1975, is much weaker than the CWC. It permits "defensive" research, which has led to suspicion that offensive research and development is being done. Efforts are currently being made to strengthen the BWC. Concern has recently been raised about the possible use of biological agents by groups or individuals to attack civilian populations.

The Anti-Personnel Landmine Convention (ALC) was opened for signature in 1997 and entered into force in 1999, setting precedents both for the speed of its ratification and for the work of nongovernmental organizations in bringing it about. The International Campaign to Ban Landmines and its leader, Jody Williams, were awarded the 1997 Nobel Peace Prize. By February 2000 the ALC had been signed by 137 governments, but not by the United States, Russia and the other states of the former USSR, and most countries of the Middle East. The ALC, in addition to banning any further production or placement of mines, calls for destroying stockpiles, removing mines from the ground, and helping landmine survivors.

Nuclear weapons were used by the United States in 1945 to destroy the Japanese cities of Hiroshima and Nagasaki. In each city, a bomb of explosive power equivalent to about 15 kilotons of TNT caused approximately 100,000 deaths within the first few days. Nuclear weapons have not been used in war since, but enormous quantities of nuclear and thermonuclear weapons have been stockpiled by the United States and the Soviet Union. Explosive tests of these weapons have been conducted by these two nations and by the United Kingdom, France, China, South Africa, and, in 1998, India and Pakistan. There have been 518 tests documented in the atmosphere, under water, or in space and, after the signing of the 1963 Limited Nuclear Test Ban Treaty, approximately 1,500 tests underground. The U.S. National Cancer Institute estimated in 1997 that the release of Iodine-131 in fallout from U.S. atmospheric nuclear test explosions was responsible for 49,000 excess cases of thyroid cancer among U.S. residents. Another study estimated that radioactive fallout from nuclear test explosions would be responsible for 430,000 cancer deaths by the year 2000. A Comprehensive Test Ban Treaty was negotiated in 1997, but a number of nations, including the United States, have refused to ratify it.

There are now approximately 35,000 nuclear weapons stockpiled in the seven nations that have declared possession—the U.S., Russia, the United Kingdom, France, China, India, and Pakistan. Israel is also widely believed to possess nuclear weapons. The declared nuclear-weapons nations agreed in the 1970 Nuclear Non-Proliferation Treaty (NPT) to work toward elimination of these weapons, but progress has been slow. The International Court of Justice in a unanimous advisory opinion in 1996 ruled that the nuclear weapons states were obligated under the NPT "to pursue in good faith . . . negotiations leading to nuclear disarmament." The International Physicians for the Prevention of Nuclear War was awarded the 1985 Nobel Peace Prize for its work to reduce the risk of nuclear weapons use by the United States and the Soviet Union. With the dissolution of the USSR, there has also been concern about leakage of nuclear weapons to other nations, to groups, and even to individuals.

THE ROLE OF HEALTH WORKERS AND ORGANIZATIONS

Physicians, nurses, and other health care personnel clearly have an ethical duty to care for the victims of war. But medical and public health workers, many believe, also have an ethical duty to prevent war and its consequences. Since membership in the armed forces of a nation seems to imply participation in a war effort, the question arises whether medical and public health personnel can ethically play such a military role.

Alternate ways for medical and public health workers to care for the casualties of war are available through organizations such as the International Red Cross, Doctors Without Borders (which received the 1999 Nobel Peace Prize), and Doctors of the World, as well as various associations that seek to alleviate the causes of war and to promote nonviolent conflict resolution. Such associations include the American Public Health Association, Physicians for Social Responsibility, Physicians for Human Rights, the International Physicians for the Prevention of Nuclear War, and Amnesty International.

Public health professionals can help to reduce and eliminate the causes of war, such as discrimination, poverty, and disease. They can educate and raise awareness about the health and social consequences of war and preparation for war; establish surveillance systems to detect wars, or the circumstances that lead to war, at an early stage; advocate for policies and treaties to ban weapons of indiscriminate destruction; encourage and support mediation and other forms of nonviolent conflict resolution; and work with all groups in society to promote a "culture of peace."

VICTOR W. SIDEL
BARRY S. LEVY

(SEE ALSO: *Ethnocentrism; Famine; Genocide; Gulf War Syndrome; Nuclear Power; Refugee Communities; Terrorism; Violence*)

BIBLIOGRAPHY

Amnesty International (1991). *Health Personnel: Victims of Human Rights Violations.* London: Author.

—— (1996). *Prescription for Change: Health Professionals and the Exposure of Human Rights Violations.* London: Author.

Arms Project of Human Rights Watch and Physicians for Human Rights (1993). *Landmines: A Deadly Legacy.* New York: Human Rights Watch.

British Medical Association (1992). *Medicine Betrayed: The Participation of Doctors in Human Rights Abuses.* London: Zed Books.

Carnegie Commission on Preventing Deadly Conflict (1997). *Preventing Deadly Conflict: Final Report.* Washington, DC: Author.

Forrow, L. F.; Blair, B. G.; Helfand, I.; Lewis, G.; Postol, T.; Sidel, V. W.; Levy, B. S.; Abrams, H.; and Cassel, C. (1998). "Accidental Nuclear War: A Post-Cold War Assessment." *New England Journal of Medicine* 338:1326–1331.

Forrow, L. F., and Sidel, V. W. (1998). "Medicine and Nuclear War: From Hiroshima to Mutual Assured Destruction to Abolition 2000." *Journal of the American Medical Association* 280:456–461.

Geiger, H. J., and Cook-Deegan, R. M. (1993). "The Role of Physicians in Conflicts and Humanitarian Crises." *Journal of the American Medical Association* 270:616–620.

Institute of Medicine (1988). *The Future of Public Health.* Washington, DC: National Academy Press.

International Physicians for the Prevention of Nuclear War (1997). *Landmines: A Global Health Crisis.* Cambridge, MA: Author.

Levy, B. S., and Sidel, V. W., eds. (1997). *War and Public Health*. New York: Oxford University Press.

Sidel, V. W. (1989). "Weapons of Mass Destruction: The Greatest Threat to Public Health." *Journal of the American Medical Association* 262:680–682.

—— (1995) "The International Arms Trade and Its Impact on Health." *British Medical Journal* 311:1677–1680.

—— (1996). "The Role of Physicians in the Prevention of Nuclear War." In *Genocide, War, and Human Survival*, eds. B C. Strozier and M. Flynn. Lanham, MD: Rowman and Littlefield Publishers.

Sidel, V. W., and Goldwyn, R. M. (1966). "Chemical and Biological Weapons—A Primer." *New England Journal of Medicine* 242:21–27.

Sidel, V. W., and Shahi, G. (1997). "The Impact of Military Activities on Development, Environment and Health." In *International Perspectives in Environment, Development and Health: Toward A Sustainable World*, eds. G. Shahi, B. S. Levy, A. Binger, T. Kjellstrom and R. Lawrence. New York: Springer.

Wright S., ed. (1990). *Preventing a Biological Arms Race*. Cambridge, MA: MIT Press.

WASTEWATER TREATMENT

Water containing human waste and excreta is generally termed "wastewater." Usually, wastewater consists of 99.9 percent water and 0.1 percent waste. In the United States, each state has a law that requires the disposal of human waste in a sanitary manner. Treatment of wastewater is required to prevent the pollution of surface waters, the pollution of groundwater, and to prevent pathogenic and microbial contamination from the use of excreta as fertilizer. Also, wastewater should be disposed of in a sanitary manner to make it inaccessible to insects that transmit disease.

Wastewater treatment consists of physical, chemical, and biological processes—either aerobic or anaerobic. The aerobic process is used most frequently. In the activated sludge process, air has to be forced into the liquid in a tank that is used to maintain aerobic microbial activity and to prevent odor. Additionally, temperature and pH must be maintained for the microbial activity.

In a municipal system the flow moves as follows: from sanitary sewer to screening and grinding process, to primary clarification, to activated sludge or trickling filter, to secondary clarification, to chlorine treatment, and finally to a water body such as a river or stream. Wastewater from the home enters a domestic or sanitary sewer—a system of pipes that collect the wastewater. The waste is then transported to a wastewater treatment plant. As it enters the plant, it flows through a bar screen, which strains out large materials. It then continues into a grit basin or chamber, where the water is slowed down enough to allow heavy or dense particles to settle out. These particles are then removed and taken to a landfill. The materials that do not settle out are ground up to prepare them to be digested by microorganisms in the treatment plant.

The wastewater then enters the primary clarifier, which allows materials to settle out. The flow of water through the clarifier is slow, allowing large amounts of suspended solids to settle at the bottom in the form of sludge. The sludge is then scraped and pumped away to allow the process to continue.

From the primary clarifier, the wastewater enters activated sludge tanks or trickling filters. Trickling filters are large areas of biological decomposition consisting of rocks that host biological organisms on their surfaces. These organisms metabolize most of the suspended solids that did not settle in the primary clarifier. The buildup on these rocks eventually sloughs off. The activated sludge tank is also used to remove waste from the wastewater. In this process, water from the primary clarifier is pumped into an aeration tank and combined with a mixture rich in bacterial growth. Pure oxygen is pumped through, allowing the decomposition of the organic materials in the wastewater. The remaining water is moved from the top of the tank, leaving sludge at the bottom.

Water from the trickling filter moves to a secondary clarifier, which settles any remaining suspended solids. The solids are then pumped into a digester, while the effluent is chlorinated and released back into a water channel, river, or stream.

MARK G. ROBSON

(SEE ALSO: *Chlorination; Sewage System; Water Quality; Water Treatment*)

BIBLIOGRAPHY

Koren, H., and Bisesi, M. (1995). *Handbook of Environmental Health and Safety*, 3rd edition, Vol. II. Boca Raton, FL: Lewis Publishers.

Morgan, M. (1997). *Environmental Health.* Madison, WI: Brown & Benchmark.

Nadakavukaren, A. (2000). *Our Global Environment*, 5th edition. Prospect Heights, IL: Waveland Press.

WATER POLLUTION

See Ambient Water Quality

WATER QUALITY

"Water quality" is a technical term that is based upon the characteristics of water in relation to guideline values of what is suitable for human consumption and for all usual domestic purposes, including personal hygiene. Components of water quality include microbial, biological, chemical, and physical aspects.

Microbial Aspects. Drinking water should not include microorganisms that are known to be pathogenic. It should also not contain bacteria that would indicate excremental pollution, the primary indicator of which are coliform bacteria that are present in the feces of warm-blooded organisms. Chlorine is the usual disinfectant, as it is readily available and inexpensive. Unfortunately, it is not fully effective, as currently used, against all organisms.

Biological Aspects. Parasitic protozoa and helminths are also indicators of water quality. Species of protozoa can be introduced into water supply through human or animal fecal contamination. Most common among the pathogenic protozoans are *Entamoeba* and *Giardia*. Coliforms are not appropriate direct indicators because of the greater resistance of these protozoans to inactivation by disinfection. Drinking water sources that are not likely to be contaminated by fecal matter should be used where possible due to the lack of good indicators for the presence or absence of pathogenic protozoa. A single mature larva or fertilized egg of parasitic roundworms and flatworms can cause infection when transmitted to humans through drinking water. The measures currently available for the detection of helminths in drinking water are not suitable for routine use.

Chemical Aspects. Chemical contamination of water sources may be due to certain industries and agricultural practices, or from natural sources. When toxic chemicals are present in drinking water, there is the potential that they may cause either acute or chronic health effects. Chronic health effects are more common than acute effects because the levels of chemicals in drinking water are seldom high enough to cause acute health effects. Since there is limited evidence relating chronic human health conditions to specific drinking-water contaminants, laboratory animal studies and human data from clinical reports are used to predict adverse effects.

Physical Aspects. The turbidity, color, taste, and odor of water can be monitored. Turbidity should always be low, especially where disinfection is practiced. High turbidity can inhibit the effects of disinfection against microorganisms and enable bacterial growth. Drinking water should be colorless, since drinking-water coloration may be due to the presence of colored organic matter. Organic substances also cause water odor, though odors may result from many factors, including biological activity and industrial pollution. Taste problems relating to water could be indicators of changes in water sources or treatment process. Inorganic compounds such as magnesium, calcium, sodium, copper, iron, and zinc are generally detected by the taste of water, and contamination with the oxygenated fuel additive MTBE has affected the taste of some water.

MARK G. ROBSON

(SEE ALSO: *Ambient Water Quality; Clean Water Act; Drinking Water; E. Coli; Pathogenic Organisms; Water Treatment; Waterborne Diseases*)

BIBLIOGRAPHY

Shelton, T. (1991). *Interpreting Drinking Water Quality Analysis–What Do the Numbers Mean?* New Brunswick, NJ: Rutgers Cooperative Extension.

World Health Organization (1985). *Guidelines for Drinking Water Quality*, Vol. 3: *Drinking Water Quality Control in Small Community Supplies.* Geneva: Author.

WATER QUALITY ACT

See Clean Water Act

WATER REUSE

"Water reuse" is the use of wastewater or water reclaimed from one application, such as municipal wastewater treatment, for another application, such as landscape watering. It is important that the reused water comply with all federal, state, and local laws and regulations. Some of the possible applications for the reuse of wastewater include industrial applications; landscape irrigation; agricultural irrigation; aesthetic uses, such as fountains in parks or cities; and fire suppression.

Several factors must be considered in any wastewater reuse program, including the quality of the water needed for the application, the identification of the wastewater source that meets this quality level, and the very practical needs of transporting this water to its new use.

The practical benefit of wastewater reuse (or reclaimed water) is that it reduces the need for surface water or groundwater. The reuse of water provides for conservation of new potable water sources as well as elimination of the need to expand treatment and processing facilities.

Water recycling is a part of water reuse. Recycling of water is the reuse of water for the same application for which it was originally used. In some cases, the recycled water requires treatment before it can be used again. The factors to be considered in a water recycling program are similar to the ones listed above for wastewater reuse. A very common example of water recycling is the circulation of cooling water. This represents a very large use of water in the United States. Water is passed through a system to lower the temperature of a heat source, then the water is discharged. Recycling the water, via a recirculating cooling system, can greatly reduce water use and still perform the cooling operation required.

MARK G. ROBSON

(SEE ALSO: *Drinking Water; Wastewater Treatment; Water Quality; Water Treatment*)

BIBLIOGRAPHY

Environmental Protection Agency (2000). *Cleaner Water Through Conservation.* Available at http://www.epa.gov/OWOW/NPS/chap3.html.

WATER TREATMENT

The goal of water treatment is to reduce or remove all contaminants that are present in the water. No water, irrespective of the original source, should be assumed to be completely free of contaminants. The most common process used for treatment of surface water and ground water consists of sedimentation, coagulation, filtration, disinfection, conditioning, softening, fluoridation, removal of tastes and odors, corrosion control, algae control, and aeration.

Sedimentation allows any coarse particles to settle out. Coagulation consists of forming flocculent particles in a liquid by adding a chemical such as alum; these particles then settle to the bottom. Filtration, as the name implies, is the passing of the water through a porous media; the amount of removal is a function of the filtering media. Disinfection kills most harmful organisms and pathogenic bacteria—chlorine is the most commonly used disinfecting agent. Softening means removal of materials that cause "hardness," such as calcium and magnesium. Corrosion is an electrochemical reaction in which metal deteriorates when it comes in contact with air, water, or soil.

In a typical municipal water treatment process, water flows through pumps to a rapid mix basin, then to a flocculation basin, to a settling basin, through filters to a clear well, then after disinfection, to storage tanks, and finally to the end users.

In areas that derive their water from rivers, pumps must be used since rivers are usually in low areas. Water enters the treatment plant at what is called the rapid-mix basin, where aluminum sulfate, polyelectrolytes, polymers, or lime and furic chloride are added as coagulants. The water flows next to the flocculation basins, where the coagulant mixes with the suspended solids. The coagulant is used to form suspended solids into clumps, or floc, which then settle out of the water. Floc forms when the particles from small solids gather to form larger particles. The water then slowly flows through settling basins where the floc settles from the water. Activated carbon is then added to the water to remove color, radioactivity, taste, and odor. Filtration then removes bacteria and turbidity from the water as it removes any remaining suspended solids and the activated carbon.

The water then enters a clear well, where additional chlorine is added to kill any pathogens which may be present. A minimum free-chlorine residual of at least 0.2 ppm is recommended in plants requiring sanitary protection through the whole water distribution system. In water supplies that are fluoridated, 1 milligram per liter of fluoride is added.

At this stage in the process, the water is potable, palatable, and ready for consumption. The water is moved into elevated tanks for storage through pumps. The water flows down from these tanks into the community.

Raw water and post-treatment water are tested for bacterial, physical, and chemical standards, particularly pH, color, and turbidity. The Safe Drinking Water Act of 1974 established maximum contaminant levels, which are the national drinking water standards. These apply to any water distribution system that serves at least twenty-five units daily. Standards may vary from state to state, but they cannot be lower than those prescribed by the federal government.

MARK G. ROBSON

(SEE ALSO: *Ambient Water Quality; Clean Water Act; Dissolved Solids; Drinking Water; Groundwater; Sanitation; Wastewater Treatment; Water Quality*)

BIBLIOGRAPHY

Koren, H., and Bisesi, M. (1997). *Handbook of Environmental Health and Safety*, Vol. II. Boca Raton, FL: Lewis Publishers.

Morgan, M. (1993). *Environmental Health*. Madison, WI: Brown & Benchmark.

WATERBORNE DISEASES

An adult human needs to drink at least 1.5 liters of water a day to replace fluid lost in urine, sweat, and respired air and to perform essential biochemical functions. Moreover, almost 90 percent of body mass is water. Water, however, can also carry dangerous pathogens and toxic chemicals into the body. The catalogue of waterborne pathogens is long, and it includes many that are well-known as well as far larger numbers of more obscure organisms. Waterborne pathogens include viruses (e.g., hepatitis A, poliomyelitis); bacteria (e.g., cholera, typhoid, coliform organisms); protozoa (e.g., *cryptosporidiosum, amebae, giardia*); worms (e.g., *schistosomia*, guinea worm); and toxins (e.g., arsenic, cadmium, numerous organic chemicals).

Water also harbors the intermediate stages of many parasites, either as free-living larvae or in some other form, and it is the vehicle for essential stages in the life cycle of many dangerous insect vectors, notably mosquitoes and blackflies.

Chemical contamination or pollution of drinking water is another serious problem—one that has become a great deal worse in the modern industrial era, due to the widespread, and often unregulated, discharge of toxic substances into rivers, lakes, and oceans.

For practical purposes, this discussion of waterborne diseases and their control focuses mainly on the pathogenic organisms for which water is a common vehicle. It is important to note that not only drinking water, but also water used for cleaning fruit, vegetables, and cooking utensils, and for washing, can convey disease. Indeed, salads that have been washed in polluted water are a frequently overlooked and rather common source of waterborne disease, responsible for an occasional outbreak of cholera or typhoid.

Water sources (springs, rivers, lakes, ponds, streams, wells, reservoirs, and rainwater runoff into tanks and cisterns) can all be contaminated by fecal matter of human or animal origin. Organic matter of other origin (dead animals, decaying vegetation) can contaminate drinking water too, in ways that range from very dangerous to merely unpleasant.

Water from suspect sources usually can be made safe to drink by boiling. Ancient empirical observation of this fact in India and China may have led to the popularity in those countries of drinking tea and other infusions made with boiling water. However, boiling is neither practical nor sensible for the treatment of large municipal water supplies. These must be protected by appropriate treatment measures—filtration and purification (generally through chlorination) that were developed mainly in the nineteenth century in the industrial nations. Provision of safe drinking water supplies has been among the most effective and important measures ever taken to advance the public's health.

The other essential components in the prevention of waterborne diseases are the sanitary disposal of sewage and the environmental control of toxic chemicals. Sanitary services are based on sewage disposal systems in most organized urban communities. Some rapidly growing suburban developments may lack adequate sanitation during their early stages, but local regulations usually prohibit occupancy until sanitation is installed and working. In rural regions and other sparsely settled localities, including campgrounds, human waste is often disposed of in septic tanks or pit privies. The combination of sanitary disposal of human sewage and the provision of safe water supplies has virtually eliminated many of the serious waterborne epidemic diseases that took such a heavy toll of life until the early years of the twentieth century. However, sanitary services break down when floods, earthquakes, and other disasters occur, and at such times it is essential to boil water to ensure that pathogens are killed. Other methods, such as the use of iodine or chloramine in tablet or powder form are sometimes used, both under emergency conditions and by backpackers and the like, but these methods are less effective than boiling.

Even with the best protective measures, however, there are occasional serious large waterborne epidemics, and innumerable small ones. Recent large epidemics include the 1993 outbreak of cryptosporidiosis in Wisconsin, which affected about 400,000 people, and several lethal outbreaks of $E.\ coli$ 0157:H7 infection, which is very dangerous because it causes kidney damage that can be fatal. Both these and other waterborne diseases are often due to pollution of public drinking water supplies by animal waste. Modern factory-farming methods generate enormous quantities of manure, and after heavy rains it is easy for runoff contaminated with animal manure to enter the water supply. Animal manure can contain the dangerous $E.\ coli$ 0157:H7 strain. Even frequent testing can fail to detect evidence of pollution in time to prevent serious waterborne outbreaks. When testing laboratories have suffered budget cuts, the staff is often downsized, making waterborne disease outbreaks more likely. Several recent outbreaks in the United States and Canada are directly attributable to this sequence of events.

Chemical pollution of water supplies presents problems of a different kind. Chemical contamination can cause acute illnesses, but more often the toxic contaminants are slow poisons, such as carcinogens, and the effects may be manifest in only a small proportion of all those who are exposed. The pollution can come to light when a cluster of cases of leukemia or some unusual variety of cancer or other illness is detected in a community, as in Woburn, Massachusetts, where ethylene chloride that had leeched into the soil contaminated groundwater that fed several wells.

Municipal water supplies should be routinely monitored by frequent bacteriological and chemical testing. Bacteriological testing focuses on coliform organisms that, if present, are not only harmful in themselves but also are a marker for other varieties of fecal contamination. Chemical pollution presents a more difficult problem because of the wide variety of chemicals that can pollute a water supply.

JOHN M. LAST

(SEE ALSO: *Ambient Water Quality; Cholera; Clean Water Act; Cryptosporidiosis; Typhoid; Water Treatment*)

WELL-BABY CLINICS

Well-baby clinics, or well-child clinics as they are commonly known, deal with the total well-being of children and family. As public health clinics, supported by tax dollars, they provide a safety net for the economically disadvantaged by offering low-cost health care. The clinics operate on a sliding-fee scale, or they may give free care to families unable to pay.

One of the important services offered by well-baby clinics is the provision of immunizations for childhood diseases such as diphtheria, pertussis, tetanus, polio, *Haemophilus influenzae* type b, hepatitis B, measles, mumps, rubella, and varicella. The clinics are responsible for tracking immunization rates in the community and notifying families when shots are due.

Families frequently ask why their children need routine health care when they have already received all of their required immunizations. The answer is simply that well-child clinics provide an array of diagnostic and preventative services. Infants are checked for growth and developmental delays. At each visit the staff will check the eyes for vision abnormalities and muscle imbalance, the ears for infection, the heart for murmurs, and the hips for developmental dysplasia. Infants are initially examined at two weeks of age. Subsequent visits are at 2, 4, 6, 9, and 12 months. Toddlers and preschoolers are seen at 15 months, 18 months, and then yearly at 2, 3, 4, 5, and 6 years. Testing is done for anemia and lead poisoning on this age group because early detection and intervention is needed to prevent damage to sensitive developing neurologic tissue. The staff also teaches anemia and lead prevention techniques. Interagency referrals are made to the Women, Infant, and Children WIC Food Program and to housing agencies when needed. These older children receive routine screening of vision, hearing, blood pressure, language, and development. When problems are detected, referrals for early intervention can then be made before school age.

School-age children are routinely examined every one to two years for school and camp physicals. Teenagers are screened for sports participation and work permits. They are also counseled on age-appropriate issues such as drug and alcohol abuse, prevention of sexually transmitted diseases, and the hazards of smoking.

Families are often not aware of available community programs and services. The staff of well-baby clinics provides referrals to other agencies that educate families on parenting skills and financial counseling. Referrals to other health-coverage programs are also often discussed. Most importantly, the staff provides parenting guidance for those with no support system in an effort to help reduce child abuse and neglect.

MARYANN C. MAY

(SEE ALSO: *Child Health Services; Immunizations; Maternal and Child Health; Screening; Women, Infants, and Children Program [WIC]*)

WELLNESS BEHAVIOR

On the surface, defining "wellness behaviors" is easy—"eat your vegetables," "go out and play with your friends," "be nice to your sister," "smoking can be hazardous to your health," "Just Say No," "don't drink and drive"—these maxims and slogans all allude to well-known healthful behaviors. If people were to follow such advice regularly, they would certainly be healthier. It is, of course, not so simple. Western medicine, shaped by physicians, has dominated health care in the United States during the past century. Most physicians are remarkably service-oriented people who want nothing more than to make people healthy. However, they are trained in curing disease, not enhancing health. As a result, health care systems focus on curing disease rather than promoting health and preventing disease. Hospitals are able to transplant vital organs, create new skin for people with burns covering a majority of their bodies, reattach severed limbs, and perform other equally miraculous procedures. Unfortunately, they do an inadequate job of keeping people healthy.

This focus is changing, however. During the second half of the twentieth century, a body of research began to emerge that provides compelling evidence that lifestyle choices make a difference between health and disease, and between life and death. Michael McGinnis and William Foege have calculated that half the deaths in the United States are caused by lifestyle-related behaviors. Their work, and that of others, has shown that over 400,000 deaths could be saved by eliminating smoking; over 300,000 through regular exercise and good nutrition; 100,000 by responsible use of alcohol; 35,000 by eliminating firearms; 30,000 through safe-sex practices; 25,000 by safer driving; and 20,000 by eliminating drug abuse. To put these numbers in perspective, tobacco causes more deaths in the United States each year than all the foreign wars in the nation's history. Lifestyle factors contribute to all of the top fifteen diseases that cause deaths in the United States.

QUALITY OF LIFE

Wellness is certainly not just avoiding death, so counting the number of deaths that healthful lifestyles could save tells only part of the story. Practicing these behaviors also improves quality of life in terms of having more energy, fewer aches and pains, better sex, and enhanced self-esteem. Such elements of health are more difficult to measure, so most scientists focus their research on objective measures such as death and disease.

There is some controversy in the interpretation of much of the available data, especially in the areas of obesity and nutrition. For example, Jeremiah Stamler estimates that obesity alone causes 240,000 to 380,000 deaths each year, while Steven Blair argues that lack of exercise, not obesity *per se*, is the more important risk factor. There are also arguments about the amount of alcohol that is optimal. After decades of debate, many scientists now believe that up to four glasses of beer or wine per week may actually be more healthful than complete abstention from alcohol for those who are not alcoholics and do not suffer from conditions that can be aggravated by alcohol. The general public is also often confused by reports about the healthfulness of specific diets. Is butter or margarine more healthy? Is beta carotene good or bad? In fact, factors at this level of detail have only a minimal impact on health. The death rate in the United States and most developed countries could be cut in half if all people could be persuaded to not use tobacco or illegal drugs; to use alcohol in moderation or not at all; exercise on a regular basis; always wear a seat belt when driving; never drink and drive; not use firearms; get plenty of sleep; practice safe sex; and eat a diet high in vegetables, fruits, and whole grains, and low in fat, sodium, and sugar. Another 20 percent of deaths could be eliminated if everyone had affordable access to health care and was diligent about getting regular medical and dental checkups, getting immunizations when needed, and taking medication as directed.

SOCIAL FACTORS

The data gets more complex when other nations of the world are examined. It is safe to say that approximately half the deaths in developed nations of the world, and possibly one-third or more of the deaths in developing nations, are caused by lifestyle-related problems. Nevertheless, the smoking rate and consumption rate of high-fat foods is higher in some European nations, though the rate of heart disease is much lower than in the United States, and very low rates of heart disease are found in Asian nations like Japan and Korea despite very high rates of smoking. The low-fat, high-vegetable diets common in these countries explain part, but not all, of the difference in heart disease rates. Within the United States, people from Hispanic backgrounds tend to have lower rates of child mortality than people from other cultures, even among those who have similar income levels and health habits. The common characteristic of all of those groups is strong social connections through extended family and networks of friends.

Findings like these are beginning to make scientists speculate that social factors are very important in determining a person's health. At least three elements of our social environment impact our health. In 1980, Robert F. Allen explained the importance of people's peers in shaping health behaviors, as well as the futility of trying to change health and other behaviors without changing the norms of the group. For example, most children start smoking cigarettes and drinking alcohol through the influence of their friends, and when they quit they often lose those friends who choose to continue. Most people who exercise as adults started when they were kids, and they often did so to be involved in neighborhood or school sports to be with their friends.

The work of Barbara Israel, Kenneth McLeroy, Michael Marmot, and others has shown the protective effect that social support provided by social networks of family and friends can have on helping avoid problems that can threaten health, as well as the effect social factors have in helping people recover from illness more quickly. In his popular book, *Love and Survival*, Dean Ornish reviewed scientific literature that showed that men who feel loved by their wives, adults who had warm relationships with their parents, and people who have a warm integrated community of friends all have lower rates of disease and death. This work has led Ornish to speculate that social factors may be as important as physical factors in determining overall health. Finally, work by Michael Marmot and others has shown that socioeconomic status, both in absolute and relative terms, has a very significant impact on health.

Can people change the social factors in their lives? They cannot choose their parents or siblings, and birth circumstances often dictate socioeconomic status. However people can choose their spouse, and they do have an influence on their children. They can also choose their friends, and, through diligent effort, can work to shape the norms of friends, organizations, and communities to influence health in a positive way. This is, however, a formidable task.

So "wellness behavior" might not be the right term. "Wellness lifestyle" may be a more accurate term but "striving for optimal health" expresses the complex set of social and behavioral factors that impact health much better.

OPTIMAL HEALTH

Inspired by the work of Bill Hettler, and recognizing the scope and complexity of all the factors that impact health, the *American Journal of Health Promotion* has suggested that people think in terms of optimal health and the factors that impact optimal health. Optimal health may be defined as "a balance of physical, emotional, social, spiritual, and intellectual health." Spiritual health includes having a sense of purpose in life, the ability to give and receive love, and feeling goodwill and charity toward others. Intellectual health is related to learning and achievements in life, which can occur through school, work, hobbies, community service, or cultural pursuits. Emotional health refers to one's mental state of being and encompasses the stresses in a person's life, how one reacts to those stresses, and the ability to relax and enjoy leisure. Rather than strive for excellence in any one area, people can best achieve a state of health by striving to achieve balance in these five areas.

Behavior alone is not the sole determinant of lifestyle; a person's environment and opportunities also play major roles in health. People may focus on different areas of optimal health as they pass through different stages in their lives, because achieving optimal health is a lifelong process. This thinking goes beyond current science, but it may provide a framework for issues to be studied in the future.

MICHAEL P. O'DONNELL

(SEE ALSO: *Behavior, Health-Related; Cultural Factors; Cultural Norms; Health Books; Health Promotion and Education; Holistic Medicine; Inequalities in Health; Lay Concepts of Health and Illness; Physical Activity; Social Determinants; Traditional Health Beliefs, Practices*)

BIBLIOGRAPHY

Allen, R. F. (1980). *Beat the System!: A Way to Create More Human Environments.* New York: McGraw-Hill.

Marmot, M., and Wilkinson, R. G. (1999). *Social Determinants of Health.* Oxford: Oxford University Press.

McGinnis, M., and Foege, W. (1993). "Actual Causes of Death." *Journal of the American Medical Association* 270(18):2208.

Ornish, D. (1998). *Love and Survival: The Scientific Basis for the Healing Power of Intimacy.* New York: HarperCollins.

Stamler, J. et al. (1999). "Death from Obesity." *Journal of the American Medical Association* 282(21):2026.

U.S. Department of Health and Human Services (1996). *Physical Activity and Exercise: A Report of the Surgeon General.* Atlanta, GA: USDHHS, National Center for Chronic Disease Prevention and Health Promotion.

WEST NILE VIRUS

See Arboviral Encephalitides

WESTERN BLOT

See Blot, Western

WESTERN EQUINE ENCEPHALITIS

See Arboviral Encephalitides

WHOOPING COUGH

See Pertussis

WIDOWHOOD

Widowhood refers to the status of a person whose spouse has died and who has not remarried. Women in this situation are referred to as widows, and men as widowers. In the United States and other Western nations, approximately 6 percent of the total population is widowed and this proportion increases to about one-third of the population sixty-five years of age or older. Recent trends indicate that widowhood is becoming less common, largely because more people either never marry or are separated or divorced.

Widowhood is commonly viewed as a life transition. A transition is a major change in life circumstances that takes place over a relatively short period of time but has lasting effects on large areas of a person's life. It requires the development of new life habits or ways of coping. Widowhood is one of the most stressful life transitions, although most people adjust successfully over time.

Most research on widowhood has focused on women, partly because widows outnumber widowers by nearly five to one. It is estimated that half of all marriages end with the death of the husband, whereas only one-fifth end with the death of the wife in Western societies, and women generally outlive men and men usually marry women who are younger than they are. Further, while most older widowed people do not remarry, widowers have remarriage rates over eight times as high as those of widows.

Different societies attach very different customs and values to widowhood, and these have a strong influence on how it is experienced. Most widows go through an intense grieving process early in widowhood, marked by feelings of depression, mood changes, disrupted sleep patterns, obsessive thoughts about the deceased, and disorientation. However, the intensity of grief usually decreases significantly within a year. Many widows and widowers begin to develop new strengths and talents and remake their social networks to include new friends and contacts. Intense grief is not required for recovery from widowhood.

CONSEQUENCES OF WIDOWHOOD FOR HEALTH AND WELL-BEING

Research on the consequences of widowhood for health and mental health is fraught with contradictory findings. Early studies found high mortality rates among widows, but recent work has not replicated these results. One of the biggest problems reported by both widows and widowers is loneliness, which may last well beyond the usual period of mourning. Symptoms of depression and decreased life satisfaction may also last for several years.

Widowhood does not appear to worsen health. However, it disrupts daily routines, especially those associated with food preparation and consumption. Widowed people commonly report decreased social participation. Among women, consequences of widowhood may include a lower income and, in older age groups, increased likelihood of nursing home placement.

One critical factor in how well the surviving spouse copes is the manner of the other spouse's death. Suicide can be devastating for the surviving spouse, and accidental death is more traumatic than death resulting from an illness. However, adjustment may also be difficult when the spouse's death follows a prolonged condition, such as Alzheimer's disease. In general, individuals are likely to cope better if they have had some time to prepare for imminent widowhood but are not exhausted by prolonged or intense caregiving.

A key concept in understanding the impacts of widowhood is that of "on-time" versus "off-time," which refer to the surviving spouse's life stage. Being widowed in later life is on-time and can be anticipated. In contrast, being widowed in early adulthood is off-time, and is both unexpected and likely to entail concurrent stresses, such as the grief of dependent children or the loss of the major source of household income.

Men are affected more by widowhood than women. Widowhood is less likely to be anticipated by men, and men are generally more dependent on their spouse for social and emotional support. A person who is devoted to his or her role as a husband or wife has a greater adjustment to make when widowed than an individual who has other valued roles.

Widowhood may be experienced as a positive transition. It may even come as a relief if the marriage was unhappy or burdensome. In comparison with married people, widowed people express less strain and a greater capacity to make plans and carry them out. Widowed individuals adjust better if they are involved in physical activity, can rely on support from family members and friends, and can develop new interests and friendships.

POLICY AND SERVICE PROVISION

Dealing with widowhood has remained largely in the private domain. Widowed people and their families are usually left to cope as best they can, with little attention from government or service providers. In contrast, other transitions commonly experienced by older people (such as retirement and becoming a caregiver), although less stressful and disruptive, have attracted considerable policy attention and service provision.

However, most older people have regular contact with their doctors, and general medical practitioners are in a good position to monitor any enduring, negative impacts of widowhood and to suggest appropriate interventions.

YVONNE D. WELLS
COLETTE J. BROWNING

(SEE ALSO: *Aging of Population; Bereavement; Gerontology; Life Expectancy and Life Tables; Women's Health*)

BIBLIOGRAPHY

Lee, G. R.; Willets, M. C.; and Seccombe, K. (1998). "Widowhood and Depression: Gender Differences." *Research on Aging* 20:611–630.

Lieberman, M. A. (1996). "Perspective on Adult Life Crises." In *Adulthood and Aging: Research on Continuities and Discontinuities,* ed. V. L. Bengtson. New York: Springer.

Lopata, H. Z. (1996). *Current Widowhood: Myths and Realities.* Thousand Oaks, CA: Sage.

Martin-Matthews, A. (1996). "Widowhood and Widowerhood." In *Encyclopedia of Gerontology,* ed. J. E. Birren. San Diego, CA: Academic Press.

McCallum, J. (1986). "Retirement and Widowhood Transitions." In *Aging and Families,* ed. H. L. Kendig. Sydney: Allen & Unwin.

Riggs, A. (1997). "Men, Friends and Widowhood: Toward Successful Ageing." *Australian Journal on Ageing* 16:182–185.

Smith, K. R., and Zick, C. D. (1996). "Risk of Mortality Following Widowhood: Age and Sex Differences by Mode of Death." *Social Biology* 43:59–71.

Wells, Y. D., and Kendig, H. L. (1997). "Health and Well-Being of Spouse Caregivers and the Widowed." *The Gerontologist* 37(5):666–674.

WINSLOW, CHARLES-EDWARD AMORY

Charles-Edward Amory Winslow (1877–1957) was a seminal figure in public health, not only in his own country, the United States, but in the wider Western world. His vision and intellectual leadership enabled him, more than anyone else, to influence the development of public health services in the United States as well as in many European nations. His inspired leadership did much to ensure that the rapidly developing industrial cities and the rural regions of the United States were adequately provided with the essential public health services of sanitation, regulation of food- and waterborne hazards to health, development of health-education programs, and education of public health specialists. In a period dominated by discoveries in bacteriology, he recognized the importance of a broader perspective on causation than that embraced by the germ theory of disease.

For forty years, from 1915 to 1945, Winslow was a professor of public health at Yale University. His teaching at Yale emphasized his holistic perspective, and he doubtless influenced many of his proteges and students, such as Joseph Goldberger, whose work on the dietary deficiency that causes pellagra may have derived in part from Winslow's teachings.

Winslow began his career as a bacteriologist, but he soon broadened his focus to embrace occupational and environmental health, housing conditions, epidemiology, public health administration, nursing, mental health, and the organization of medical care. Winslow's legacy includes several monographs that have become classics of public health and epidemiology, including *The Evolution and Significance of the Modern Public Health Campaign* (1923), *The Conquest of Epidemic Disease* (1943), and *The History of American Epidemiology* (1952).

JOHN M. LAST

(SEE ALSO: *Goldberger, Joseph*)

WOMEN, INFANTS, AND CHILDREN PROGRAM (WIC)

The Special Supplemental Nutrition Program for Women, Infants, and Children (WIC) provides nutritious food, nutrition education, breastfeeding support, and referral to health care and social services for low-income, nutritionally at risk, pregnant, and postpartum women, and for infants and children under the age of five.

WIC was funded at $4 billion for 2001, serving about 7.2 million women and young children. WIC operates nationwide through 1,800 local health departments, community health centers, hospitals, and health or social-service agencies. Some thirty inter-tribal organizations operate WIC programs, and the program also operates in Puerto Rico and in several U.S. territories. The United States Department of Agriculture operates WIC at the federal level, and state health departments administer the program in conjunction with local agencies.

WIC services include foods containing nutrients that are often lacking in the diets of low-income pregnant women and young children; nutrition assessment and nutrition education; and referral to health insurance and social programs like food stamps. WIC promotes breastfeeding through classes and individual counseling done by peer counselors and lactation consultants. In many communities, WIC operates closely with health programs for women and children including immunization programs. Public health issues such as smoking and obesity are incorporated into the WIC educational efforts of many agencies.

Numerous evaluations have found that WIC improves health status and reduces medical costs. Studies have found that women who participate in WIC have longer pregnancies leading to fewer premature births; WIC lowers the incidence of late fetal deaths by up to one-third; WIC contributes to decreases in anemia; every dollar invested in WIC for pregnant women produces $1.92 to $4.21 in Medicaid savings; and that WIC increases prenatal and well-child care use.

STEFAN HARVEY

(SEE ALSO: *Child Health Services; Maternal and Child Health; Nutrition; Poverty; Women's Health*)

WOMEN'S HEALTH

Despite obvious differences between women and men—biologically, psychologically, and socially—the concept of viewing the totality of women's health as different from men's health arose in Western medicine only in the last two decades of the twentieth century. As recently as the 1980s, students in most Western medical schools were taught that, except for issues related directly to reproductive anatomy and function, women were medically identical to men. According to this belief system, medical research could be carried out on men, and the results could simply be applied to women. As a result, only health care providers who specialized in areas related to reproduction were expected to be knowledgeable about issues particular to women.

In order to understand the modern definition of women's health, it is important to understand the history of how women's health care has been viewed by the medical and medical research establishments. Traditionally, the health of women has been seen as synonymous with maternal or reproductive health. Clearly, the Western medical profession's view of women's health as "maternal health" was concordant with societal mores that valued women mainly for their ability to bear children. However, until well into the twentieth century, the major causes of illness and death in women did, in fact, relate to reproductive issues. Childbirth and sexually transmitted diseases, including cervical cancer, have been the most important health issues for women in all ages and places—except in the West and certain other countries in the twentieth century. Prior to 1900, the majority of elderly persons in the United States were men, reflecting the toll that childbearing took on the health of women.

In 1970 the book *Our Bodies, Ourselves* became a touchstone of the women's health movement. Authored by a group of women participating in a course on health, sexuality, and childbearing, the book emphasizes the importance of women attaining knowledge about their health and being active participants in health care in both an individual and societal sense. *Our Bodies, Ourselves* also considers the social context of health, including effects of sexism, racism, and financial pressures on the health of women. Throughout the 1970s, major focuses of the women's health movement included reproductive freedom, understanding health in a broader social context, and a critical orientation toward the medical establishment.

In the 1980s, women's health advocates began to argue for a broader definition of women's health and increased participation of women in research studies. A major new focus became changing the medical establishment. The reasons for this change in orientation, particularly toward the participation by women in research studies, were complex. They included, but were not limited to, the growing number of women living beyond their reproductive years and the growing number of women reaching positions of influence within academic medicine.

In 1983 the United States Public Health Service commissioned a task force on women's health. This task force broadly defined women's health issues to include not only reproductive and social issues, but also biological differences between men and women. The modern field of women's health includes the study of illnesses and conditions that are unique to women, more common or serious in women, have distinct causes or manifestations in women, or have different outcomes or treatments in women. Since the 1980s, research on gender differences in health and disease has had important implications for the treatment and prevention of a variety of common serious illnesses, including heart disease, stroke, lung cancer, depression, colon cancer, and dementia. Research in all these areas is ongoing.

Integral to this new expanded view of women's health has been a change in how medical research has been viewed by the public. In the 1970s, the focus of women's health advocates in the United States was on "protecting" women from potential abuses by seeking to avoid their inclusion in medical research studies. It should be noted that women were excluded from medical research during this time because of a variety of factors, and not solely, or even mainly, because of popular advocacy. Medical research was conducted almost exclusively by male physicians, and because most research scientists believed that effects of the reproductive cycle of women might lead to unreliable research results, most supported the belief that research should be conducted on men and then applied to women. Even most medical research on rats during this period was conducted using male rats.

However, by the 1980s, women's health advocates had realized that because women were being excluded from research studies, knowledge about the diagnosis and treatment of a wide variety of common diseases in women lagged far behind knowledge of diseases in men. A major focus of the women's health movement in the 1980s and 1990s was improving knowledge about disease in women by promoting the inclusion of women in research studies, mainly through mandating inclusion of women in federally funded research studies.

A greater understanding of the factors influencing women's health from a biological perspective has been paralleled by a greater understanding of the psychosocial and societal factors that affect women's health status. As an example, research published in the early 1990s showed that because women were more likely than men to require ongoing, rather than episodic, treatment for their health conditions, federally sponsored insurance in the United States (Medicare) actually covered less overall health costs for women than for men. Differences in employment patterns also result in fewer women being medically insured than men, strongly affecting access to health care and health status. Research on domestic violence, which disproportionately victimizes women, underlined the short- and long-term health effects of what had previously been considered either a nonissue or a law enforcement issue.

Some have suggested that the term "women's health" be replaced by the term "gender-based medicine," in part to reflect that medical research that promotes a greater understanding of the effect of gender on health benefits both women and men. However, others believe that the term "women's health" is most accurate, since it incorporates not only biomedical issues, but also the psychosocial and societal factors that ultimately influence the overall health status of women.

The field of women's health seeks to promote an understanding of the biological and psychosocial factor affecting women's health, and to integrate this understanding into public health initiatives, including training of health care providers. Recognition by the medical research establishment of the need to study health and disease in women as well as men has been essential to this new paradigm. Despite the strong influence of biological factors, psychosocial issues still remain the single most important determinant of health status for many women.

JANET P. PREGLER

(SEE ALSO: *Domestic Violence; Gender and Health; Maternal and Child Health; Reproduction; Women, Infant, and Children Program [WIC]*)

BIBLIOGRAPHY

The Boston Women's Health Book Collective (1998). *Our Bodies, Ourselves for the New Century.* New York: Simon and Schuster.

Clancy, C. M., and Massion, C. T. (1992). "American Women's Health Care." *Journal of the American Medical Association* 269:1918–1920.

Council on Graduate Medical Education (1995). *Fifth Report: Women in Medicine.* Washington, DC: U.S. Department of Health and Human Services.

Haseltine, F. P., and Greenberg-Jacobson, B. (1997). *Women's Health Research: A Medical and Policy Primer.* Washington, DC.: Health Press International.

Healy, B. (1995). *A New Prescription for Women's Health.* New York: Penguin.

Schroeder, P. (1999). *24 Years of House Work and the Place Is Still a Mess: My Life in Politics.* Kansas City, MO: Andrews McMeel Publishing.

Walzer Leavitt, J. (1999). *Women and Health in America.* Madison, WI: University of Wisconsin Press.

WORKMEN'S COMPENSATION

See Occupational Safety and Health

WORKPLACE SMOKING POLICIES AND PROGRAMS

Worksite smoking policies aim mainly to protect nonsmokers from environmental tobacco smoke (ETS), while the objective of worksite cessation programs is to help employees who do smoke (and sometimes their family members, too) give up the habit. Together, these two elements form a worksite tobacco-control program.

Worksite smoking policies began with an early concern for protection of equipment, such as computers, and for employee safety, such as those working around natural gas. Following the 1986 *Surgeon General's Report on the Health Consequences of Involuntary Smoking,* the rate of adoption of restrictive smoking policies increased. With the classification of ETS as a "Group A" carcinogen by the Environmental Protection Agency in 1993, it became a major risk and liability issue for worksites.

In 1999, 79 percent of worksites with fifty or more employees were smoke-free, or limited smoking to separately ventilated areas, a large increase from 27 percent in 1985. All occupational groups are not equally protected, however. In a 1992–1993 national survey, blue-collar and service workers, who have higher smoking rates than that of the total population, reported a percentage of smoke-free worksites well below the national average.

Policies that ban smoking are more effective than restrictive policies, as they reduce exposure to ETS for all employees. In addition, such policies may influence smokers to cut down or quit, are easier to implement and enforce, and decrease maintenance costs.

A secondary effect of restrictive smoking policies is their impact on employee smoking behavior. There is consistent evidence that restrictive policies lead to a reduction of cigarettes smoked at work (a median reduction of 3.4 per day in one review article). The evidence that these policies influence smoking employees to quit, however, is inconclusive. Researchers have estimated that smoke-free workplaces are currently responsible for a 2 percent decrease in cigarette consumption in the United States (a decrease of 9.7 billion cigarettes), and that if all worksites were smoke-free, a 4.1 percent decrease (20.9 billion cigarettes) would occur.

In 1992, 40 percent of worksites with fifty or more employees offered smoking cessation programs. The rationale for corporate sponsorship of smoke cessation programs has been to decrease health care demand and to reduce health care costs, as smokers have been shown to have higher than average health care costs, and to increase productivity, as smoking has been associated with absenteeism and reduced productivity. A recent economic analysis, using current data for the background quit rate, participation and cessation rates of programs, absenteeism, on-the-job productivity, employee turnover rates, and the health effects of smoking, showed an average positive cost-benefit ratio of 1.75 five years after a program began, and increasing to 8.89 after twenty-five years.

A review of studies evaluating the effectiveness of smoking cessation programs between 1968 and 1994 found median quit rates for cessation groups to be 23 percent, while those for minimal treatment programs were 10.1 percent. Competitions and incentives were found to boost cessation rates, although how much was unclear due to methodological flaws. Comprehensive programming that included smoking was successful in reducing smoking in twelve of nineteen studies reviewed. A meta-analysis of long-term (over twelve months) cessation rates from twenty controlled cessation trials at worksites found a weighted average quit rate of 13 percent, with higher rates from longer interventions, those that used employee time as well as work time, and those in smaller worksites.

The worksite provides a unique opportunity to create interventions for the total population of smoking employees. However, most cessation programs attract only those smokers who are motivated both to quit and to use the particular format of the program. Thus, participation rates are low. Better marketing and tailoring of programs would increase participation. Of particular importance is the tailoring of programs to different stages of change. Many smokers have no intention to quit or are merely thinking about it; these employees require a different intervention, one that emphasizes the benefits of quitting and decreases the perceived positive outcomes of smoking and negative outcomes of quitting. Media communication, through employee newsletters, for example, is a good format for this and can be part of a comprehensive cessation intervention that reaches smokers at all stages of change.

To augment worksite programming, corporate health-insurance benefits should include nicotine replacement therapy and other recommended pharmacotherapy, and programs should be coordinated with managed-care providers' offerings of tobacco assessment and counseling. Internally,

physical activity, nutrition, and stress management programs will assist smokers to quit and to stay abstinent.

NELL H. GOTTLIEB

(SEE ALSO: *Absenteeism; Addiction and Habituation; Environmental Tobacco Smoke; Occupational Safety and Health; Smoking Behavior; Smoking Cessation; Smoking: Indoor Restrictions; Tobacco Control*)

BIBLIOGRAPHY

Association for Worksite Health Promotion, U.S. Department of Health and Human Services, and William M. Mercer, Inc. (2000). *1999 National Worksite Health Promotion Survey.* Northbrook, IL: Association for Worksite Health Promotion.

Brownson, R. C.; Eriksen, M. P.; Davis, R. M.; and Warner, K. E. (1997). "Environmental Tobacco Smoke: Health Effects and Policies to Reduce Exposure." *Annual Review Public Health* 18:163–165.

Centers for Disease Control and Prevention, Office on Smoking and Health; Wellness Council of America; and American Cancer Society (1997). *Making Your Workplace Smokefree. A Decision Maker's Guide.* Atlanta, GA: Author. Available at http://www.cdc.gov/tobacco/research_data/environmental/etsguide.htm.

Centers for Disease Control and Prevention (1997). *Chronology: Significant Developments Related to Smoking and Health 1964–1996.* Available at http://www.cdc.gov/tobacco/chron96.htm.

Chapman, S.; Borland, R.; Scollo, M.; Brownson, R. C.; Dominello, A.; and Woodward, S. (1999). "The Impact of Smoke-Free Workplaces on Declining Cigarette Consumption in Australia and the United States." *American Journal of Public Health* 89:1018–1023.

Eriksen, M. P., and Gottlieb, N. H. (1998). "A Review of the Health Impact of Smoking Control at the Workplace." *American Journal of Health Promotion* 13(2):83–104.

Fiore, M. D.; Bailey, W. C.; Cohen, S. J. et al. (2000). *Treating Tobacco Use and Dependence: A Clinical Practice Guideline.* Rockville, MD: U.S. Department of Health and Human Services, Public Health Service.

Fisher, E. J.; Glasgow, R. E.; and Terborg, J. R. (1990). "Worksite Smoking Cessation: A Meta-analysis of Long-Term Quit Rates from Controlled Studies." *Journal of Occupational Medicine* 32(5):429–439.

Gerlach, K. K.; Shopland, D. R.; Hartman, A. M.; Gibson, J. T.; and Pechacek, T. F. (1997). "Workplace Smoking Policies in the United States: Results from a

National Survey of More Than 100,000 Workers." *Tobacco Control* 6:199–206.

Gottlieb, N. H. (2001). "Tobacco Control and Cessation." In *Health Promotion in the Worksite,* 3rd edition, ed. M. P. O'Donnell. Albany, NY: Delmar Publishers.

Heaney, C. A., and Goetzel, R. Z. (1997). "A Review of Health-Related Outcomes of Multi-component Worksite Health Promotion Programs." *American Journal Health Promotion* 11(4):290–308.

Nelson, D. E.; Emont, S. L.; Brackbill, R. M.; Cameron, L. L.; Peddicord, J.; and Fiore, M. C. (1994). "Cigarette Smoking Prevalence by Occupation in the United States. A Comparison between 1978–1980 and 1987–1990." *Journal of Occupational Medicine* 36(5): 516–525.

Prochaska, J. O.; Redding, C. A.; and Evers, K. E. (1997). "The Transtheoretical Model and Stages of Change." In *Health Behavior and Health Education: Theory, Research, and Practice,* 2nd edition, eds. K. Glanz, F. M. Lewis, and B. K. Rimer. San Francisco: Jossey-Bass.

U.S. Department of Health and Human Services (1986). *The Health Consequences of Involuntary Smoking. A Report of the Surgeon General.* Washington, DC: U.S. Government Printing Office.

—— (1993). *1992 National Survey of Worksite Health Promotion Activities: Summary Report.* Washington, DC: USDHHS, U.S. Public Health Service, Office of Disease Prevention and Health Promotion.

Warner, K. E.; Smith, R. J.; Smith, D. G.; and Fries, B. E. (1996). "Health and Economic Implications of a Work-Site Smoking Cessation Program: A Simulation Analysis." *Journal of Occupational and Environmental Medicine* 38(10):981–992.

WORKSITE DRUG TESTING

Because of the growing use of illicit drugs and the abuse of prescription drugs and alcohol in modern society, an extensive program of worksite drug testing has developed. Workers who abuse drugs are much more likely to injure themselves and put fellow workers at risk, and many companies now require preemployment drug screening as a tool to keep those who have been abusing drugs out of the workplace. Drug testing can be done for the use of illegal drugs, for the abuse of legal drugs for which a person does not have an appropriate medical need and prescription, or for abuse of alcohol.

Not only has the number of companies that use drug screening risen dramatically over the years, but organizations such as the United States Armed Forces also have regularly implemented intake drug testing. Many legal protections guarantee employment in spite of having evidence of illness, but drug abuse is not covered in the same way, and employment may be legally denied for failure to pass a drug test.

In addition to preemployment drug testing, many corporations employ repetitive drug testing; and in some work settings, such as in the transportation area, random drug testing may be carried out for all workers engaged in certain activities. Also, when there is an accident in transportation, or in many other work settings, an immediate post-accident drug test is often done. In such instances, the results can lead to disciplinary or legal action.

Drug testing and evaluation must follow strict legal guidelines. Specially designated medical officials, called Medical Review Officers (MRP), review results and simply report that an individual has either passed or failed a drug screen; they are barred from revealing to anyone, including the police, which substance or substances were detected. Drug testing generally utilizes urine samples. However, blood tests and hair analysis may also be used. Workers have legal rights with regard to the taking of urine specimens, and these are safeguarded by elaborate collection and handling procedures. All personnel involved must conform to rigid guidelines, with a proper "chain-of-custody" being followed. This means that specimens must be obtained under close supervision, including visual inspection and temperature measurement, and put into sealed containers with the person from whom the specimen has been taken signing for it. Each person handling the specimen must sign for it along the way.

Substance abuse is characterized by either the use of illegal drugs, or the used of prescription drugs for which one has no prescription. Initial screening tests, which are relatively insensitive, must be further validated by the use of more specific and accurate test measurements. Such secondary testing must be carried out to verify, or disprove, the findings of the relatively insensitive screening tests most commonly used.

ARTHUR L. FRANK

(SEE ALSO: *Alcohol Use and Abuse; Occupational Safety and Health; Substance Abuse, Definition of*)

BIBLIOGRAPHY

Olden, K. (1997). "Substance Abuse and Employee Assistance Programs." In *Occupational and Environmental Medicine,* 2nd edition, ed. J. LaDou. Stamford, CT: Appleton and Lange.

WORLD BANK

Ensuring adequate levels of basic health and nutrition lies at the heart of poverty reduction and economic development, which are the cornerstones of the World Bank's mission. While much of the world has experienced notable health gains, the health, nutrition, and population challenges for most developing countries remain great in the twenty-first century:

- Six communicable diseases—HIV/AIDS (human immunodeficiency virus/ acquired immunodeficiency syndrome), malaria, tuberculosis, measles, diarrheal disease, and acute respiratory infection— account for more than half of the global communicable disease burden.

- HIV/AIDS threatens the future progress of many countries, particularly in Africa where health care systems are stretched beyond their limits.

- Two million children die each year from vaccine-preventable diseases, and over half of the child mortality in low-income countries is linked to malnutrition.

- Cancer, heart disease, and injuries represent a growing proportion of the disease burden in many countries, and tobacco-related illness and death threaten more people, particularly women and young people.

- More than 500,000 maternal deaths occur each year, and more than one-third of all pregnancies are believed to be unwanted or mistimed.

- Environmental degradation poses a serious threat to health in much of the world, and the ability of populations to fight poverty and improve well-being.

Addressing these challenges requires approaches which transcend regional or organizational boundaries and embrace the active participation of communities. Together with sustained improvements in education (particularly for girls), the environment, and the availability of roads and safe water supplies, better health care can be achieved.

The World Bank's objectives for its work in health, nutrition, and population (HNP) are to assist countries in improving the HNP outcomes of poor people and protecting the population from the impoverishing effects of illness, malnutrition, and high fertility; enhancing the performance of health care systems; and securing sustainable health care financing.

The bank works together with countries in achieving these objectives in several complementary ways. First, the World Bank is the single largest source of HNP financing for developing countries. From 1970 through 2000, the bank has offered $16 billion in loans to more than one hundred countries. Second, the World Bank provides technical and policy advice on a wide range of topics in HNP, from health-system reform to maternal and child health and nutrition. The bank also supports governments in the formulation of poverty-reduction strategies that stress the role of human capital in general, and health status in particular, in fighting poverty. Third, the bank mobilizes and maintains partnerships with countries, nongovernmental organizations (NGOs), private enterprises, bilateral donors, foundations, and other agencies. Fourth, knowledge management and sharing, including dissemination of the bank's analytical work, are also critical.

The bank's work in health emphasizes the interconnectedness between ill health and poverty. Recent work has supported improvements in the equity and efficiency of health systems through changing how health care providers are paid, how resources are allocated, and engaging private providers in publicly funded service provisions. Support is also directed towards upgrading infrastructure and equipment, training health personnel, and strengthening policymaking and capacity building.

In public health, the bank focuses on five priority areas: HIV/AIDS, malaria, tuberculosis, maternal/child health and nutrition, and tobacco control. Recent work in the economics of tobacco control is helping to demonstrate to governments that taxation, together with other measures such as advertising bans, can significantly reduce smoking and save lives without permanent negative effects on the economy. Support for immunization programs continues to expand through the bank's partnership with the Global Alliance for Vaccines and Immunization.

Recognizing that malnutrition takes an enormous toll on health and well-being, the bank committed about $2 billion to support nutrition activities from 1976 through 2000. The multisectoral approach adopted in these activities encompasses community- and school-based programs, with an emphasis on communication for behavior change, food fortification programs, and food policy reforms.

From 1970 through 2000, the bank supported more than 239 population and reproductive health projects in 87 countries. These activities help to address the impoverishing effects of unplanned pregnancy and maternal mortality, and to ensure that the vital needs of women, children, and adolescents are met. The bank's work links population policy with poverty reduction and human development through an approach which integrates family planning, maternal health, and the prevention and treatment of sexually transmitted infections, including HIV/AIDS.

SABRINA HUFFMAN

(SEE ALSO: *Family Planning Behavior; HIV/AIDS; International Development of Public Health; International Nongovernmental Organizations; Maternal and Child Health; Poverty; Reproduction*)

BIBLIOGRAPHY

World Bank (2001). *World Development Report 2000–2001: Attacking Poverty*. New York: Oxford University Press.

—— (2001). *The World Bank Annual Report 2000*. Washington, DC: Author.

World Bank Group (1997). *Health, Nutrition, and Population Sector Strategy Paper*. Washington, DC: Author.

WORLD HEALTH ORGANIZATION

The World Health Organization (WHO) was created in 1948 by member states of the United Nations (UN) as a specialized agency with a broad mandate for health. The WHO is the world's leading health organization. Its policies and programs have a far-reaching impact on the status of international public health.

Defined by its constitution as "the directing and coordinating authority on international health work," WHO aims at "the attainment by all peoples of the highest possible standard of health." Its mission is to improve people's lives, to reduce the burdens of disease and poverty, and to provide access to responsive health care for all people.

RESPONSIBILITIES AND FUNCTIONS

WHO's responsibilities and functions include assisting governments in strengthening health services; establishing and maintaining administrative and technical services, such as epidemiological and statistical services; stimulating the eradication of diseases; improving nutrition, housing, sanitation, working conditions and other aspects of environmental hygiene; promoting cooperation among scientific and professional groups; proposing international conventions and agreements on health matters; conducting research; developing international standards for food, and biological and pharmaceutical products; and developing an informed public opinion among all peoples on matters of health.

WHO operations are carried out by three distinct components: the World Health Assembly, the executive board, and the secretariat. The World Health Assembly is the supreme decision-making body, and it meets annually, with participation of ministers of health from its 191 member nations. In a real sense, the WHO is an international health cooperative that monitors the state of the world's health and takes steps to improve the health status of individual countries and of the world community.

The executive board, composed of thirty-two individuals chosen on the basis of their scientific and professional qualifications, meets between the assembly sessions. It implements the decisions and policies of the assembly.

The secretariat is headed by the director general, who is elected by the assembly upon the nomination of the board. The headquarters of the WHO is in Geneva. The director general, however, shares responsibilities with six regional directors, who are in turn chosen by member states of their respective regions. The regional offices are located in Copenhagen for Europe, Cairo for the eastern Mediterranean, New Delhi for Southeast Asia, Manila for the western Pacific, Harare for Africa, and Washington D.C. for the Americas. Their regional directors, in turn, choose the WHO representatives at the country level for their respective regions. There are 141 WHO country offices, and the total number of WHO staff, as of 2001, stands at 3,800. WHO is the only agency of the UN system with such a decentralized structure. The Pan American Health Organization (PAHO) existed before the birth of WHO and serves as WHO's regional office for the Americas.

The founding fathers of the UN purposely set aside a network of specialized agencies with their own assemblies, intending that technical cooperation among member states would be free of the political considerations of the UN itself. It has not always worked out this way, however. WHO could not escape entirely the political fights that occurred in the specialized agencies, and the assembly's deliberations have often reflected the political currents of the time.

The decentralized structure of WHO has added a political dimension that has its pluses and minuses. Many of the resources are assigned to the regional centers, which better reflect regional interests. On the other hand, the regional directors, as elected officials, can act quite independently—and occasionally they do. This has given rise to the impression that there are several WHOs.

Moreover, because the regional directors are elected, they need to give consideration to the requirements of reelection. Since the regional directors choose country representatives in their regions, the dynamics of personnel interaction in WHO's administration is quite unique in the UN system. Regional control over country offices is strong, leaving the WHO country representatives with limited authority or leeway for program implementation.

ACCOMPLISHMENTS AND CHALLENGES

The second half of the twentieth century saw remarkable gains in global health, spurred by rapid economic growth and unprecedented scientific advances. WHO has played a very pivotal role in setting health policies, as well as providing technical cooperation to its member states. Life expectancy rose from 48 years in 1955 to 69 years in 1985. During the same period, the infant mortality rate fell from 148 per 1000 live births to below 59 per 1000. Population growth has been slowed dramatically in many of the most populous countries. Smallpox, the ancient scourge, has disappeared. Other successes include the control of lice-borne typhus and yaws. Polio and guinea worms are on the verge of total elimination. A number of other communicable and tropical diseases, including onchocerciasis and schistosomiasis, are in retreat. With universal salt iodization in place, the prospect of virtually eliminating iodine deficiency disorders (IDD), the major cause for brain damage among young children, is also in sight.

Absolute poverty is still spreading in many parts of the world, however. Disparities in health and wealth are growing between and within countries. More than one billion people are without the benefits of modern medical science. One out of five persons in the world has no access to safe drinking water. Infectious diseases alone account for 13 million deaths a year, most of them in the developing countries. Seventy percent of the poor are women. The chance of an expectant mother in the world's poorest country dying of childbirth is 500 times greater than her counterpart in the richest country.

Excessive consumption and pollution practices have produced profound climatic changes that impact on the environment and the health of human beings. Globalization of trade and marketing has led to a sharp increase in the use of tobacco, alcohol, and high fat foods, along with unhealthy lifestyles.

THE EARLY YEARS OF WHO

Initially, WHO devoted much of its resources to the fight against the major communicable diseases. Mass campaigns were waged against malaria, trachoma, yaws, and typhus, among others. Malaria turned out to be a more complex problem than anticipated, and early efforts at eradication had to be scaled back to the level of control. Efforts to improve maternal and child health services included the training of traditional birth attendants—an approach advocated by UNICEF,

WHO's close partner in all child-health projects—to reduce infant and maternal deaths. WHO also followed up on the work done by its predecessor organizations on sanitary conventions. It adopted, in 1951, the International Sanitary Regulations, later (in 1971) renamed the International Health Regulations.

Beginning in the 1960s, WHO began an effort to extend health services to rural populations. In 1974, recognizing the underutilization of existing technologies to fight childhood diseases, WHO launched an expanded immunization program against polio, measles, diphtheria, whooping cough, tetanus, and tuberculosis.

HFA AND PHC

Widespread dissatisfaction with health services in the later 1960s and early 1970s led to an effort to find an alternative approach to standard health care, and eventually the joint WHO/UNICEF conference in Alma-Ata in 1979.

The goal of Health for All (HFA), adopted by member states at the 1977 World Health Assembly, called for the attainment by all people of the world of a level of health that will permit them to lead a socially and economically productive life. In 1978, WHO and UNICEF cosponsored the historic International Conference on Primary Health Care (PHC) in Alma-Ata, at which the international development community adopted PHC as the key to attaining the goal of Health for All by the year 2000.

PHC, as defined at the Alma-Ata conference, called for a revolutionary redefinition of health care. Instead of the traditional "from-the-top-down" approach to medical service, it embraced the principles of social justice, equity, self-reliance, appropriate technology, decentralization, community involvement, intersectoral collaboration, and affordable cost. The Alma-Ata Declaration on PHC envisaged a minimum package of eight elements: (1) education concerning prevailing health problems and the methods of preventing and controlling them; (2) promotion of food supply and proper nutrition; (3) an adequate supply of safe water and basic sanitation; (4) maternal and child health, including family planning; (5) immunization against the major infectious diseases; (6) prevention and control of locally endemic diseases; (7) appropriate treatment of common diseases and injuries; and (8) provision of essential drugs. Where appropriate, the employment of lay health workers from the community should be trained to tackle specific tasks, including education, and to provide first-level care, with appropriate referrals to secondary and tertiary health facilities.

Though few, if any, countries have successfully followed all the precepts of PHC as enunciated at Alma-Ata, PHC has since provided the philosophical linchpin for virtually all subsequent international health activities. In the 1960s and early 1970s, community health workers and traditional birth attendants were grudgingly accepted by many, though only as second-class health care providers, and they were scorned by others, especially by some traditionally trained allopathic medical practitioners. With Alma-Ata, however, plus the exemplary success of the work of "barefoot doctors" in China, PHC precepts and programs became respectable.

ERADICATION OF SMALLPOX

After an exhaustive and intensive effort, the last cases of smallpox were identified and treated in East Africa. In 1979 a global commission certified the worldwide eradication of this ancient scourge. The cost over the decade-long campaign came to $300 million, a small price to pay for the elimination of the disease, for which the annual cost of vaccination worldwide was close to $1 billion. No ordinary victory, this was humankind's first conquest of a deadly malady, and a clear demonstration that investment in health begets economic benefit as well as humanitarian relief.

GLOBAL STRATEGY FOR HFA

In 1979 the World Health Assembly adopted the Global Strategy for HFA, which was subsequently endorsed by the UN General Assembly. The UN resolution was the health community's attempt to mobilize the world community at large to take collaborative actions to improve the status of the world's health. The main thrust of the strategy was the development of a health-system infrastructure, starting with PHC, for the delivery of countrywide programs that would reach the entire population.

The strategy called for the application of the principles of the Alma-Ata Declaration and the development of the minimum package of the eight PHC elements.

HFA was conceived as a process leading to progressive improvement in the health of people and not as a single finite target, though some indicators were recommended. It aims at social justice, with health resources evenly distributed and essential health service accessible to everyone, with full community involvement.

While member states all voted to adopt HFA via PHC, implementation lagged far behind, as economic crises loomed and political and military conflicts flared. Natural disasters also intervened. The rapid rise of the urban poor and weaknesses in the organization and management of health services resulted in waste and misuse of meager resources. Above all, poverty, its deep-rooted causes unresolved, undermined various efforts in the slow march towards HFA.

CSDR, BAMAKO, AND ARI

In the early 1980s, UNICEF launched its Child Survival and Development Revolution (CSDR) with four inexpensive interventions: growth monitoring, oral rehydration, breastfeeding, and immunization programs (commonly referred to as GOBI). After some initial reservation, and with assurances that GOBI efforts would be within the context of PHC, WHO became an active player in CSDR, which has made impressive inroads in reducing infant deaths, especially through the immunization campaign and the oral rehydration program for the control of diarrhea, which also benefited from water and sanitation programs.

WHO also joined UNICEF in launching the Bamako Initiative in the 1980s, which aimed at the provision of essential drugs and their rational use in the context of PHC, initially in African countries but later expanded to other regions. The initiative introduced the element of cost recovery as well as community management of drug supplies and sales. Indeed, in spite of the retrogressive economic situation in Africa south of the Sahara in the 1980s, infant mortality and life expectancy continued to improve gradually in Africa. These gains, however, have since been brutally reversed by the spread of HIV/AIDS.

The 1980s also saw WHO initiating a broad-scale attack against acute respiratory infections (ARI), a major cause of child mortality, and implementing the Safe Motherhood program, designed to reduce maternal deaths—which stood at 500,000 avoidable deaths, almost all in the developing countries. In these efforts, WHO was joined by UNICEF and the World Bank, which had begun to turn some of its attention to the social aspects of development. In the later 1990s, the Integrated Management of Childhood Illness program was launched to bring together a number of programs for a more rational approach.

Though there was progress, the PHC implementation was found to be limited to a number of countries and some specific areas. The principles of PHC, however, were found to be the only viable option even in the most difficult circumstances, with some adjustment of the approaches and strategies necessary in country-specific situations. The effort to introduce district-level PHC did succeed in bringing the services closer to the people who need them.

THE HIV/AIDS PANDEMIC

Although HIV/AIDS first raised its ugly head in the public eye in North America, it soon became clear that the AIDS epidemic was to become a pandemic. Under pressure from WHO, a number of governments, and various developments agencies, the pharmaceutical industry has agreed to allow the price of AIDS treatment drugs to drop from around $15,000 a year per patient in the industrialized countries to $350 in the developing countries. This will encourage more people to come forward for screening in some countries, and in other countries, with help from international organizations, programs of treatment are now a possibility. However, the principal way to fight AIDS is still prevention through education and behavioral change, as work towards an effective vaccine is making very slow progress. While no part of the world is free of the AIDS threat, AIDS spread fast and wide in Africa, especially in countries south of the Sahara. In Asia, where the population pools are much greater, the number of HIV/AIDS cases is expected to exceed that of Africa by 2005.

In fighting AIDS, development agencies of the UN system have joined together to form UNAIDS, in which WHO plays the lead technical role. The pandemic is now such a serious threat to entire societies that it has been brought to the UN Security Council as a matter of grave security concern.

YEAR 2000 GOALS

In 1990, WHO joined with UNICEF in urging the UN Summit for Children to set Year 2000 goals. These goals included increased immunization rates; reduction of infant, under five, and maternal mortality rates; water and sanitation, as well as education for all; the reduction of malnutrition; and the elimination of micronutrient disorders.

After the end of the Cold War, the hope for a "peace dividend" from disarmament did not materialize. On the contrary, with a few exceptions, since that time the volume of development funds from the industrialized countries has shrunk. The 2001 session of the UN General Assembly is likely to be disappointing in its review of the summit goals. The water, sanitation, and education for all goals will certainly fall far short of target. There is still hope, however, for the elimination of polio and guinea worms, as well as the virtual elimination of iodine deficiency disorders.

HEALTH PROMOTION AND OTHER ACTIVITIES

In 1982 WHO undertook a reorientation of health education, designed to expand its community approach and include communication theories and practice. In 1987 the term "health education" was changed to "health promotion" to denote a broader, ecological approach to the work of facilitating "informed choices" by people on health matters.

The first international consultation on this subject was held in Ottawa in 1986, followed by consultations in Adelaide in 1988, Sundsvall in 1991, and Jakarta in 1997. WHO's new approach calls for broader societal involvement, and in the eastern Mediterranean region, member nations adopted social mobilization as the strategy for health promotion. Individual programs, such as the tuberculosis and micronutrient elimination programs, adopted similar stances.

WHO publishes a number of technical journals, the most important of which is the *WHO Bulletin*, and maintains a media and public relations unit. Every year, World Health Day is observed on April 7, the day, in 1948, when WHO came into being. Each World Health Day is devoted to a particular theme, and material is made available for member states to commemorate the day with a program focus.

Noteworthy, but less publicized, activities of WHO include its worldwide efforts in mental health, oral health, food safety (including the FAO/WHO Codex Alimentarius Commission), health in the work place, elder care, chemical safety, veterinary health, cancer, cardiovascular diseases, and health and the environment. Its essential drug program has had a major impact on the rational use of medicines in developing countries.

WHO maintains a network of collaborating centers, which engage in work in various specific fields. It also maintains a working relationship with a large number of nongovernmental organizations involved in health and development. These organizations are accredited and approved by the World Health Assembly.

YEAR 2020 GOALS

The World Health Assembly has adopted the following set of new goals to be reached by, or before, 2020:

- By 2005, health equity indices will be used within and between countries as a basis for promoting and monitoring equity in health.

- By 2010, transmission of Chagas' disease will be interrupted, and leprosy will be eliminated.

- By 2020, maternal mortality rates will be halved; the worldwide burden of disease will be substantially decreased by reversing the current trends of incidence and disability caused by tuberculosis, malaria, HIV/AIDS, tobacco-related diseases, and violence; measles will be eradicated; and lymphatic filariasis eliminated.

- By 2020, all countries will have made major progress in making available safe drinking water, adequate sanitation, food and shelter in sufficient quantity and quality; all countries will have introduced and be actively managing monitoring strategies that strengthen health-enhancing lifestyles and weaken health-damaging ones, through a combination of regulatory, economic, educational, organization-based, and community-based programs.

- By 2005, member states will have operational mechanisms for developing, implementing, and monitoring policies that are consistent with the HFA policy.

- By 2010, appropriate global and national health information, surveillance, and alert systems will be operational; research policies and institutional mechanisms will be operational at global, regional, and country levels; and all people will have access throughout their lives to comprehensive, essential, quality health care, supported by essential public health functions.

WHO has also launched a series of initiatives, including programs to roll back malaria, stop the spread of tuberculosis, fight the AIDS pandemic, and curtail tobacco use. A breakthrough in the drastic reduction of the cost of AIDS treatment drugs is likely to impact the AIDS fight. Negotiation for a tobacco-control convention may lead to greater success for WHO's Tobacco-Free Initiative. With additional resources from private foundations, WHO, in partnership with the World Bank and UNICEF, has launched an ambitious Global Alliance for Vaccines and Immunization (GAVI). Malnutrition, which accounts for nearly half of the 10.5 million deaths each year among preschool children, will continue to be a priority item in the years to come.

WHO has also undergone a number of reorganizations, the latest resulting in nine clusters, each covering a number of programs.

In addition to the two clusters on management and governing bodies, the program clusters are: communicable diseases, noncommunicable diseases, sustainable development and health environments, family and community health, evidence and information for policy, health technology and pharmaceuticals, and social change and mental health.

DIRECTORS GENERAL

There have been a total of five directors general. Dr. Brock Chisholm, a psychiatrist from Canada, was the first. He was succeeded by Dr. Marcolino Candau of Brazil, who ran the organization for twenty years. Dr. Halfdan Mahler, a tuberculosis specialist from Denmark, took the helm after Candau. Mahler oriented the organization towards development, launched the PHC movement, and confronted the infant formula and pharmaceutical industries on health grounds. After fifteen years, he was succeeded by Dr. Hiroshi Nakajima of Japan, who ran the organization for ten years. The current director general is Dr. Gro Harlem Brundtland, a physician from Norway and a former prime minister of that country. Brundtland has placed considerable emphasis on advocacy at the political level.

JACK CHIEH-SHENG LING

(SEE ALSO: *Alma-Ata Declaration; Barefoot Doctors; Blood-Borne Diseases; Communicable Disease Control; Famine; Global Burden of Disease; Health Promotion and Education; HIV/AIDS; Immunizations; Infant Mortality Rate; International Health; Iodine; Maternal and Child Health; Poverty; Sanitation in Developing Countries; Smallpox; Thyroid Disorders; Tropical Infectious Diseases; UNICEF; Waterborne Diseases; World Bank*)

WORMS

See Dracunculosis *and* Trichinosis

Y

YEARS OF POTENTIAL LIFE LOST (YPLL)

The statistic known as "years of potential life lost" (YPLL) is a measure of the relative impact of various diseases and other lethal forces on a population. It is a useful way to draw attention to the loss of expected years of life due to deaths in childhood, adolescence, and early adult life. Injury-related deaths that affect predominantly young males cause as many lost years of potential life expectancy as cancer, which is mainly a disease of older people, even though cancer may cause more deaths. For instance, in Canada in 1993, injuries killed 10,286 people and cancer killed 25,687 people—yet cancer caused 302,585 YPLL, whereas injuries caused 336,593 YPLL.

JOHN M. LAST

(SEE ALSO: *Life Expectancy and Life Tables*)

YELLOW FEVER

Yellow fever, a member of the genus *Flavivirus*, is an arboviral infection found throughout Africa and South America. It is transmitted primarily by the bite of the *Aedes aegypti* mosquito and also by *Haemogogus* mosquitoes in South America.

Though yellow fever caused epidemics in the United States and Europe in earlier centuries, today it exists only in Africa and Central and South America.

There are two main cycles of transmission of yellow fever: the sylvatic, or jungle, cycle; and the urban cycle. In the sylvatic cycle, the infection is maintained between monkeys and mosquitoes. A human entering the jungle environment (e.g., loggers, hunters) is at risk if bitten by an infected mosquito. Urban yellow fever occurs when the virus is introduced into urban centers, for example by migrant laborers arriving from rural regions. The domestic mosquito, *A. aegypti*, then carries the infection from person to person. In contrast to jungle yellow fever, where only small numbers of individuals are at risk, urban yellow fever epidemics may be quite extensive.

An intermediate cycle has also been described in Africa in areas where there is increased contact between humans, monkeys, and mosquitoes, such as at the edges of forested areas; this is a likely source of larger urban outbreaks.

Following the bite of an infective mosquito, the incubation period is three to six days. Although some cases may be asymptomatic or very mild, most cases are characterized by sudden onset of fever, chills, myalgias, backache, headache, nausea, and vomiting. Relative bradycardia (Faget's sign) is common, as are leukopenia and proteinuria. This early stage lasts three to five days, at which point the majority of patients will recover. Approximately 15 percent will relapse within twenty-four hours and develop a stage of "intoxication" characterized by a reoccurrence and worsening of the above symptoms. Jaundice appears (hence the name "yellow fever"), and patients develop a bleeding tendency marked by blood in the vomit and stool, bruising, and bleeding from mucous membranes. Kidney failure is common. The mortality rate for this stage is over 50 percent. Treatment is supportive as there is no specific antiviral agent available.

As the clinical presentation of yellow fever is similar to that of other viral hemorrhagic fevers, the diagnosis should be confirmed in a laboratory. Diagnosis can be made by culture of the virus or by finding viral antigen in blood or liver tissue. It is also possible to identify virus-specific antibodies in blood.

A live, attenuated vaccine against yellow fever is over 95 percent effective and confers protection for ten years. As it is a live vaccine, it is contraindicated in infants under the age of six months, in pregnant women, and in immunocompromised individuals. It should be used with caution in anyone with a history of egg allergy.

The best method for control of yellow fever is mass vaccination of susceptible populations. Although the World Health Organization advocates including the yellow fever vaccine in the Expanded Programme of Immunization (EPI) for children, most countries use the vaccine only in outbreak situations, a strategy that has not proven to be very effective in controlling the disease.

MARTHA FULFORD
JAY KEYSTONE

(SEE ALSO: *Communicable Disease Control; Epidemics; Vector-Borne Diseases*)

BIBLIOGRAPHY

Desowitz, R. (1997). *Who Gave Pinta to the Santa Maria? Torrid Diseases in a Temperate World.* New York: W. W. Norton & Company.

Halstead, S. (1998). "Emergence Mechanisms in Yellow Fever and Dengue." *Emerging Infections 2*, eds. W. M. Scheld, W. A. Craig, and J. M. Hughes. Washington, DC: ASM Press.

Robertson, S. E.; Hull, B. P.; Tomori, O.; et al. (1998). "Yellow Fever: A Decade of Re-emergence." *Journal of the American Medical Association* 276:1157–1162.

Tomori, O. (1999). "Impact of Yellow Fever on the Developing World." *Advances in Virus Research* 53:5–34.

World Health Organization (1998). "Yellow Fever." *Bulletin of the World Health Organization* 76(Supp. 2):158–159.

YOUTH RISK BEHAVIOR SURVEILLANCE SYSTEM

The Youth Risk Behavior Surveillance System (YRBSS) is a social epidemiologic surveillance system established by the U.S. Centers for Disease Control and Prevention (CDC) in order to monitor health-risk behaviors among high school students, evaluate the impact of national and local efforts to prevent health-risk behaviors, and monitor progress toward achieving *Healthy People 2000* and *Healthy People 2010* objectives.

The YRBSS includes national, state, and local school-based surveys of high school students. The national Youth Risk Behavior Surveys (YRBS), representing a national sample of students, were conducted in 1990, 1991, 1993, 1995, 1997, and 1999, and continue to be conducted on a periodic basis. Special surveys include the 1995 National College Health Risk Behavior Survey and the 1998 National Alternative High School YRBS. The School Health Policies and Programs Study (SHPPS) assesses school health policies and programs at the state, district, school, and classroom levels.

The YRBSS provides prevalence estimates of six categories of priority health-risk behaviors: (1) behaviors that contribute to unintentional and intentional injuries; (2) tobacco use; (3) alcohol and other drug use; (4) sexual behaviors that contribute to unintended pregnancy and sexually transmitted diseases; (5) unhealthy diet behaviors; and (6) physical inactivity. Data and documentation are available for all years of the national YRBS, and for both the 1995 National College Health Risk Behavior Survey and the 1998 National Alternative High School YRBS. Fact sheets and brochures on specific topics are also available. Numerous informational products are available from the CDC.

DAWN M. UPCHURCH

(SEE ALSO: *Centers for Disease Control and Prevention; Risk Assessment, Risk Management; Surveillance; Surveys*)

BIBLIOGRAPHY

Centers for Disease Control and Prevention (2000). *Youth Risk Behavior Surveillance–1999*. Washington, DC: Government Printing Office. Available at http://www.cdc.gov/nccdphp/dash/yrbs/index.htm.

Kolbe, L.; Kann, L.; and Collins, J. (1993). "Overview of the Youth Risk Behavior Surveillance System." *Public Health Report* 108 (Supp. 1):2–10.

Z

ZERO POPULATION GROWTH

Zero population growth occurs when there is neither a net growth nor a net decline in population, but rather a steady state in which the numbers added by annual births and immigration exactly balance the numbers who die and emigrate each year. Zero population growth is the ideal to which nations (and the world as a whole) should aspire in the interests of achieving long-term environmental sustainability.

JOHN M. LAST

(SEE ALSO: *Demography; Population at Risk; Population Growth; Population Policies*)

ZOONOSES

Zoonoses, or zoonotic diseases, are caused by infectious agents that are transmissible under natural circumstances from vertebrate animals to humans. Zoonoses may arise from wild or domestic animals or from products of animal origin. Zoonoses have been known since early hystorical times. There are biblical references to plague, a bacterial zoonosis mainly transmitted to humans by fleas; and some historians contend that a disease first described by Thucydides during the Plague of Athens (430–425 B.C.E.) was typhus, a louse-borne zoonosis (Zinsser). Certain zoonoses, such as yellow fever, malaria, and rabies, are well known to the general public, but a vast number of lesser-known zoonoses exist in limited cycles in different parts of the world. There are undoubtedly many zoonoses lurking in nature that have the potential to cause serious public health consequences if introduced into humans. This is, in fact, what may be our greatest concern about zoonoses—not the diseases that we know they are capable of causing, but the hidden potential of what diseases might arise in the future. Examples that foster our concern include the emergence of AIDS (acquired immunodeficiency syndrome) from nonhuman primates, which has developed into one of the most significant infectious disease threats in the world today, and the crossing of the species barrier of certain influenza virus strains that have led to large human pandemics. Diseases such as AIDS and influenza have their origins as zoonoses, but they subsequently adapted to human-to-human transmission.

There are a number of different types of microbial agents that cause zoonotic diseases, and various ways humans can become infected with these agents. This may best be explained by a few examples: (1) Lyme disease, a bacterial disease transmitted via the bite of an infected tick; (2) rabies, a viral disease acquired by the bite of an infected animal; (3) Ebola hemorrhagic fever, a viral disease spread by infected blood, tissues, secretions, or excretions; (4) hantaviral disease, a disease contracted by inhaling air contaminated with virus-infected excreta from rodents; (5) leptospirosis, a bacterial disease usually transmitted to humans through contact with urine from infected animals; (6) brucellosis, a bacterial disease contracted by ingestion of unpasteurized milk; and (7) cat-scratch disease, a disease contracted through bites or licks of infected cats.

Enteric bacteria such as *Salmonella* and *Escherichia coli* and parasites such as *Cryptosporidium* and *Giardia* are responsible for major food-borne and waterborne disease outbreaks around the world, and recently the nonmicrobial, transmissible agent of bovine spongiform encephalopathy (mad cow disease) appears to have crossed over to humans to produce a degenerative neurological disease known as variant Creutzfeldt-Jakob disease.

There has been a disturbing trend of reemergence of previously recognized zoonoses that were believed to be under control. This has been coupled with the emergence of new zoonotic diseases. Numerous factors may account for this, including: (1) alteration of the environment, affecting the size and distribution of certain animal species, vectors, and transmitters of infectious agents to humans; (2) increasing human populations causing an increased level of contact between humans and infected animals; (3) industrialization of foods of animal origin—that is, changes in food processing and consumer nutritional habits; (4) increasing movements of people, as well as an increased trade in animals and animal products; and (5) decreasing surveillance and control of some of the major zoonoses. Some supposedly "new zoonoses" have been around for a long time but have simply not been recognized. For example, several types of hantaviruses are transmitted by rodents such as deer mice and can cause the disease known as hantavirus pulmonary syndrome. This disease has likely been around for decades, if not centuries, but human cases were first documented only in 1993. In addition, global warming has the potential to broaden the geographic distribution and abundance of arthropods as well as the vertebrate hosts in which some zoonoses persist.

There is no single clinical picture that can be drawn of zoonoses, given the diverse group of microorganisms that are capable of causing zoonotic diseases. A partial list of symptoms may include some, but not all, of the following: fever (sometimes hemorrhagic), headache, rash, muscle aches, arthritis, respiratory distress (sometimes pneumonia), abdominal pain, vomiting, diarrhea, jaundice, cardiac abnormalities, and neurological involvement ranging from stiff neck to meningitis

or encephalitis. The course of disease varies between different zoonotic pathogens but can be more severe in the very young or very old, or in individuals who are immunocompromised. Many zoonoses can be treated with antimicrobial drugs, but there are few drugs that can be used to successfully treat viral zoonoses. Treatment for a known or suspected exposure to a viral zoonosis such as rabies involves administration of immune globulin, whereas only supportive treatment can be offered for many other viral zoonoses.

Vaccines are available for the general public for a small number of zoonoses, such as Japanese encephalitis and yellow fever, and on a limited basis for individuals perceived to be at occupational or recreational risk. In addition, chemoprophylactic regimens such as antimalarial drugs are recommended for travellers to high disease-risk areas. The risk of contracting vector-borne diseases can be reduced by avoidance of areas infested by arthropods, use of insect repellents, and appropriate clothing (the less skin exposed the better). Occasionally it is possible to reduce zoonotic disease risks by decreasing the abundance of certain reservoir hosts such as rodents. Individuals should also not drink untreated water or unpasteurized milk. Areas containing potentially contaminated animal material such as rodent excreta should be cleaned using appropriate disinfectants. Patients with diseases such as Ebola virus should be kept in strict isolation. Diseases such as tularemia and leptospirosis may be contracted by handling infected animal tissue, so trappers should use gloves when handling dead animals.

The disease incidence and pattern of occurrence of zoonoses varies greatly between different regions within a country and between countries. In general, zoonoses do not occur in large numbers in the industrialized world. Because of this relative infrequency of occurrence, some zoonotic infections may be overlooked and underdiagnosed.

Certain individuals may be at greater risk for contracting zoonoses. These include people with occupational exposure, such as veterinarians, farmers, and slaughterhouse workers, or individuals who participate in outdoor recreational activities, such as hunters. The best defense against contracting zoonoses is education. Individuals should be aware of the respective zoonoses that may be circulating in their environment and the times of year of greatest risk for contracting these zoonoses. This type of information is generally available from public health departments and veterinarians, and can also be found on the Internet.

HARVEY ARTSOB

(SEE ALSO: *Communicable Disease Control; Ecosystems; Epidemics; Epidemiology; Vector-Borne Diseases; Veterinary Public Health; and articles on diseases mentioned herein*)

BIBLIOGRAPHY

Lederberg, J.; Shope, R. E.; and Oaks, S. C. (1992). *Emerging Infections. Microbial Threats to Health in the United States.* Washington, DC: National Academy Press.

Meslin, F. X. (1997). "Global Aspects of Emerging and Potential Zoonoses: A WHO Perspective." *Emerging Infectious Diseases,* Vol. 3. Geneva: World Health Organization.

Zinsser, H. (1934). *Rats, Lice, and History.* Boston: Little, Brown.

Appendix

Prayer of Maimonides

Prayer attributed to Maimonides (Rabbi Moshe ben Maimon, 1135–1204 <c.<e.), a physician born in Moorish Cordoba, Spain. The text is also available via the Internet: http://www.fordham.edu/halsall/source/rambam-oath.html.

The eternal providence has appointed me to watch over the life and health of Thy creatures. May the love for my art actuate me at all time; may neither avarice nor miserliness, nor thirst for glory or for a great reputation engage my mind; for the enemies of truth and philanthropy could easily deceive me and make me forgetful of my lofty aim of doing good to Thy children.

May I never see in the patient anything but a fellow creature in pain.

Grant me the strength, time, and opportunity always to correct what I have acquired, always to extend its domain; for knowledge is immense and the spirit of man can extend indefinitely to enrich itself daily with new requirements.

Today he can discover his errors of yesterday and tomorrow he can obtain a new light on what he thinks himself sure of today. Oh, God, Thou has appointed me to watch over the life and death of Thy creatures; here am I ready for my vocation and now I turn unto my calling.

The Oath of Hippocrates

I swear by Apollo the physician, and Aesculapius, and Health, and All-heal, and all the gods and goddesses, that, according to my ability and judgment, I will keep this Oath and this stipulation to reckon him who taught me this Art equally dear to me as my parents, to share my substance with him, and relieve his necessities if required; to look upon his offspring in the same footing as my own brothers, and to teach them this art, if they shall wish to learn it, without fee or stipulation; and that by precept, lecture, and every other mode of instruction, I will impart a knowledge of the Art to my own sons, and those of my teachers, and to disciples bound by a stipulation and oath according to the law of medicine, but to none others. I will follow that system of regimen which, according to my ability and judgment, I consider for the benefit of my patients, and abstain from whatever is deleterious and mischievous. I will give no deadly medicine to any one if asked, nor suggest any such counsel; and in like manner I will not give to a woman a pessary to produce abortion. With purity and with holiness I will pass my life and practice my Art. I will not cut persons laboring under the stone, but will leave this to be done by men who are practitioners of this work. Into whatever houses I enter, I will go into them for the benefit of the sick, and will abstain from every voluntary act of mischief and corruption; and, further from the seduction of females or males, of freemen and slaves. Whatever, in connection with my professional practice or not, in connection with it, I see or hear, in the life of men, which ought not to be spoken of abroad, I will not divulge, as reckoning that all such should be kept secret. While I continue to keep this Oath unviolated, may it be granted to me to enjoy life and the practice of the art, respected by all men, in all times! But should I trespass and violate this Oath, may the reverse be my lot!

SOURCE: Hippocrates, *Works*, vol. 1:299–301, trans., Francis Adams. New York: Loeb. Available on the Internet: http://www.humanities.ccny.cuny.edu/history/reader/hippoath.htm.

Declaration of Alma-Ata

The document below is available via the Internet: http://www.who.int/hpr/docs/almaata.html.

INTERNATIONAL CONFERENCE ON PRIMARY HEALTH CARE, ALMA-ATA, USSR, 6–12 SEPTEMBER 1978

The International Conference on Primary Health Care, meeting in Alma-Ata this twelfth day of September in the year nineteen hundred and seventy-eight, expressing the need for urgent action by all governments, all health and development workers, and the world community to protect and promote the health of all the people of the world, hereby makes the following Declaration:

I
The Conference strongly reaffirms that health, which is a state of complete physical, mental and social well-being, and not merely the absence of disease or infirmity, is a fundamental human right and that the attainment of the highest possible level of health is a most important worldwide social goal whose realization requires the action of many other social and economic sectors in addition to the health sector.

II
The existing gross inequality in the health status of the people, particularly between developed and developing countries as well as within countries, is

politically, socially and economically unacceptable and is, therefore, of common concern to all countries.

III

Economic and social development, based on a New International Economic Order, is of basic importance to the fullest attainment of health for all and to the reduction of the gap between the health status of the developing and developed countries. The promotion and protection of the health of the people is essential to sustained economic and social development and contributes to a better quality of life and to world peace.

IV

The people have the right and duty to participate individually and collectively in the planning and implementation of their health care.

V

Governments have a responsibility for the health of their people which can be fulfilled only by the provision of adequate health and social measures. A main social target of governments, international organizations, and the whole world community in the coming decades should be the attainment by all peoples of the world by the year 2000 of a level of health that will permit them to lead a socially and economically productive life. Primary health care is the key to attaining this target as part of development in the spirit of social justice.

VI

Primary health care is essential health care based on practical, scientifically sound and socially acceptable methods and technology made universally accessible to individuals and families in the community through their full participation and at a cost that the community and country can afford to maintain at every stage of their development in the spirit of self-reliance and self-determination. It forms an integral part both of the country's health system, of which it is the central function and main focus, and of the overall social and economic development of the community. It is the first level of contact of individuals, the family, and community with the national health system bringing health care as close as possible to where people live and work, and constitutes the first element of a continuing health care process.

VII

Primary health care:

1. reflects and evolves from the economic conditions and sociocultural and political characteristics of the country and its communities and is based on the application of the relevant results of social, biomedical and health services research, and public health experience;

2. addresses the main health problems in the community, providing promotive, preventive, curative, and rehabilitative services accordingly;

3. includes at least: education concerning prevailing health problems and the methods of preventing and controlling them; promotion of food supply and proper nutrition; an adequate

supply of safe water and basic sanitation; maternal and child health care, including family planning; immunization against the major infectious diseases; prevention and control of locally endemic diseases; appropriate treatment of common diseases and injuries; and provision of essential drugs;

4. involves, in addition to the health sector, all related sectors and aspects of national and community development, in particular agriculture, animal husbandry, food, industry, education, housing, public works, communications, and other sectors; and demands the coordinated efforts of all those sectors;

5. requires and promotes maximum community and individual self-reliance and participation in the planning, organization, operation, and control of primary health care, making fullest use of local, national, and other available resources; and to this end develops through appropriate education the ability of communities to participate;

6. should be sustained by integrated, functional and mutually supportive referral systems, leading to the progressive improvement of comprehensive health care for all, and giving priority to those most in need;

7. relies, at local and referral levels, on health workers, including physicians, nurses, midwives, auxiliaries, and community workers as applicable, as well as traditional practitioners as needed, suitably trained socially and technically to work as a health team and to respond to the expressed health needs of the community.

VIII

All governments should formulate national policies, strategies, and plans of action to launch and sustain primary health care as part of a comprehensive national health system and in coordination with other sectors. To this end, it will be necessary to exercise political will, to mobilize the country's resources, and to use available external resources rationally.

IX

All countries should cooperate in a spirit of partnership and service to ensure primary health care for all people since the attainment of health by people in any one country directly concerns and benefits every other country. In this context the joint WHO/UNICEF report on primary health care constitutes a solid basis for the further development and operation of primary health care throughout the world.

X

An acceptable level of health for all the people of the world by the year 2000 can be attained through a fuller and better use of the world's resources, a considerable part of which is now spent on armaments and military conflicts. A genuine policy of independence, peace, détente, and disarmament could and should release additional resources that could well be devoted to peaceful aims and in particular to the acceleration of social and economic development of which primary health care, as an essential part, should be allotted its proper share.

The International Conference on Primary Health Care calls for urgent and effective national and international action to develop and implement primary health care throughout the world, and particularly in developing countries, in a spirit of technical cooperation and in keeping with a New International Economic Order. It urges governments, WHO and UNICEF, and other international organizations, as well as multilateral and bilateral agencies, non-governmental organizations, funding agencies, all health workers and the whole world community to support national and international commitment to primary health care and to channel increased technical and financial support to it, particularly in developing countries. The Conference calls on all the aforementioned to collaborate in introducing, developing, and maintaining primary health care in accordance with the spirit and content of this Declaration.

Declaration of the Fifth ASEAN Health Ministers

Proclaimed at the Fifth ASEAN Health Ministers Meeting in Yogyakarta, Indonesia, April 28–29, 2000. Below, some portions of the Declaration have been excerpted and others summarized. The full text of the Declaration is available via the Internet: http://www.asean. or.id/function/ahmm_dec.htm.

"WE, the Ministers of Health of ASEAN Member Countries, representing Brunei Darussalam, the Kingdom of Cambodia, the Republic of Indonesia, the Lao People's Democratic Republic, Malaysia, the Union of Myanmar, the Republic of the Philippines, the Republic of Singapore, the Kingdom of Thailand, and the Socialist Republic of Viet Nam;

"RECALLING that the ASEAN Vision 2020, adopted by the 2nd Informal Summit held in Kuala Lumpur in December 1997, envisioned ASEAN as a concert of Southeast Asian nations, outward looking, living in peace, stability, and prosperity, bonded together in partnership in dynamic development and in a community of caring societies;

"SUPPORTIVE of the need to promote social development and address the social impact of the financial and economic crisis as outlined in the Hanoi Plan of Action (HPA) implementing ASEAN Vision 2020 and adopted during the 6th ASEAN Summit held in Hanoi in December 1998;

"RESPONDING to the call of the Hanoi Declaration adopted by the Sixth ASEAN Summit held in Hanoi in December 1998 that we shall, together, make sure that our people are assured of adequate medical care and access to essential medicines and that cooperation shall be stepped up in the control and prevention of communicable diseases, including HIV/AIDS;

"FULLY AWARE that, despite significant progress made in uplifting the quality of life of individuals in our region, health problems continue to be associated with poverty and are increasingly associated with urbanisation, industrialisation, environmental pollution, lifestyle diseases, and stress-related conditions;

"RECOGNIZING the need to prepare the health sector for the challenges and opportunities arising from globalisation and trade liberalisation;

"ENCOURAGED by the notable progress made by the ASEAN Sub-Committee on Health and Nutrition and the ASEAN Task Force on AIDS in formulating action plans and programmes and in implementing regional activities on health, despite funding constraints;

"DO HEREBY AGREE, IN THE SPIRIT OF ASEAN SOLIDARITY AND MUTUAL ASSISTANCE, TO STRENGTHEN ASEAN COOPERATION ON HEALTH TO MEET THE CHALLENGES OF THE NEW MILLENNIUM, BY ADOPTING THE FOLLOWING FRAMEWORK:"

Guiding Principles

1. "Emphasize health as a fundamental right of our peoples;

2. "Health development is a shared responsibility and must involve greater participation and empowerment of the people, communities, and institutions;

3. "ASEAN cooperation shall strive to achieve social justice and equity in health development and solidarity in action towards a healthy paradigm that emphasizes health promotion and disease prevention;

4. "Political commitment to strengthen and intensify ASEAN cooperation in health development and to mobilise resources at the national, regional, and international levels must derive from the highest level of policy and governance;

5. "ASEAN cooperation in health development must be guided by well-defined and focused strategic policies which emphasize the regional perspective and value-added element in all undertakings, while keeping in mind the specific development requirements of Member Countries; and

6. "The organizational machinery for pursuing ASEAN cooperation in health development must be strengthened to achieve better coordination and integration across related development sectors."

Mission

The Declaration states the mission of the signatory nations to include strengthening regional cooperation to ensure health, advocating to promote increased awareness of health issues, and ensuring the availability of health care and health-related products and services.

Strategies

The Declaration specifies various strategies to support these goals, including "greater emphasis on health promotion and disease prevention" and the intensification of "human resources development."

Program of Action

A series of steps are outlined in order to carry out the goals and principles of the Declaration, including the implementation of existing ASEAN plans and programs, an effort to "address the impact of globalisation/trade liberalisation on the health sector," and strengthening the mechanisms for collaboration among the ASEAN nations.

Universal Declaration of Human Rights

On December 10, 1948 the General Assembly of the United Nations adopted and proclaimed the Universal Declaration of Human Rights [Resolution 217 A]. Following this historic act the Assembly called upon all member countries to publicize the text of the Declaration and "to cause it to be disseminated, displayed, read and expounded principally in schools and other educational institutions, without distinction based on the political status of countries or territories." Below, some portions of the Declaration have been excerpted and others summarized. The full text of the Declaration is available via the Internet: http://www.un.org/Overview/rights.html.

PREAMBLE

"Whereas recognition of the inherent dignity and of the equal and inalienable rights of all members of the human family is the foundation of freedom, justice and peace in the world,

"Whereas disregard and contempt for human rights have resulted in barbarous acts which have outraged the conscience of mankind, and the advent of a world in which human beings shall enjoy freedom of speech and belief and freedom from fear and want has been proclaimed as the highest aspiration of the common people,

"Whereas it is essential, if man is not to be compelled to have recourse, as a last resort, to rebellion against tyranny and oppression, that human rights should be protected by the rule of law,

"Whereas it is essential to promote the development of friendly relations between nations,

"Whereas the peoples of the United Nations have in the Charter reaffirmed their faith in fundamental human rights, in the dignity and worth of the human person, and in the equal rights of men and women and have determined to promote social progress and better standards of life in larger freedom,

"Whereas Member States have pledged themselves to achieve, in co-operation with the United Nations, the promotion of universal respect for and observance of human rights and fundamental freedoms,

"Whereas a common understanding of these rights and freedoms is of the greatest importance for the full realization of this pledge,

"Now, therefore, THE GENERAL ASSEMBLY proclaims THIS UNIVERSAL DECLARATION OF HUMAN RIGHTS as a common standard of achievement for all peoples and all nations, to the end that every individual and every organ of society, keeping this Declaration constantly in mind, shall strive by teaching and education to promote respect for these rights and freedoms and by progressive measures, national and international, to secure their universal and effective recognition and observance, both among the peoples of Member States themselves and among the peoples of territories under their jurisdiction.

Article 1.
"All human beings are born free and equal in dignity and rights. They are endowed with reason and conscience and should act towards one another in a spirit of brotherhood.

Article 2.
"Everyone is entitled to all the rights and freedoms set forth in this Declaration, without distinction of any kind, such as race, color, sex, language, religion, political or other opinion, national or social origin, property, birth, or other status. Furthermore, no distinction shall be made on the basis of the political, jurisdictional, or international status of the country or territory to which a person belongs, whether it be independent, trust, non-self-governing, or under any other limitation of sovereignty.

Article 3.
"Everyone has the right to life, liberty and security of person.

Article 4.
"No one shall be held in slavery or servitude; slavery and the slave trade shall be prohibited in all their forms.

Article 5.
"No one shall be subjected to torture or to cruel, inhuman, or degrading treatment or punishment."

Articles 6–11.
All persons are equal before the law and are entitled to equal legal protection including a lack of discrimination, access to legal tribunals, freedom from arbitrary arrest and/or detention, and the right to the presumption of innocence.

Articles 12–21.
All persons have a right to privacy, to nationality and asylum, and to political participation; as well as freedom of movement and association and freedom of thought, conscience, and religion.

Article 22.
"Everyone, as a member of society, has the right to social security and is entitled to realization, through national effort and international co-operation and in accordance with the organization and resources of each State, of the economic, social, and cultural rights indispensable for his dignity and the free development of his personality.

Article 23.
"(1) Everyone has the right to work, to free choice of employment, to just and favorable conditions of work, and to protection against unemployment. (2) Everyone, without any discrimination, has the right to equal pay for equal work. (3) Everyone who works has the right to just and favorable remuneration ensuring for himself and his family an existence worthy of human dignity, and supplemented, if necessary, by other means of social protection.

(4) Everyone has the right to form and to join trade unions for the protection of his interests.

Article 24.

"Everyone has the right to rest and leisure, including reasonable limitation of working hours and periodic holidays with pay.

Article 25.

"(1) Everyone has the right to a standard of living adequate for the health and well-being of himself and of his family, including food, clothing, housing and medical care, and necessary social services, and the right to security in the event of unemployment, sickness, disability, widowhood, old age, or other lack of livelihood in circumstances beyond his control. (2) Motherhood and childhood are entitled to special care and assistance. All children, whether born in or out of wedlock, shall enjoy the same social protection."

Articles 26–28.

All persons have a right to education and full participation in the cultural life of the community.

Article 29.

"(1) Everyone has duties to the community in which alone the free and full development of his personality is possible. (2) In the exercise of his rights and freedoms, everyone shall be subject only to such limitations as are determined by law solely for the purpose of securing due recognition and respect for the rights and freedoms of others and of meeting the just requirements of morality, public order, and the general welfare in a democratic society. (3) These rights and freedoms may in no case be exercised contrary to the purposes and principles of the United Nations.

Article 30.

"Nothing in this Declaration may be interpreted as implying for any State, group or person any right to engage in any activity or to perform any act aimed at the destruction of any of the rights and freedoms set forth herein."

World Scientists' Warning to Humanity

The Warning was written on November 18, 1992 and was subsequently signed by over 1,500 scientists from all countries. The full text of the Warning appears below. It is also available via the Internet: http://www.ucsusa.org/about/warning.html.

INTRODUCTION

Human beings and the natural world are on a collision course. Human activities inflict harsh and often irreversible damage on the environment and on critical resources. If not checked, many of our current practices put at serious risk the future that we wish for human society and the plant and animal kingdoms, and may so alter the living world that it will be unable to sustain life in the manner that we know. Fundamental changes are urgent if we are to avoid the collision our present course will bring about.

THE ENVIRONMENT

The environment is suffering critical stress:

The Atmosphere
Stratospheric ozone depletion threatens us with enhanced ultra-violet radiation at the Earth's surface, which can be damaging or lethal to many life forms. Air pollution near ground level and acid precipitation are already causing widespread injury to humans, forests and crops.

Water Resources
Heedless exploitation of depletable ground water supplies endangers food production and other essential human systems. Heavy demands on the world's surface waters have resulted in serious shortages in some 80 countries, containing 40% of the world's population. Pollution of rivers, lakes, and ground water further limits the supply.

Oceans
Destructive pressure on the oceans is severe, particularly in the coastal regions which produce most of the world's food fish. The total marine catch is now at or above the estimated maximum sustainable yield. Some fisheries have already shown signs of collapse. Rivers carrying heavy burdens of eroded soil into the seas also carry industrial, municipal, agricultural, and livestock waste—some of it toxic.

Soil
Loss of soil productivity, which is causing extensive land abandonment, is a widespread byproduct of current practices in agriculture and animal husbandry. Since 1945, 11% of the Earth's vegetated surface has been degraded—an area larger than India and China combined—and per capita food production in many parts of the world is decreasing.

Forests
Tropical rain forests, as well as tropical and temperate dry forests, are being destroyed rapidly. At present rates, some critical forest types will be gone in a few years and most of the tropical rain forest will be gone before the end of the next century. With them will go large numbers of plant and animal species.

Living Species
The irreversible loss of species, which by 2100 may reach one third of all species now living, is especially serious. We are losing the potential they hold for providing medicinal and other benefits, and the contribution that genetic diversity of life forms gives to the robustness of the world's biological systems and to the astonishing beauty of the Earth itself.

Much of this damage is irreversible on a scale of centuries or permanent. Other processes appear to pose additional threats. Increasing levels of gases in the atmosphere from human activities, including carbon dioxide released from fossil fuel burning and from deforestation, may alter climate on a global scale. Predictions of global warming are still uncertain—with projected effects ranging from tolerable to very severe—but the potential risks are very great.

Our massive tampering with the world's interdependent web of life—coupled with the environmental damage inflicted by deforestation, species loss, and climate change—could trigger widespread adverse effects, including unpredictable collapses of critical biological systems whose interactions and dynamics we only imperfectly understand.

Uncertainty over the extent of these effects cannot excuse complacency or delay in facing the threat.

POPULATION

The Earth is finite. Its ability to absorb wastes and destructive effluent is finite. Its ability to provide food and energy is finite. Its ability to provide for growing numbers of people is finite. And we are fast approaching many of the Earth's limits. Current economic practices which damage the environment, in both developed and underdeveloped nations cannot be continued without the risk that vital global systems will be damaged beyond repair.

Pressures resulting from unrestrained population growth put demands on the natural world that can overwhelm any efforts to achieve a sustainable future. If we are to halt the destruction of our environment, we must accept limits to that growth. A World Bank estimate indicates that world population will not stabilize at less than 12.4 billion, while the United Nations concludes that the eventual total could reach 14 billion, a near tripling of today's 5.4 billion. But, even at this moment, one person in five lives in absolute poverty without enough to eat, and one in ten suffers serious malnutrition.

No more than one or a few decades remain before the chance to avert the threats we now confront will be lost and the prospects for humanity immeasurably diminished.

WARNING

We the undersigned, senior members of the world's scientific community, hereby warn all humanity of what lies ahead. A great change in our stewardship of the Earth, and the life on it, is required if vast human misery is to be avoided and our global home on this planet is not to be irretrievably mutilated.

WHAT WE MUST DO

Five inextricably linked areas must be addressed simultaneously:

1. We must bring environmentally damaging activities under control to restore and protect the integrity of the Earth's systems we depend on. We must, for example, move away from fossil fuels to more benign, inexhaustible energy sources to cut greenhouse gas emissions and the pollution of our air and water. Priority must be given to the development of energy sources matched to Third World needs—small scale and relatively easy to implement. We must halt deforestation, injury to and loss of agricultural land, and the loss of terrestrial and marine plant and animal species.

2. We must manage resources crucial to human welfare more effectively. We must give high priority to efficient use of energy,

water, and other materials, including expansion of conservation and recycling.

3. We must stabilize population. This will be possible only if all nations recognize that it requires improved social and economic conditions, and the adoption of effective, voluntary family planning.

4. We must reduce and eventually eliminate poverty.

5. We must ensure sexual equality, and guarantee women control over their own reproductive decisions.

DEVELOPED NATIONS MUST ACT NOW

The developed nations are the largest polluters in the world today. They must greatly reduce their overconsumption, if we are to reduce pressures on resources and the global environment. The developed nations have the obligation to provide aid and support to developing nations, because only the developed nations have the financial resources and the technical skills for these tasks.

Acting on this recognition is not altruism, but enlightened self-interest: whether industrialized or not, we all have but one lifeboat. No nation can escape from injury when global biological systems are damaged. No nation can escape from conflicts over increasingly scarce resources. In addition, environmental and economic instabilities will cause mass migrations with incalculable consequences for developed and undeveloped nations alike.

Developing nations must realize that environmental damage is one of the gravest threats they face, and that attempts to blunt it will be overwhelmed if their populations go unchecked. The greatest peril is to become trapped in spirals of environmental decline, poverty, and unrest, leading to social, economic, and environmental collapse.

Success in this global endeavor will require a great reduction in violence and war. Resources now devoted to the preparation and conduct of war— amounting to over $1 trillion annually—will be badly needed in the new tasks and should be diverted to the new challenges.

A new ethic is required—a new attitude towards discharging our responsibility for caring for ourselves and for the Earth. We must recognize the Earth's limited capacity to provide for us. We must recognize its fragility. We must no longer allow it to be ravaged. This ethic must motivate a great movement, convince reluctant leaders and reluctant governments and reluctant peoples themselves to effect the needed changes.

The scientists issuing this warning hope that our message will reach and affect people everywhere. We need the help of many.

- We require the help of the world community of scientists—natural, social, economic, political;
- We require the help of the world's business and industrial leaders;
- We require the help of the world's religious leaders; and

- We require the help of the world's peoples.

We call on all to join us in this task.

The Convention on the Rights of the Child

The Convention was adopted and opened for signature, ratification, and accession by General Assembly resolution 44/25 of November 20, 1989. It entered into force September 2, 1990. Below, some portions of the Convention have been excerpted and others summarized. The full text of the Convention is available via the Internet: http://www.unicef.org/crc/fulltext.htm.

PREAMBLE

"The States Parties to the present Convention,

"Considering that, in accordance with the principles proclaimed in the Charter of the United Nations, recognition of the inherent dignity and of the equal and inalienable rights of all members of the human family is the foundation of freedom, justice and peace in the world,

"Bearing in mind that the peoples of the United Nations have, in the Charter, reaffirmed their faith in fundamental human rights and in the dignity and worth of the human person and have determined to promote social progress and better standards of life in larger freedom,

"Recognizing that the United Nations has, in the Universal Declaration of Human Rights and in the International Covenants on Human Rights, proclaimed and agreed that everyone is entitled to all the rights and freedoms set forth therein, without distinction of any kind, such as race, colour, sex, language, religion, political or other opinion, national or social origin, property, birth, or other status,

"Recalling that, in the Universal Declaration of Human Rights, the United Nations has proclaimed that childhood is entitled to special care and assistance,

"Convinced that the family, as the fundamental group of society and the natural environment for the growth and well-being of all its members and particularly children, should be afforded the necessary protection and assistance so that it can fully assume its responsibilities within the community,

"Recognizing that the child, for the full and harmonious development of his or her personality, should grow up in a family environment, in an atmosphere of happiness, love, and understanding,

"Considering that the child should be fully prepared to live an individual life in society and brought up in the spirit of the ideals proclaimed in the Charter of the United Nations and in particular in the spirit of peace, dignity, tolerance, freedom, equality, and solidarity,

"Bearing in mind that the need to extend particular care to the child has been stated in the Geneva Declaration of the Rights of the Child of 1924 and in the Declaration of the Rights of the Child adopted by the General

Assembly on 20 November 1959 and recognized in the Universal Declaration of Human Rights, in the International Covenant on Civil and Political Rights (in particular in articles 23 and 24), in the International Covenant on Economic, Social and Cultural Rights (in particular in article 10), and in the statutes and relevant instruments of specialized agencies and international organizations concerned with the welfare of children,

"Bearing in mind that, as indicated in the Declaration of the Rights of the Child, 'the child, by reason of his physical and mental immaturity, needs special safeguards and care, including appropriate legal protection, before as well as after birth,'

"Recalling the provisions of the Declaration on Social and Legal Principles relating to the Protection and Welfare of Children, with Special Reference to Foster Placement and Adoption Nationally and Internationally; the United Nations Standard Minimum Rules for the Administration of Juvenile Justice (The Beijing Rules); and the Declaration on the Protection of Women and Children in Emergency and Armed Conflict,

"Recognizing that, in all countries in the world, there are children living in exceptionally difficult conditions and that such children need special consideration,

"Taking due account of the importance of the traditions and cultural values of each people for the protection and harmonious development of the child,

"Recognizing the importance of international cooperation for improving the living conditions of children in every country, in particular in the developing countries,

"Have agreed as follows:"

PART I

Articles 1–5
The Convention states the terms and scope of the agreement, including that in all matters addressed "the best interests of the child shall be a primary consideration."

Articles 6–11
The Convention stipulates certain basic rights of all children, foremost amongst which is the right to life and subsidiary rights to a name, identity, family, and nationality. In keeping with these rights, the Convention requires that all parties to the agreement take measures to "combat the illicit transfer and non-return of children abroad."

Articles 12–17
Continuing the enumeration of rights held by children, the Convention names the freedoms of thought, speech, conscience, and religion, as well as the freedoms of privacy and assembly.

Articles 18–27
In order to support the exercise of the rights recognized by the Convention, the parties agree to encourage and, as needed, regulate activities pertaining to the parenting and care of the child, including the physical safety of the

child, foster care and adoption, mental and physical disability, health care, and social and economic security.

Articles 28–31

The Convention recognizes each child's right to education, participation in his or her culture, and play, and encourages measures to support that right.

Articles 32–39

The Convention names and recognizes the child's right to be free from various forms of exploitation and abuse, including physical and sexual abuse, economic and sexual exploitation, exposure to addictive drugs, and warfare.

Articles 40–41

The Convention names and establishes measures to support the various rights of the child before national penal courts.

PART II

Articles 42–45

The Convention stipulates various measures by which the parties to the agreement will promulgate and support the above articles of the Convention.

PART III

Articles 46–54

The Convention stipulates the procedure by which the Convention will be presented to and ratified by the parties to the agreement, and be thereafter administered by the Secretary General of the United Nations.

European Charter on Environment and Health

Proclaimed at the First European Conference on Environment and Health, Frankfurt-am-Main, Federal Republic of Germany, December 7–8, 1989. Below, some portions of the Charter have been excerpted and others summarized. The full text of the Charter is available via the Internet: http://www.who.dk/policy/ehchart.htm.

PREAMBLE

"In the light of WHO's [World Health Organization] strategy for health for all in Europe, the report of the World Commission on Environment and Development and the related Environmental Perspective to the Year 2000 and Beyond (resolutions 42/187 and 42/186 of the United Nations General Assembly) and World Health Assembly resolution WHA42.26,

- "Recognizing the dependence of human health on a wide range of crucial environmental factors,

- "Stressing the vital importance of preventing health hazards by protecting the environment,

- "Acknowledging the benefits to health and well-being that accrue from a clean and harmonious environment,

- "Encouraged by the many examples of positive achievement in the abatement of pollution and the restoration of a healthy environment,
- "Mindful that the maintenance and improvement of health and well-being require a sustainable system of development,
- "Concerned at the ill-considered use of natural resources and man-made products in ways liable to damage the environment and endanger health,
- "Considering the international character of many environmental and health issues and the interdependence of nations and individuals in these matters,
- "Conscious of the fact that, since developing countries are faced with major environmental problems, there is a need for global cooperation,
- "Responding to the specific characteristics of the European Region, and notably its large population, intensive industrialization, and dense traffic,
- "Taking into account existing international instruments (such as agreements on protection of the ozone layer) and other initiatives relating to the environment and health,

"The Ministers of the Environment and of Health of the Member States of the European Region of WHO, meeting together for the first time at Frankfurt-am-Main on 7 and 8 December 1989, have adopted the attached European Charter on Environment and Health and have accordingly agreed upon the principles and strategies laid down therein as a firm commitment to action. In view of its environmental mandate, the Commission of the European Communities was specially invited to participate and, acting on behalf of the Community, also adopted the Charter as a guideline for future action by the Community in areas which lie within Community competence."

Entitlements and responsibilities

1. "Every individual is entitled to:

   - an environment conducive to the highest attainable level of health and well-being;
   - information and consultation on the state of the environment, and on plans, decisions, and activities likely to affect both the environment and health;
   - participation in the decision-making process.

2. "Every individual has a responsibility to contribute to the protection of the environment, in the interests of his or her own health and the health of others.

3. "All sections of society are responsible for protecting the environment and health as an intersectoral matter involving many disciplines; their respective duties should be clarified.

4. "Every public authority and agency at different levels, in its daily work, should cooperate with other sectors in order to resolve problems of the environment and health.

5. "Every government and public authority has the responsibility to protect the environment and to promote human health within the area under its jurisdiction, and to ensure that activities under its jurisdiction or control do not cause damage to human health in other states. Furthermore, each shares the common responsibility for safeguarding the global environment.

6. "Every public and private body should assess its activities and carry them out in such a way as to protect people's health from harmful effects related to the physical, chemical, biological, microbiological, and social environments. Each of these bodies should be accountable for its actions.

7. "The media play a key role in promoting awareness and a positive attitude towards protection of health and the environment. They are entitled to adequate and accurate information and should be encouraged to communicate this information effectively to the public.

8. "Nongovernmental organizations also play an important role in disseminating information to the public and promoting public awareness and response."

Principles for Public Policy

1. "Good health and well-being require a clean and harmonious environment in which physical, psychological, social, and aesthetic factors are all given their due importance. The environment should be regarded as a resource for improving living conditions and increasing well-being.

2. "The preferred approach should be to promote the principle of 'prevention is better than cure.'

3. "The health of every individual, especially those in vulnerable and high-risk groups, must be protected. Special attention should be paid to disadvantaged groups.

4. "Action on problems of the environment and health should be based on the best available scientific information.

5. "New policies, technologies, and developments should be introduced with prudence and not before appropriate prior assessment of the potential environmental and health impact. There should be a responsibility to show that they are not harmful to health or the environment.

6. "The health of individuals and communities should take clear precedence over considerations of economy and trade.

7. "All aspects of socioeconomic development that relate to the impact of the environment on health and well-being must be considered.

8. "The entire flow of chemicals, materials, products, and waste should be managed in such a way as to achieve optimal use of natural resources and to cause minimal contamination.

9. "Governments, public authorities, and private bodies should aim at both preventing and reducing adverse effects caused by potentially hazardous agents and degraded urban and rural environments.

10. "Environmental standards need to be continually reviewed to take account of new knowledge about the environment and health and of the effects of future economic development. Where applicable such standards should be harmonized.

11. "The principle should be applied whereby every public and private body that causes or may cause damage to the environment is made financially responsible (the polluter pays principle).

12. "Criteria and procedures to quantify, monitor, and evaluate environmental and health damage should be further developed and implemented.

13. "Trade and economic policies and development assistance programmes affecting the environment and health in foreign countries should comply with all the above principles. Export of environmental and health hazards should be avoided.

14. "Development assistance should promote sustainable development and the safeguarding and improvement of human health as one of its integral components."

Strategic Elements

The Charter states that "the environment should be managed as a positive resource for human health and well-being," and stipulates that "comprehensive strategies" be undertaken to achieve that end. Among those strategies the Charter specifies: the responsibility of public and private bodies to promulgate and implement appropriate regulations, the establishment of control measures and safety standards to reduce health risks, the use of appropriate technologies, and the creation of information systems and contingency plans to monitor and respond to health risks. The Charter also recommends a multi-disciplinary approach to epidemiological surveillance and "greater attention to all aspects of environmental health."

Priorities

The Charter specifies that governments and other public authorities should "pay particular attention" to a number of issues of the environment and health. Those issues include: "global disturbances of the environment," urban development, drinking water, microbiological and chemical safety of food, and the environmental impact of various fuels, chemicals, and wastes.

The Way Forward

The Charter states that member states of the European Region and the WHO Regional Office for Europe should undertake various actions, including: reversing negative trends in environmental health, increasing regional cooperation, strengthening international mechanisms for assessing potential hazards to health, and establishing a European Advisory Committee on the Environment and Health.

Introduction to *Healthy People 2010*

Described as "a comprehensive, nationwide health promotion and disease prevention agenda," Healthy People 2010: Understanding and Improving Health *"is designed to serve as a roadmap for improving the health of all people in the United States during the first decade of the 21st century." Below is the complete text of the introduction. Available via the Internet: http://www.health.gov/healthypeople/document/.*

INTRODUCTION

Healthy People 2010 presents a comprehensive, nationwide health promotion and disease prevention agenda. It is designed to serve as a roadmap for improving the health of all people in the United States during the first decade of the 21st century.

Like the preceding Healthy People 2000 initiative—which was driven by an ambitious, yet achievable, 10-year strategy for improving the nation's health by the end of the 20th century—Healthy People 2010 is committed to a single, overarching purpose: promoting health and preventing illness, disability, and premature death.

THE HISTORY BEHIND THE HEALTHY PEOPLE 2010 INITIATIVE

Healthy People 2010 builds on initiatives pursued over the past two decades. In 1979, *Healthy People: The Surgeon General's Report on Health Promotion and Disease Prevention* provided national goals for reducing premature deaths and preserving independence for older adults. In 1980, another report, *Promoting Health/Preventing Disease: Objectives for the Nation,* set forth 226 targeted health objectives for the Nation to achieve over the next 10 years.

Healthy People 2000: National Health Promotion and Disease Prevention Objectives, released in 1990, identified health improvement goals and objectives to be reached by the year 2000. The Healthy People 2010 initiative continues in this tradition as an instrument to improve health for the first decade of the 21st century.

THE DEVELOPMENT OF HEALTHY PEOPLE 2010 GOALS AND OBJECTIVES

Healthy People 2010 represents the ideas and expertise of a diverse range of individuals and organizations concerned about the nation's health. The Healthy People Consortium—an alliance of more than 350 national organizations and 250 State public health, mental health, substance abuse, and environmental agencies—conducted three national meetings on the development of Healthy People 2010. In addition, many individuals and organizations gave testimony about health priorities at five Healthy People 2010 regional meetings held in late 1998.

On two occasions—in 1997 and in 1998—the American public was given the opportunity to share its thoughts and ideas. More than 11,000 comments on draft materials were received by mail or via the Internet from individuals in every State, the District of Columbia, and Puerto Rico. All the comments received during the development of Healthy People 2010 can be viewed on the Healthy People Web site: http://www.health.gov/healthypeople/.

The final Healthy People 2010 objectives were developed by teams of experts from a variety of Federal agencies under the direction of Health and Human Services Secretary Donna Shalala, Assistant Secretary for Health and Surgeon General David Satcher, and former Assistant Secretaries for Health. The process was coordinated by the Office of Disease Prevention and Health Promotion, U.S. Department of Health and Human Services.

THE GOALS OF HEALTHY PEOPLE

Healthy People 2010 is designed to achieve two overarching goals:

- Increase quality and years of healthy life.
- Eliminate health disparities.

These two goals are supported by specific objectives in 28 focus areas. Each objective was developed with a target to be achieved by the year 2010.

THE RELATIONSHIP BETWEEN INDIVIDUAL AND COMMUNITY HEALTH

Over the years, it has become clear that individual health is closely linked to community health—the health of the community and environment in which individuals live, work, and play. Likewise, community health is profoundly affected by the collective beliefs, attitudes, and behaviors of everyone who lives in the community.

Indeed, the underlying premise of Healthy People 2010 is that the health of the individual is almost inseparable from the health of the larger community and that the health of every community in every State and territory determines the overall health status of the Nation. That is why the vision for Healthy People 2010 is "Healthy People in Healthy Communities."

HOW HEALTHY PEOPLE 2010 WILL IMPROVE THE NATION'S HEALTH

One of the most compelling and encouraging lessons learned from the Healthy People 2000 initiative is that we, as a nation, can make dramatic progress in improving the nation's health in a relatively short period of time. For example, during the past decade, we achieved significant reductions in infant mortality. Childhood vaccinations are at the highest levels ever recorded in the United States. Fewer teenagers are becoming parents. Overall, alcohol, tobacco, and illicit drug use is leveling off. Death rates for coronary heart disease and stroke have declined. Significant advances have been made in the diagnosis and treatment of cancer and in reducing unintentional injuries.

But we still have a long way to go. Diabetes and other chronic conditions continue to present a serious obstacle to public health. Violence and abusive behavior continue to ravage homes and communities across the country.

Mental disorders continue to go undiagnosed and untreated. Obesity in adults has increased 50 percent over the past two decades. Nearly 40 percent of adults engage in no leisure time physical activity. Smoking among adolescents has increased in the past decade. And HIV/AIDS remains a serious health problem, now disproportionately affecting women and communities of color.

Healthy People 2010 will be the guiding instrument for addressing these and emerging health issues, reversing unfavorable trends, and expanding past achievements in health.

THE KEY ROLE OF COMMUNITY PARTNERSHIPS

Community partnerships, particularly when they reach out to nontraditional partners, can be among the most effective tools for improving health in communities.

For the past two decades, Healthy People has been used as a strategic management tool for the federal government, states, communities, and many other public- and private-sector partners. Virtually all states, the District of Columbia, and Guam have developed their own Healthy People plans modeled after the national plan. Most states have tailored the national objectives to their specific needs.

Businesses; local governments; and civic, professional, and religious organizations also have been inspired by Healthy People to print immunization reminders, set up hotlines, change cafeteria menus, begin community recycling, establish worksite fitness programs, assess school health education curriculums, sponsor health fairs, and engage in myriad other activities.

EVERYONE CAN HELP ACHIEVE THE
HEALTHY PEOPLE 2010 OBJECTIVES

Addressing the challenge of health improvement is a shared responsibility that requires the active participation and leadership of the federal government, states, local governments, policymakers, health care providers, professionals, business executives, educators, community leaders, and the American public itself. Although administrative responsibility for the Healthy People 2010 initiative rests in the U.S. Department of Health and Human Services, representatives of all these diverse groups shared their experience, expertise, and ideas in developing the Healthy People 2010 goals and objectives.

Healthy People 2010, however, is just the beginning. The biggest challenges still stand before us, and we all have a role in building a healthier nation.

Regardless of your age, gender, education level, income, race, ethnicity, cultural customs, language, religious beliefs, disability, sexual orientation, geographic location, or occupation, Healthy People 2010 is designed to be a valuable resource in determining how you can participate most effectively in improving the nation's health. Perhaps you will recognize the need to be a more active participant in decisions affecting your own health or the health of your children or loved ones. Perhaps you will assume a leadership role in promoting healthier behaviors in your neighborhood or community. Or perhaps you will use your influence and social stature to advocate for and implement policies and programs that can improve dramatically the health of dozens, hundreds, thousands, or even millions of people.

SOURCE: U.S. Department of Health and Human Services (November 2000). *Healthy People 2010: Understanding and Improving Health*, 2nd edition. Washington, DC: U.S. Government Printing Office.

Ottawa Charter for Health Promotion

Proclaimed at the First International Conference on Health Promotion Ottawa, Canada, November 17–21, 1986. Below, some portions of the Charter have been excerpted and others summarized. The full text of the Charter is available via the Internet: http://www.who.dk/policy/ottawa.htm.

Health Promotion

"Health promotion is the process of enabling people to increase control over, and to improve, their health. To reach a state of complete physical, mental, and social well-being, an individual or group must be able to identify and to realize aspirations, to satisfy needs, and to change or cope with the environment. Health is, therefore, seen as a resource for everyday life, not the objective of living. Health is a positive concept emphasizing social and personal resources, as well as physical capacities. Therefore, health promotion is not just the responsibility of the health sector, but goes beyond healthy lifestyles to well-being.

Prerequisites for Health

"The fundamental conditions and resources for health are peace, shelter, education, food, income, a stable ecosystem, sustainable resources, social justice, and equity. Improvement in health requires a secure foundation in these basic prerequisites.

Advocate

"Good health is a major resource for social, economic, and personal development and an important dimension of quality of life. Political, economic, social, cultural, environmental, behavioral, and biological factors can all favor health or be harmful to it. Health promotion action aims at making these conditions favorable through advocacy for health.

Enable

"Health promotion focuses on achieving equity in health. Health promotion action aims at reducing differences in current health status and ensuring equal opportunities and resources to enable all people to achieve their fullest health potential. This includes a secure foundation in a supportive environment, access to information, life skills, and opportunities for making healthy choices. People cannot achieve their fullest health potential unless they are able to take control of those things which determine their health. This must apply equally to women and men.

Mediate

"The prerequisites and prospects for health cannot be ensured by the health sector alone. More importantly, health promotion demands coordinated action by all concerned: by governments, by health and other social and economic sectors, by nongovernmental and voluntary organizations, by local authorities, by industry, and by the media. People in all walks of life are involved as individuals, families, and communities. Professional and social groups and health personnel have a major responsibility to mediate between differing interests in society for the pursuit of health.

"Health promotion strategies and programs should be adapted to the local needs and possibilities of individual countries and regions to take into account differing social, cultural, and economic systems."

Health Promotion Action Means

The Charter defines health promotion in terms of the following activities: building healthy public policy in the full range of administrative and legislative action; creating supportive environments via a socioecological approach to health; strengthening community action and democratic planning processes; developing personal skills via education; and reorienting health services toward health promotion in addition to curative services.

Moving into the Future

Citing caring, holism, and ecology as central issues, the signatories to the Charter pledged to promote health in various ways, including: advocating a clear political commitment to health and equity in all sectors; counteracting trends and products that harm health; reorienting health services toward health promotion; recognizing health and its maintenance as a major social investment.

Call for International Action

The Charter concludes with a statement calling on the World Health Organization and other international bodies to advocate the promotion of health.

The Nuremberg Code

Below is an excerpt from the Nuremberg Code. The complete text is available via the Internet: http://www.ushmm.org/research/doctors/Nuremberg_Code.htm.

Permissible Medical Experiments

The great weight of the evidence before us is to the effect that certain types of medical experiments on human beings, when kept within reasonably well-defined bounds, conform to the ethics of the medical profession generally. The protagonists of the practice of human experimentation justify their views on the basis that such experiments yield results for the good of society that are unprocurable by other methods or means of study. All agree, however, that certain basic principles must be observed in order to satisfy moral, ethical, and legal concepts:

1. The voluntary consent of the human subject is absolutely essential. This means that the person involved should have legal capacity to give consent; should be so situated as to be able to

exercise free power of choice, without the intervention of any element of force, fraud, deceit, duress, over-reaching, or other ulterior form of constraint or coercion; and should have sufficient knowledge and comprehension of the elements of the subject matter involved as to enable him to make an understanding and enlightened decision. This latter element requires that before the acceptance of an affirmative decision by the experimental subject there should be made known to him the nature, duration, and purpose of the experiment; the method and means by which it is to be conducted; all inconveniences and hazards reasonably to be expected; and the effects upon his health or person which may possibly come from his participation in the experiment. The duty and responsibility for ascertaining the quality of the consent rests upon each individual who initiates, directs, or engages in the experiment. It is a personal duty and responsibility which may not be delegated to another with impunity.

2. The experiment should be such as to yield fruitful results for the good of society, unprocurable by other methods or means of study, and not random and unnecessary in nature.

3. The experiment should be so designed and based on the results of animal experimentation and a knowledge of the natural history of the disease or other problem under study that the anticipated results will justify the performance of the experiment.

4. The experiment should be so conducted as to avoid all unnecessary physical and mental suffering and injury.

5. No experiment should be conducted where there is an a priori reason to believe that death or disabling injury will occur; except, perhaps, in those experiments where the experimental physicians also serve as subjects.

6. The degree of risk to be taken should never exceed that determined by the humanitarian importance of the problem to be solved by the experiment.

7. Proper preparations should be made and adequate facilities provided to protect the experimental subject against even remote possibilities of injury, disability, or death.

8. The experiment should be conducted only by scientifically qualified persons. The highest degree of skill, and care should be required through all stages of the experiment of those who conduct or engage in the experiment.

9. During the course of the experiment the human subject should be at liberty to bring the experiment to an end if he has reached the physical or mental state where continuation of the experiment seems to him to be impossible.

10. During the course of the experiment the scientist in charge must be prepared to terminate the experiment at any stage, if he

has probable cause to believe, in the exercise of the good faith, superior skill, and careful judgment required of him, that a continuation of the experiment is likely to result in injury, disability, or death to the experimental subject.

SOURCE: *Trials of War Criminals before the Nuremberg Military Tribunals under Control Council Law No. 10,* vol. 2 (1949). Washington, DC: U.S. General Printing Office.

Annotated Bibliography

This bibliography is divided into three sections. The first two contain important historical and modern works on public health, from 2000 <B.<C.<E. to the present. These works are presented chronologically so as to give a sense of the development of public health, and of the various disciplines that make up the field. The third section is devoted to works on the history of health, medicine, and public health. These are listed in alphabetical order, by author. It is hoped that this annotated bibliography will aid the reader in understanding the extraordinary progress of the field of public health.

CLASSICS OF PUBLIC HEALTH AND MEDICINE

Code of Hammurabi. This code, dating from c. 2000 <B.<C.<E., is among the oldest extant medical documents. It suggests ways to stay healthy, and includes rules of behavior and fee schedules for the priest-physicians of ancient Babylon, providing interesting insights into Babylonian civilization. It is summarized in H. E. Sigerist, *History of Medicine*, Vol. 1, *Primitive and Archaic Medicine* (New York: Oxford University Press, 1951).

Hippocrates. "Airs, Waters, Places" and "On Epidemics," in *Hippocratic Writings*, ed. G. R. Lloyd (New York: Penguin, 1978). The surviving documents from the medical school of Hippocrates of Cos, located at Epidaurus c. 440–330 <B.<C.<E., reveal some of the best features of classical Greek civilization. They cover many aspects of medicine, including clinical descriptions of diseases, as well as the oath that is still used as the foundation for good medical conduct and much teaching of medical ethics. "Airs, Waters, Places" was the first text on environmental health; it includes ideas on how individuals and communities can protect good health. "On Epidemics" contains many good descriptions of contagious and other diseases of public health importance.

Regimen Sanitas Salernitarum. Translated by P. Parente as *The Regime of Health of the Medical School of Salerno* (New York: Vantage, 1967). First published in 1484, the material gathered in this text of the Salerno medical school dates from the late thirteenth century and consists of double-rhymed Latin hexameters describing many sensible dietetic and hygienic precepts, including avoidance of overeating and the desirability of personal cleanliness.

Fracastorius (Girolamo Fracastoro). *De contagione* (Venice: Lucaeantonij Iuntae Florentini, 1546). Translated by W. C. Wright as *On Contagion* (New York and London: Putnam, 1930). This is the first systematic description of ways infection can be transmitted—by direct contact, via infected items such as clothing and utensils, or by droplets, as in coughing and sneezing. Fracastorius did not, however, identify vector-borne transmission or the role of contaminated water and food. Fracastorius also wrote a mock-heroic poem, *Syphilis, sive morbis gallicus* (1530), about a swineherd, Syphilis, afflicted with the disease that ever since has carried his name. Fracastorius recognized that this disease is sexually transmitted and he suggested that diseases might be transmitted by invisible particles, and was therefore ahead of his time in hinting at a "germ theory" of disease.

Graunt, John. *Natural and Political Observations, Mentioned in a Following Index, and Made upon the Bills of Mortality* (London, 1662; reprint, North Stratford, NH: Ayer Company Publishers, 1975). Graunt was the first to use records of deaths and their causes to analyze the state of a population's health. His analysis of the London population showed that male mortality rates were higher than those of females at all ages from birth onward, revealed urban-rural differences in mortality rates, and showed the fluctuations of those rates due to epidemics, notably of the plague. Graunt's work was the founding text for the science of vital statistics.

Petty, William. *An Essay Concerning the Multiplication of Mankind; Together with Another Essay on Political Arithmetic* (London and Dublin: 1682). Petty's work emulated Graunt's. He examined records of ages and causes of death in London, Dublin, and other cities, emphasizing the economic implications of premature deaths among those who produced the nation's wealth.

Halley, Edmund. "An Estimate of the Degrees of Mortality of Mankind, Drawn from Curious Tables of the Births and Funerals at the City of Breslaw, with an Attempt to Ascertain the Price of Annuities upon Lives." *Philosophical Transactions of the Royal Society* 17(1683):596–610. An important advance in vital statistics, this work provided the foundation for life insurance and the work of actuaries.

Ramazzini, Bernardino. *De morbis artificum diatriba* (Modena: 1713). Translated by W. C. Wright as *Diseases of Workers* (New York: Academy of Medicine, 1964). A descriptive catalogue of the illnesses—mostly attributable to exposure on the job—commonly found among workers in many occupations. This is the first text on occupational medicine.

Lind, James. *A Treatise of the Scurvy* (Edinburgh: 1753; reprint, Edinburgh: University of Edinburgh Press, 1953). This work is often cited as the earliest example of a clinical trial. Lind used pairs of sailors who were allocated various dietary regimens to demonstrate that small daily doses of lime juice prevented the onset of scurvy on long sea voyages. Lind thus showed also that this disease was not contagious but associated with a dietary deficiency.

Frank, Johan Pieter. *System einer vollständigen medicinischen Polizey* (Vienna and Budapest: 1779). Translated by E. Lesky as *A System of Complete Medical Police* (Baltimore, MD: Johns Hopkins University Press, 1976). Frank's massive, multivolume work discusses many aspects of personal and public health and prescribes rules and laws for such practices as city cleanliness, the inspection of food premises, and the regulation of prostitution. It also contains many suggestions about diet and lifestyle. It is the foundation text for public health law and adopts a paternalist approach that has prevailed until at least the middle of the twentieth century.

Jenner, Edward. *An Inquiry into the Causes and Effects of the Variolae Vaccinae* (London: 1798; reprint, London: Dawsons, 1966). Jenner describes his successful experiment with cowpox vaccine in this short book, which may be the most important single work in the field of public health published anywhere in the past millennium. This work led directly to the World Health Organization campaign responsible for the eradication of smallpox, among the most deadly of all the contagious epidemic diseases, less than two hundred years later.

Malthus, Thomas. *An Essay on the Principle of Population, or a View of Its Past and Present Effects on Human Happiness with an Inquiry into Our Prospects Respecting the Future Removal or Mitigation of the Evils Which It Occasions* (London: J. Johnson, 1798; reprint, Cambridge: Cambridge University Press, 1992). Malthus uses simple arithmetical calculations to show that human reproductive rates would sooner or later outstrip the capacity of food supplies to sustain the numbers in the population. His method is sound, but his predictions of imminent famine are invalid because he does not allow for the increases in food production in the Americas and Australia in the nineteenth century. All that may have been wrong is his time scale: The Malthusian crisis could yet overtake humanity.

Louis, Pierre Charles Alexandre. *Recherches anatomico-pathologiques sur la phtisie* (Paris: C. Gabon, 1825). Translated by W. H. Walshe as *Researches on Phthisis: Anatomical, Pathological, and Therapeutical* (London: Sydenham Society, 1844). This work and others by Louis laid the foundations for statistical analysis of medical data and was instrumental in establishing the science of medical statistics.

Henle, Friedrich Gustav Jacob. *Von den Miasmen und Contagien* (Berlin: 1840). Translated by G. Rosen as *On Miasmata and Contagia* (Baltimore, MD: Johns Hopkins University Press, 1938). Henle's critical analysis of the characteristics of contagion is among the works that stimulated the rise of the germ theory of disease.

Chadwick, Edwin. *Report on the Sanitary Condition of the Labouring Population of Great Britain* (London: Her Majesty's Stationery Office, 1842; reprint, Edinburgh: University of Edinburgh Press, 1965). A monumental work by a dedicated civil servant, Chadwick's report describes the appalling and unsanitary conditions under which the vast majority of people lived in the new cities that grew up in the early phases of the Industrial Revolution. This work set the scene for new legislation regulating housing conditions, and was thus seminal in transforming sanitary and hygienic conditions that were the most important single contributing factor for the improvements in public health in the second half of the nineteenth century in Britain and in other industrial nations that followed Britain's lead.

Holmes, Oliver Wendell. "The Contagiousness of Puerperal Fever." *New England Quarterly Journal of Medicine and Surgery* 1(1842):503–540. Holmes, a Boston physician, published in this paper the evidence that women in child labor who were attended by physicians who washed their hands before attending them were much less likely to get puerperal fever, which at that time caused many maternal deaths soon after childbirth. Unfortunately, most of his colleagues ignored his findings and women continued to die of this preventable obstetric disaster.

Shattuck, Lemuel. *Report to the Committee of the City Council Appointed to Obtain the Census of Boston for the Year 1845* (Boston: 1846; reprint, New York: Arno Press, 1976). This work is a comprehensive census assessment of the city of Boston in the mid-nineteenth century, a landmark in statistical census data and its contribution to public health. It includes twenty-two sections on various features of Boston's population and living conditions, including birthplace, water supply, education, health, occupation, wealth, marriages, and deaths.

Semmelweis, Ignaz. *Die Aetiologie, der Begriff und die Prophylaxis des Kindbetfiebers* (Pest, Wien, and Leipzig: C.A. Hartleben's Verlags-Expedition, 1861). Translated by F. P. Murphy as *The Etiology, the Concept, and the Prophylaxis of Childbed Fever* (Birmingham, AL: Classics of Medicine Library, 1981). Semmelweis's work is among the first uses of epidemiological methods to establish the causal relationship of behavior (e.g., personal hygiene) to occurrence of a deadly disease, puerperal sepsis, which was killing many women whose child labor was supervised by physicians who did not wash their hands. These findings, like those of Holmes, were rejected by the conservative medical establishment in Vienna. However,

Semmelweis's work, published fifteen years after he wrote it, is epidemiologically excellent.

Drake, Daniel. *A Systematic Treatise, Historical, Etiological, and Practical on the Principal Diseases of the Interior Valley of North America* (Philadelphia, PA: Lippincott, Grambo, & Co., 1854; reprint, New York: Franklin Burt Publisher, 1971). A classic of early American medicine, initially published in installments from 1850 through 1854, this is a descriptive account of the findings from a survey Drake conducted to investigate the health and sanitation problems encountered by pioneering settlers as they colonized the American West.

Shattuck, Lemuel, et al. *Report of the Sanitary Commission of Massachusetts* (1850; reprint, Cambridge: Harvard University Press, 1950). The American replication of Chadwick's report, this work was likewise instrumental in leading to improved public health in the industrial heartland of the United States in the late nineteenth century.

Snow, John. *On the Mode of Communication of Cholera* (London: Churchill, 1855). This monograph describes Snow's rigorous logical analysis of the facts that led him to conduct his epidemiological investigations establishing the role of drinking water polluted with sewage in the transmission of the agent that causes cholera. It is a seminal work on epidemiology that can still be used to teach the subject today.

Darwin, Charles. *On the Origin of Species by Means of Natural Selection; or, The Preservation of Favoured Races in the Struggle for Life* (London: John Murray, 1859; reprint, Cambridge: Harvard University Press, 1990). The most significant work on human biology of the past millennium. Darwin presents evidence that establishes beyond any doubt that living creatures, including humans, have undergone prolonged evolutionary changes extending over several billion years since life first appeared on Earth. Humans have been shown by subsequent paleontological discoveries to have evolved over the past 4 million to 6 million years.

Nightingale, Florence. *Notes on Hospitals* (London: Longman 1863; reprint, New York: Garland, 1989). Nightingale, famous as the founder of modern nursing practice, was a major figure in public health and vital statistics, a member of the London Epidemiological Society, and a prominent social reformer. In this, her most important book, she describes and discusses hygienic design of hospitals and outlines the ways in which records of patient care in hospitals could be used to compile sickness statistics.

Galton, Francis. *Hereditary Genius: An Inquiry into its Laws and Consequences* (London: Macmillan, 1869; reprint, New York: St. Martins, 1978). A classic of human genetics that treats the topic with attention to mathematical probabilities, this work has become a template for later works on biostatistics, such as Karl Pearson's equally significant work, *The Grammar of Science* (New York: Charles Scribner's Sons, 1895; reprint, Gloucester, MA: Peter Smith, 1969).

Farr, William. *Vital Statistics; a Memorial Volume of Selections from the Reports and Writings of William Farr*, ed. N. A. Humphreys (London: The Sanitary Institute, 1885; reprint, Metuchen, NJ: Scarecrow Press, 1975). Farr's many contributions to vital statistics and epidemiology are scattered throughout his annual reports and other writings. Humphreys compiled them in this commemorative volume.

Pasteur, Louis. *Oeuvres* (Paris: Masson, 1922–1939). Pasteur's scientific papers appeared over many years in the mid- to late-nineteenth century. Summaries in English are found in a 1952 biography by René Dubos, *Louis Pasteur: Freelance of Science* (Boston: Little, Brown).

Koch, Robert. *Gesammelte Werke* (Leipzig: G. Thieme, 1912). Koch's prolific publications are scattered among many sources and are not readily accessible. Several summary accounts of his life and work are available. Koch made his major discoveries, including the tubercle bacillus and the cholera vibrio, in the 1880s. One good recent account in English, with summaries of key contributions, appears in Alfred S. Evans, *Causation and Disease* (New York: Plenum, 1993), pp. 18–31.

Virchow, Rudolph Ludwig Karl. *Gesammelte Abhandlungen aus dem Gebiete der öffentlichen Medicin und der Seuchenlehre* (Berlin: A. Hirschwald, 1879). Translated by R. Rather as *Collected Essays on Public Health and Epidemiology* (Canton, MA: Science History Publications, 1985). This two-volume collection contains many of Virchow's most important contributions to public health, mostly dating from the last three decades of the nineteenth century.

Finlay, Carlos Eduardo. *Fiebre amarilla experimental* (Havana: Manzana Central, 1904). Translated by R. Matas as *The Mosquito Hypothetically Considered as an Agent in the Transmission of Yellow Fever Poison* (Chapel Hill, NC: Delta Omega Society, 1989). This work by the great Cuban physician and epidemiologist Finlay led to the work undertaken by Finlay and Walter Reed that elucidated the epidemiology of yellow fever.

Simon, John. *English Sanitary Institutions Reviewed in Their Course of Development and in Some of Their Political and Social Relations* (London: Cassell, 1890; reprint, New York: Johnson Reprint Company, 1970). Simon was the first Chief Medical Officer of England and Wales, a physician, and a public health specialist. Of his many books, this best summarizes his life's work and his professional outlook.

Ross, Ronald. "The Role of the Mosquito in the Evolution of the Malaria Parasite." *Lancet* 2(1898):488–489. Among Ross's numerous publications, this is the most important, being the first description of the essential role of mosquitoes in the transmission of malaria.

Goldberger, Joseph. *Goldberger on Pellagra*, ed. M. Terris (Baton Rouge: Louisiana State University Press, 1964). This is a collection of Goldberger's papers on pellagra, a common seasonal disease in the southern United States in the late nineteenth and early twentieth centuries. Goldberger, sometimes with coauthors, wrote many papers describing his research, establishing that dietary deficiency of vitamin B_2 caused pellagra.

Sheppard-Towner Act. In passing the Sheppard-Towner Act (the Infant and Maternity Act of 1921), the U.S. Congress made funds available, to be matched by the states, to assist in developing maternal and child health programs throughout the country. Opposition by medical associations and others to this "intrusion" of the federal government into medical care led to the act's lapse in 1927, but the precedent led to its reestablishment in the 1935 Social Security Act.

Winslow, Charles-Edward Amory. *The Evolution and Significance of the Modern Public Health Campaign* (New Haven, CT: Yale University Press, 1923). A seminal work on the framework of organized public health services, this volume set the scene for public health in the industrial nations, especially in the United States, throughout much of the remainder of the twentieth century. Winslow was one of the leading creative thinkers in public health in the early twentieth century.

Sydenstricker, Edgar. *The Challenge of Facts; Selected Public Health Papers of Edgar Sydenstricker*, ed. R. V. Kasius (New York: Prodist, 1974). Sydenstricker was one of the leading figures in American public health in the late nineteenth and early twentieth centuries, during which time he brought to the discipline a renewed intellectual rigor combined with epidemiological insights.

Frost, Wade Hampton. *Papers of Wade Hampton Frost, M.D.; A Contribution to Epidemiological Methods*, ed. K. F. Maxcy (New York: Commonwealth Fund, 1977). Frost (1880–1938), the leading epidemiologist of his time, was a professor and head of epidemiology at the Johns Hopkins University School of Hygiene and Public Health.

Fleming, Alexander. "On the Antibacterial Action of Cultures of a Penicillium, with Special Reference to Their Use in the Isolation of B Influenzae." *British Journal of Experimental Pathology* 10(1929):226–236. The paper reports Fleming's original observation, which led to the development by Fleming, Howard Florey, and Ernst Chain of penicillin, the first true antibiotic.

Watson, James D., and Crick, Francis H. "Molecular Structure of Nucleic Acids: A Structure for Deoxyribose Nucleic Acid." *Nature* 171(4356)(1953):737–738. This is the first paper describing the molecular structure of DNA, from which the science of molecular genetics and the human genome project have developed.

IMPORTANT MODERN MONOGRAPHS, REPORTS, AND OTHER DOCUMENTS

Sinclair, Upton. *The Jungle* (New York: Doubleday, Page, and Co., 1906). A striking exposé of the grossly unsanitary conditions that prevailed in the slaughtering segment of the meat industry, Sinclair's work aroused public revulsion, prompted political action to clean up the situation, and inspired the century-long campaign in the United States for pure food.

Beveridge, Sir William. *Social Insurance and Allied Services* (London: His Majesty's Stationery Office, 1942). As chairman of the writing committee, Beveridge organized this report that became the blueprint for the British National Health Service. Much of what Beveridge recommended was implemented by the Labour government that took office in the United Kingdom near the end of World War II.

Commission on Chronic Illness. *Chronic Illness in the United States*, Vol.1, *Prevention* (Cambridge, MA: Harvard University Press, 1957). This is the first volume of a four-volume set of reports on major health problems in the United States with causes other than infectious pathogens. The first volume explains the concepts of primary and secondary prevention and emphasizes the importance of prevention as the best way to control these conditions. Volume 2 of the Commission's report deals with long-term care, Volume 3 considers chronic illness in a rural community, and Volume 4 addresses chronic illness in a large city.

Morris, Jeremy N. *Uses of Epidemiology* (Edinburgh and London: E. and S. Livingstone, 1957). This modern medical classic summarizes the evidence on causes of many noncommunicable diseases, notably coronary heart disease, lung cancer, chronic bronchitis, and the chronic disabling disorders of bones and joints. Later editions update the evidence, but the essential ideas are all contained in this first edition.

Dubos, René J. *Mirage of Health: Utopias, Progress, and Biological Change* (New York: Harper, 1959). This book emphasizes the incompatibility of complete freedom from disease with the process of living. It was one of the early works concerning the limitations of medicine in the search for the solution of all health problems.

Carson, Rachel. *Silent Spring* (Boston: Houghton Mifflin, 1962). A foundation text of the modern environmental movement, Carson's book is a passionate plea to desist from using pesticides that kill insect species with which humans are interdependent.

Royal College of Physicians. *Smoking and Health* (London: Royal College of Physicians, 1962). The work by the Royal College of Physicians was the first authoritative report by a responsible national organization to identify cigarette smoking as a causal agent of lung and other respiratory cancers. This document drew upon all the work published up to that time and was in most respects a more cogent statement than the American one that followed it two years later.

U.S. Public Health Service. *Smoking and Health, Report of the Advisory Committee to the Surgeon General of the Public Health Service* (Washington, DC: U.S. Government Printing Office, 1964). This document is the first American report on the epidemic of cigarette addiction and its causal relationship to cancer. The report was followed by annual reports that continued for many years, reinforcing and adding to the original evidence and demonstrating that tobacco smoking is also a major risk factor for coronary heart disease, emphysema, and various forms of cancer. These subsequent reports also addressed the addictive nature of nicotine and many other harmful consequences of tobacco use in any form.

Roemer, Milton I. *The Organization of Medical Care under Social Security* (Geneva: International Labour Office, 1969). A masterly survey of how collective (generally tax-supported) payment for medical care was arranged in many nations.

President's Committee on Health Education. *Report of the President's Committee on Health Education* (New York: New York Public Affairs Institute, 1973). Appointed by President Richard M. Nixon, the committee recommended establishing a national focal point for health education. The report led to the passage of the National Health Information and Health Promotion Act of 1976, which launched health education programs in Public Health Service agencies.

Lalonde, Marc. *A New Perspective on the Health of Canadians: A Working Document* (Ottawa: 1974). An epochal report (drafted mainly by two career civil servants, Hubert Laframboise and D. D. Gellman, under the direction of Lalonde, then Minister for National Health and Welfare), this document has shaped public health policy in Canada and many other countries.

Sheps, Cecil G. *Higher Education for Public Health: A Report of the Milbank Memorial Fund Commission* (New York: Prodist, 1976). This report constitutes a prescription, written under the commission's chair Sheps, for improved teaching of the sciences and arts of public health.

U.S. Public Health Service, Office of the Surgeon General. *Healthy People: The Surgeon General's Report on Health Promotion and Disease Prevention* (Washington, DC: U.S. Government Printing Office, 1979). This comprehensive overview of the state of health of the American people was the first report by the U. S. Surgeon General on health promotion and disease prevention.

U.S. Public Health Service. *Promoting Health, Preventing Disease: Objectives for the Nation* (Washington, DC: U.S. Department of Health and Human Services, 1980). A necessary sequel to *Healthy People*, this document spelled out actions needed to improve health, with target dates by which measurable improvements could be achieved. It is a benchmark document.

Working Group on Inequalities in Health. *Report of the Working Group on Inequalities in Health* (London: Department of Health and Social Services, 1980). Known as the Black Report, the document was commissioned in the late 1970s by the Labour government of Britain, was submitted to the Conservative government led by Margaret Thatcher, and was subsequently suppressed for political reasons. It was published in 1982 as *Inequalities in Health* (London: Penguin) under the names of two of the members of the working group, Peter Townsend and Nick Davidson. (Sir Douglas Black, who had chaired the group, was unable to add his name because of the official position he held, but the report has always been identified with him.) This report was the first definitive statement of the underlying social and economic reasons that in many countries chronic illness, disability, and premature death do not affect all people equally, but disproportionately affect those in the lowest socioeconomic strata.

Barkan, Ilyse D. "Industry Invites Regulation: The Passage of the Pure Food and Drug Act of 1906." *American Journal of Public Health* 75(1)(1985):18–26. An account of

Annotated Bibliography

how the continuing effort in the United States to safeguard food and drugs was initiated following the disclosure of the commercial production of adulterated and unsanitary food, particularly the public outrage following the publication of Upton Sinclair's *The Jungle.*

National Academy of Sciences, Institute of Medicine. *The Future of Public Health* (Washington, DC: National Academy Press, 1988). An important review, this report is constructively critical of the way public health services were conducted in the United States.

Guinta, Marguerite A., and Allegrante, John P. "The President's Committee on Health Education: A 20-Year Retrospective on Its Politics and Policy Impact." *American Journal of Public Health* 82(1992):1033–1041. This article analyzes the committee's origins, methods, and impact on subsequent developments during the period in which national health policy began to emphasize health promotion.

U.S. Public Health Service, Office on Smoking and Health. *Reducing the Consequences of Smoking–Twenty-Five Years of Progress: A Report of the Surgeon General* (Rockville, MD: U.S. Department of Health and Human Services, 1989). This review of the twenty-five years since the Surgeon General's report of 1964 summarizes the voluminous evidence of and reviews the progress made in the effort to control the smoking epidemic. All the annual reports of the Surgeon General on the health consequences of smoking are worth studying.

U.S. Preventive Services Task Force. *Guide to Clinical Preventive Services: An Assessment of the Effectiveness of 169 Interventions* (Washington, DC: U.S. Public Health Service, Office of Disease Prevention and Health Promotion, 1989). This report is an evidence-based critical analysis of ways to promote good health and prevent many important common diseases, such as various kinds of cancer. It was followed by several others, including, in 1994, the *Clinicians' Handbook of Preventive Services: Putting Prevention into Practice* (Washington, DC: U.S. Department of Health and Human Services).

Airhihenbuwa, Collins O. *Health and Culture: Beyond the Western Paradigm* (Thousand Oaks, CA: Sage Publications, 1995). This book challenges some of the assumptions about health and health promotion that are a product of Western history and culture, drawing contrasts with African history and health concepts.

World Commission on Environment and Development. *Our Common Future: The World Commission on Environment and Development* (Oxford: Oxford University Press, 1987). This commission was headed by Gro Harlem Brundtland, then prime minister of Norway and later director of the World Health Organization. The report, also known as the Brundtland Report, provides the basic arguments concerning the need for sustainable development of the planet and the interconnectedness of global processes of economic and social development with the planetary biosphere.

Rose, Geoffrey A. *The Strategy of Preventive Medicine* (Oxford: Oxford University Press, 1992). A slim volume that expands on ideas first presented in Rose's 1985 paper, "Sick Individuals and Sick Populations" (*International Journal of Epidemiology* 14:32–38), this book emphasizes the importance of dealing with both individuals and groups to control public health problems.

Canadian Task Force on the Periodic Health Examination. *Canadian Guide to Clinical Preventive Health Care* (Ottawa: Minister of Supply and Services, 1994). The Canadian Task Force preceded the U.S. Preventive Services Task Force. In its first report, in 1979, the task force introduced the concept of the hierarchy of evidence, assigning the highest rank to evidence based on randomized controlled trials. This and subsequent work by the Canadian Task Force led to the development of evidence-based medicine.

U.S. Department of Health and Human Services, Office of the Surgeon General. *Physical Activity and Health: A Report of the Surgeon General* (Atlanta, GA: Centers for Disease Control and Prevention, 1996). A comprehensive review of the evidence that physical activity helps to promote good health for most people.

U.S. Public Health Service Functions Project. *The Public Health Service: An Agenda for the Twenty-First Century* (Washington, DC: U.S. Public Health Service, 1997). At the beginning of the new millennium, the Public Health Service outlined the major public health tasks for the twenty-first century. These tasks are substantially different from those put forward at the beginning of the twentieth century.

U.S. Public Health Service. *Healthy People 2010: The Surgeon General's Report on Health Promotion and Disease Prevention* (Washington, DC: U.S. Department of Health and Human Services, 2001). This is the third such decennial planning document, following those in 1980 (for 1990) and in 1990 (for 2000), setting forth goals and specific health objectives for the United States. The 2010 statement includes two broad goals: to increase the quality and years of healthy life, and to eliminate health disparities among and between racial, ethnic, and other groups. It is available online at http://www.health.gov/healthypeople/Document/.

World Health Organization. *World Health Report* (Geneva: WHO). In addition to statistical summaries and overviews of prominent world public health problems, this annual publication is subtitled to indicate the areas emphasized each year. It is available online at http://www.who.int.

WORKS ON THE HISTORY OF HEALTH, MEDICINE, AND PUBLIC HEALTH

Ackerman, Evelyn B. *Health Care in the Parisian Countryside, 1800–1914* (New Brunswick, NJ: Rutgers University Press, 1990). This examination of how the French rural population perceived and dealt with illness gives insights into the social history of health in the nineteenth century. Separate chapters deal with public health efforts, cholera epidemics, and the bacteriological revolution.

Brockington, C. Fraser. *A Short History of Public Health*, 2nd edition (London: Churchill, 1966). This good brief historical review gives more emphasis to contributions by British and European public health workers.

Brodeur, Paul. *The Asbestos Hazard* (New York: New York Academy of Sciences, 1980). In this book aimed at workers and the general population, Brodeur provides an overview of the history of asbestos use and the diseases that it causes. He discusses the pioneering work of Irving Selikoff and his colleagues at Mt. Sinai Medical School. The international scope of the problem is described, as is the resistance that needed to be overcome before the start of concerted public health efforts.

Bullough, Bonnie, and Rosen, George. *Preventive Medicine in the United States, 1900–1990: Trends and Interpretations* (Canton, MA: Science History, 1992). This review of progress through most of the twentieth century is well referenced, with emphasis on public health and some discussion of trends in clinical preventive medicine.

Chesler, Ellen. *Woman of Valor: Margaret Sanger and the Birth Control Movement in America* (New York: Simon & Schuster, 1992). Sanger persistently posed the question: Whose body is it? She brought her nursing experience to the Lower East Side of New York City and, in 1916, opened the first birth control clinic in the United States. After several weeks, the police raided it and put Sanger in jail. She went on to spearhead the birth control movement through her writings, lectures, and international conferences.

Curtain, Philip D. *Death by Migration: Europe's Encounter with the Tropical World in the Nineteenth Century* (Cambridge: Cambridge University Press, 1989). Curtain provides an account of the interaction of susceptible populations with pathogens to which they had little or no (inherited) resistance.

Fee, Elizabeth, and Acheson, Roy M., eds. *A History of Education in Public Health* (Oxford: Oxford University Press, 1991). A comprehensive survey, this history includes an account of the rise of schools of public health in the United States and elsewhere.

Garrett, Laurie. *The Coming Plague: Newly Emerging Diseases in a World out of Balance* (New York: Farrar, Straus, and Giroux, 1994). A comprehensive survey of new and emerging infections by a first-class science reporter, this book about possible "future history" is highly recommended.

Garrison, Fielding H. *An Introduction to the History of Medicine*, 4th edition (Philadelphia, PA: Saunders, 1929). The definitive work on the history of medicine, this book is still as reliable as it was when first written.

Greenwood, Major. *Medical Statistics from Graunt to Farr* (Cambridge: Cambridge University Press, 1948; reprint, New York: Arno Press, 1977) and *Some British Pioneers of Social Medicine* (Oxford: Oxford University Press, 1948; reprint, Freeport, NY: Books for Libraries, 1970). These are two short works on the history of aspects of public health by the great pioneer epidemiologist who taught at the London School of Hygiene and Tropical Medicine in the 1930s and 1940s.

Hamilton, Alice. *Exploring the Dangerous Trades* (Boston: Northeastern University Press, 1985). An autobiography by a pioneer woman in occupational health, the work describes her personal and professional experiences during a lifetime of work in occupational health and industrial hygiene.

Hamlin, Christopher. *The Science of Impurity: Water Analysis in Nineteenth Century Britain* (Berkeley, CA: University of California Press, 1991). A history of early water science, this book places the sanitation issues of Great Britain during that formative period of public health into historical, philosophical, and social science perspectives.

Lilienfeld, Abraham M., ed. *Times, Places, and Persons; Aspects of the History of Epidemiology* (Baltimore, MD: Johns Hopkins University Press, 1980). These proceedings of a colloquium on the history of epidemiology contain addresses by many leading figures in the field.

Major, Ralph H., ed. *Classic Descriptions of Disease, with Biographical Sketches of the Authors*, 3rd edition (Springfield, IL: Charles C. Thomas, 1978). This work is a useful anthology of the first systematic descriptions of many important and common diseases.

McKeown, Thomas. *The Origins of Human Disease* (Oxford: Blackwell, 1988). McKeown presents a thoughtful survey of biological, ecological, and behavioral determinants of infections, cancer, heart disease, and other ailments.

McNeill, William H. *Plagues and Peoples* (New York: Doubleday, 1976). This study provides an excellent brief account of the impact of epidemic diseases and food shortages on the health status of people, as well as the influence of these plagues on the rise and fall of civilizations.

Mullan, Fitzhugh. *Plagues and Politics: The Story of the United States Public Health Service* (New York: Basic Books, 1989). A well-written history of the major problems and events in the development of the lead federal health agency in the United States, this work is authored by a public health physician with a good sense of history.

Porter, Dorothy. *Health, Civilization, and the State: A History of Public Health from Ancient to Modern Times* (London: Routledge, 1999). This recent contribution to the field is more comprehensive than the work of either Rosen or Brockington.

Powell, John H. *Bring out Your Dead: The Great Plague of Yellow Fever in Philadelphia in 1793* (Philadelphia: University of Pennsylvania Press, 1993). This book is a historical account of the impact of a yellow fever epidemic that claimed the lives of over 10 percent of the population of Philadelphia and caused its virtual evacuation. The extraordinary and mostly unsuccessful measures taken to combat the epidemic were based on competing schools of thought as to the cause, none of which appreciated the importance of the mosquito vector.

Rosen, George. *A History of Public Health* (New York: MD Publications, 1958; reprint, Baltimore, MD: Johns Hopkins University Press, 1991). Rosen presents a good brief historical survey of public health, particularly for its coverage of American contributions.

—— *From Medical Police to Social Medicine: Essays on the History of Health Care* (New York: Science History Publications, 1974). This work traces the philosophical and conceptual development of personal preventive care services.

Sigerist, Henry. E. *A History of Medicine* (Oxford and New York: Oxford University Press, 1958–1961). The most ambitious work ever conceived on the history of medicine, it was intended to be a massive, multivolume scholarly treatise. Unfortunately, Sigerist, a physician, philosopher, and medical historian, died before he could complete more than these two introductory volumes: *Primitive and Archaic Medicine* (Vol. 1) and *Early Greek, Hindu, and Persian Medicine* (Vol. 2). There is considerable emphasis on public health and preventive medical aspects throughout, as well as a masterly account of the complex interactions of medicine and human society in early civilizations.

—— *Henry Sigerist on the History of Medicine*, ed. F. Marti-Ibanez (New York: MD Publications, 1960). Sigerist is a towering figure in the history of medicine. For the general reader, this is probably the most accessible work among his prolific output.

Winslow, Charles-Edward Amory. *The Conquest of Epidemic Disease: A Chapter in the History of Ideas* (Princeton, NJ: Princeton University Press, 1943; reprint, Madison: University of Wisconsin Press, 1980). This book, probably more so than the same author's history of American epidemiology, traces the development of understanding about causes, methods of spread, and control of epidemic communicable diseases.

Zinsser, Hans. *Rats, Lice and History* (Boston: Little, Brown, 1935). A classic in the history of medicine, this is an eminent bacteriologist's racy account of the impact of epidemics, especially typhus, on the outcome of wars through the ages.

Outline of Contents

II. COMMUNICABLE DISEASES

A. MAJOR COMMUNICABLE DISEASES AND THEIR MEANS OF SPREAD

1. GENERAL

Carrier

Common Vehicle Spread

Contagion

Cross Infection

Emerging Infectious Diseases

Epidemics

Epidemic Theory: Herd Immunity

Filth Diseases

Infection (see Antisepsis and Sterilization; Contagion)

Tropical Infectious Diseases

Tropical Medicine (see Tropical Infectious Diseases)

Tularemia

Viral Infections (see Communicable Diseases)

Zoonoses

2. PERSON-TO-PERSON SPREAD

A. RESPIRATORY EXCHANGE

Acute Respiratory Diseases

Bronchitis

Chicken Pox and Shingles

Common Cold (see Acute Respiratory Disease)

Diphtheria

German Measles (see Rubella)

Herpes Zoster (see Chicken Pox and Shingles)

Infantile Paralysis (see Poliomyelitis)

Influenza

Measles

Mumps

Pertussis

Poliomyelitis

Rubella

Shingles (see Chicken Pox and Shingles)

Smallpox

Streptococcal Infection

Tuberculosis

Varicella (see Chicken Pox and Shingles)

Whooping Cough (see Pertussis)

B. DURING SEXUAL ACTIVITY

AIDS (see HIV/AIDS)

Chlamydia

Genital Herpes

Gonorrhea

HIV/AIDS

Human Papillomavirus Infection

Prostitution

Sexually Transmitted Diseases

Syphilis

C. OTHER PERSONAL CONTACT

Cytomegalovirus Disease

Leprosy

Ophthalmia Neonatorum

Smallpox

Staphylococcal Infection

3. SPREAD VIA FOOD AND/OR WATER

Botulism

Bovine Spongiform Encephalopathy

Brucellosis

Campylobacter Infection

Cholera

Cryptosporidiosis

Diarrhea (see Food-Borne Diseases; Waterborne Diseases)

Dracunculosis

Food-Borne Diseases

Mad Cow Disease (see Bovine Spongiform Encephalopathy; Transmissible Spongiform Encephalopathy)

Regulations Affecting Restaurants

Restaurants (see Regulations Affecting Restaurants)

Salmonellosis

Shigellosis

Transmissible Spongiform Encephalopathy

Trichinosis

Typhoid

Typhoid Mary

Waterborne Diseases

Worms (see Dracunculosis; Trichinosis)

4. SPREAD BY INSECT VECTORS

Arboviral Encephalitides

Black Death

Bubonic Plague (see Plague)

Chagas Disease (see Trypanosomiasis)

Eastern Equine Encephalitis (see Arboviral Encephalitides)

Encephalitis (see Arboviral Encephalitides)

Leishmaniasis

Malaria

Index

ISBN 0-02-865353-X

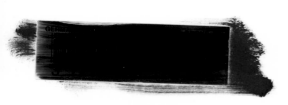

For Reference

Not to be taken from this room

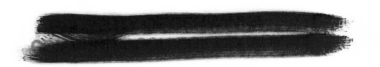